TARGET–NEET PG

(Review of NEET–PG 2020 Paper–Model Questions with Solved Explanatory Answers)

Dr. T. ARUN BABU
MD Pediatrics (JIPMER), DAA (CMC Vellore), MBA (HM)
Fellow in Neonatal Perinatal Medicine (Canada)
Associate Professor and Head, Department of Pediatrics
All India Institute of Medical Sciences (AIIMS)
Mangalagiri – 522 503
Website: www.drarunbabu.in

Peepee Publishers and Distributors (P) Ltd.®

TARGET–NEET PG

Published by
Pawaninder P. Vij and Anupam Vij

Peepee Publishers and Distributors (P) Ltd.
Head Office: 160, Shakti Vihar, Pitam Pura, Delhi-110 034 (India)

Correspondence Address:
7/31, First Floor, Ansari Road, Daryaganj
New Delhi-110 002 (India)
Ph: 41512412, 23246245, 9811156083
e-mail: peepee160@yahoo.co.in
e-mail: peepee160@gmail.com
www.peepeepub.com
join us on facebook.com/pp.publishers

First Edition: 2021

ISBN: 978-81-8445-287-7

DEDICATION

To my Parents, Teachers,
my wife Dr. Sharmila,
my kids Akshaya and Akash

DISCLAIMER

PREFACE

The NEET PG exam is the single largest medical entrance exam in India, which decides the future of thousands of budding medicos. As we all know, the exam conducting team, the pattern of exam and type of MCQs keep changing every year. It is extremely important for a PG aspirant to be aware of these changes in examination pattern and recent trends about questions being asked in various subjects to outshine their competitors. Most of these exams have direct repeats and favourite topic repeats every-time, which play a crucial role in deciding your rank. On reviewing the most recent NEET PG exam pattern which is there for last 2 years (single session/same paper pattern), it is very obvious there are only few books available in the market specifically targeting this recent pattern exam.

This book was edited with the sole purpose of guiding aspirants to crack the recent NEET PG. This book includes collection of model MCQs from the most recent 2020 exam. The important advantage of this book is that the students will be aware of the recent trends in questions asked and can strategize their preparations accordingly. This book will give PG aspirants the cutting edge required to excel in this exam.

We have put in tremendous effort to make sure that all the questions discussed in the book are accurate. Questions have been solved using references from standard textbooks/articles and a detailed background theory has been included. Numerous tables and illustrations are included for easy understanding and long-term retention. MCQs have been solved by a team of qualified and experienced subject experts from various reputed institutes of India. *For controversial questions, every attempt has been made to trace the source textbook or article and solve the questions.* Every subject MCQs have references, Tablets, Magical Points, Illustrations and Flowcharts for the better understanding and authenticity. All Highlighted points are essential for answering repeat questions in forthcoming exams.

I would like to express our sincere gratitude to all the contributors, for their hard work and commitment which has led to this high quality content. We wish to thank our publishers, Mr. Pawaninder Paul Vij and Mr. Anupam Vij, the Directors of Peepee Publishers and Distributors (P) Ltd, for their support and special interest on this project. I would also like to thank our publishing team for their relentless efforts in releasing this book in a short notice. I am deeply indebted to students for their overwhelming support, feedback and critical appraisal on our previous projects. I am looking forward to hear your feedback on this book and am fully committed in bringing out better editions in the future. "Our happiness lies in your success" and the only path for success is "Persistence" and "Hard work". Have faith in yourselves and Almighty God. All the best!

T. Arun Babu

Website: *www.drarunbabu.in*
Email: *babuarun.t@gmail.com*

> **"Books are infinite in number and time is short. The secret of knowledge is to take what is essential."**
>
> –*Swami Vivekananda*

ACKNOWLEDGEMENTS

Mr. Thirunavukkarasu D, Government School English Lecturer (Retd), Puducherry.
Mrs. Sampurnam, Principal (Retd), SSVHSS, Puducherry.
Mr. Vijayan D, Cash Officer (Retd), SBI, Puducherry.
Mrs. Sagoundala, Under Secretary (Retd), Government of Puducherry.
Mr. Srinivasan@Babu, PWD, Puducherry.
Mr. Dhinesh Shankar, MCA Team Leader, EDS Emphasis, Chennai.
Mr. Rajkumar, System Engineer, Apple, CA, USA.

Sincere Thanks to:

- Director and CEO, AIIMS, Mangalagiri
- Dean, AIIMS, Mangalagiri
- Medical Superindentent, AIIMS, Mangalagiri

Write to Us:

Any observations, suggestions, criticisms are welcome. Write to the author at babuarun.t@gmail.com

Errata

Please visit *www.drarunbabu.in and www.peepeepub.com*

Follow Author in Facebook: *www.facebook.com/targetjipmer/ and www.facebook.com/targetneetpg/ Dr Arun Babu's Pediatrics Discussion group*

CONTRIBUTORS

Dr. T Arun Babu, MD Pediatrics (JIPMER), DAA (CMC), Fellow NPM (Canada)
Associate Professor and I/C Head, Department of Pediatrics
All India Institute of Medical Sciences (AIIMS)
Mangalagiri, Andhra Pradesh – 522 503
(Chief Editor)

Dr. Dhivyalakshmi, MD Anatomy (JIPMER)
Senior Resident, Department of Anatomy
JIPMER, Puducherry
(Anatomy)

Dr. Jean Fredrick, MD Physiology
Assistant Professor
Department of Physiology
Mahatma Gandhi Medical College and Research Institute
(MGMC&RI), Pillaiyarkuppam, Puducherry
(Physiology)

Dr. Usha S Adiga, MBBS MD PhD
Professor, Department of Biochemistry
KS Hegde Medical Academy
Mangalore, Karnataka.
(Biochemistry)

Dr. Arundhathi S, MD Pathology
Associate Professor and I/C Head, Department of Pathology
All India Institute of Medical Sciences (AIIMS)
Mangalagiri, Andhra Pradesh – 522 503
(Pathology)

Dr. A Sivaranjini, MD Microbiology
Assistant Professor
Rajah Muthiah Medical College and Hospital
Annamalai University, Chidambaram
Tamil Nadu
(Microbiology)

Dr. Madhav Rao, MD Pharm (JIPMER)
Associate Professor, Department of Pharmacology
All India Institute of Medical Sciences (AIIMS)
Mangalagiri, Andhra Pradesh – 522 503
(Pharmacology)

Dr. Yatiraj Singi, MD Forensic Medicine
Professor, Department of Forensic Medicine
Sree Mookambika Institute of Medical Sciences
Kulasekharam, District Kanya Kumari, TN
(Forensic Medicine)

Dr. Priyanka Choudhary, MD Community Medicine
Senior Resident, Department of Community Medicine
PGIMS, Rohtak, Haryana
(Preventive and Social Medicine)

Dr. Satvinder Singh Bakshi, MS ENT (JIPMER), DNB
Associate Professor and I/C Head
Department of Otorhinolaryngology
All India Institute of Medical Sciences (AIIMS)
Mangalagiri, Andhra Pradesh – 522 503
(ENT)

Dr. Venipriya, MS Ophthalmology
Senior Resident, Department of Ophthalmology
Indira Gandhi Medical College and Research Institute
(IGMC&RI)
Puducherry - 605 009
(Ophthalmology)

Dr. Soumya Sathyan, MD General Medicine
Consultant Physician
Moulana Hospital
Perintalmanna
(Medicine)

Dr. Naresh Kumar P, MS Gen Surgery
Associate Professor and I/C Head, Department of Surgery
All India Institute of Medical Sciences (AIIMS)
Mangalagiri, Andhra Pradesh – 522 503
(Surgery)

Dr. Sharmila Arun Babu, MS OBG (JIPMER)
Additional Professor and I/C Head, Department of Obstetrics and Gynecology
All India Institute of Medical Sciences (AIIMS)
Mangalagiri, Andhra Pradesh – 522 503
(Obs and Gyne)

Dr. Dinesh Kumar, MD Pediatrics
Assistant Professor, Department of Pediatrics
JIPMER, Karaikal, Puducherry – 605009
(Pediatrics)

Dr. Mukul Mohindra, MS (Ortho), DNB, MNAMS, Dip. SICOT (Belgium)
Fellow National Board (Arthroscopy and Sports Medicine)
Sports Injury Center, Safdarjung Hospital and VMM College
New Delhi
(Orthopedics)

Dr. Prabhakaran N, MD Dermatology (JIPMER), DNB
Assistant Professor, Department of Dermatology
All India Institute of Medical Sciences (AIIMS)
Mangalagiri, Andhra Pradesh – 522 503
(Dermatology)

Dr. Sangeeta Dhanger, DA, DNB, MNAMS
Assistant Professor, Department of Anesthesiology
Indira Gandhi Medical College and Research Institute
(IGMC&RI)
Puducherry – 605009
(Anesthesiology)

Dr. Prudhvinath Reddy N, MD
Assistant Professor, Department of Radiology
All India Institute of Medical Sciences (AIIMS)
Mangalagiri, Andhra Pradesh – 522 503
(Radiology)

Dr. Arul Varman, MD Psychiatry (JIPMER)
Assistant Professor, Department of Psychiatry
Indira Gandhi Medical College and Research Institute
(IGMC&RI), Puducherry – 605009
(Psychiatry)

EDITORIAL ASSISTANCE

Gaurang Narayan, MBBS
Indira Gandhi Medical College and Research Institute
(IGMC&RI), Puducherry – 605009

Padmapriya, MD Pathology
Resident, Department of Pathology
Andhra Medical College
Visakhapatnam – 605009

CONTENTS

ANATOMY

1. The reason for the long left recurrent laryngeal nerve is the persistence of which arch artery?

(a) 3rd arch
(b) 4th arch
(c) 6th arch
(d) 2nd arch

Explanation:

- After disappearance of the distal part of the sixth aortic arch on right side, the right recurrent laryngeal nerve hooks around the right subclavian artery.
- On the left, the nerve remains in place and hooks around the ligamentum arteriosum which develops from the distal part of left sixth aortic arch.

Arteries	Source of development
Arch of aorta	• **Aortic sac** (ventral part) • Left horn of aortic sac • **Left fourth** arch artery
Brachiocephalic artery	• **Right horn** of aortic sac
Right subclavian artery	• Proximal part from **right fourth arch artery** and • Distal part from **right seventh cervical intersegmental artery**
Left subclavian artery	• **Left seventh cervical intersegmental artery**
Common carotid artery	• **Third arch artery** proximal to the external carotid artery bud
Internal carotid artery	• **Third arch artery** distal to the external carotid bud and • Cranial part of **dorsal aorta** distal to the attachment of third arch artery
External carotid artery	• Bud from **third arch artery**
Pulmonary arteries	• Part of the **sixth arch artery** between pulmonary trunk and • Branch to lung bud on each side
Descending aorta	• Proximal part from **left dorsal aorta** distal to attachment of fourth arch artery and • Distal part from **fused dorsal aortae** forming **single median artery**

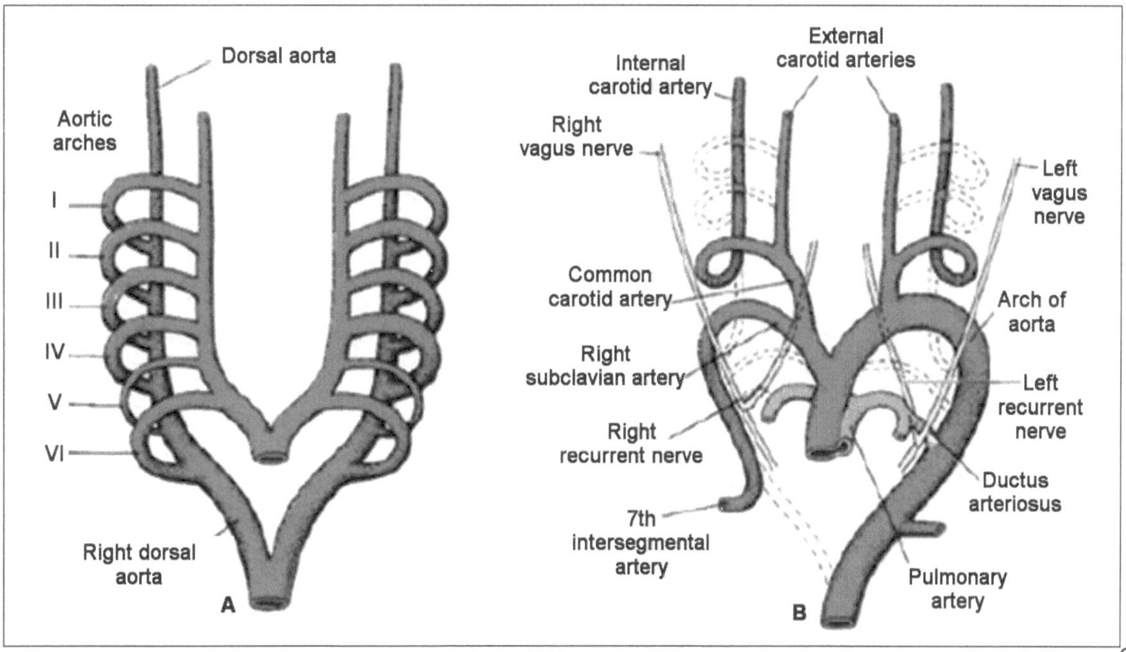

Contd.

Contd.

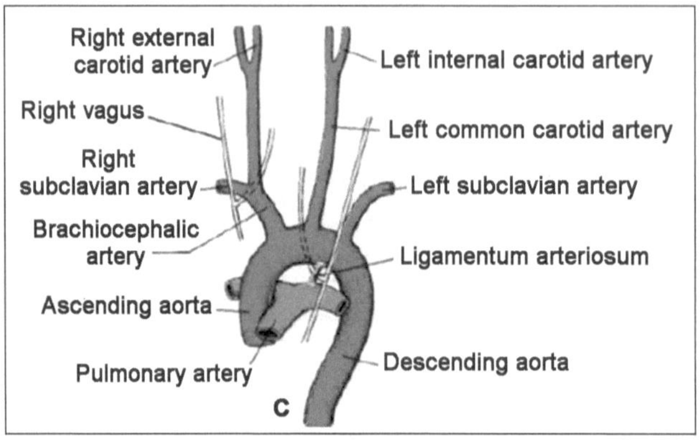

Ans: (c) 6th arch

Ref: *Langman's Medical Embryology, 12th Edition, Page 187-188; Vishram Singh, Clinical Embryology, Page 215*

2. A patient presented with the extension of the MCP joint and flexion of IP. Which muscle is most likely affected?

(a) Interossei and lumbricals
(b) Extensor digitorum
(c) Abductor pollicis longus
(d) Abductor pollicis brevis

Explanation:

- The case presented here seems to be **claw hand** where **intrinsic muscles** of the **hand** is affected.
- Ulnar nerve is called as nerve of **fine movements** as it innervates **most of the intrinsic muscles** of the **hand.**
- **Median nerve** through **recurrent branch** supplies **1st and 2nd lumbricals** and **thenar group of muscles except deep head of flexor pollicis brevis.**
- **Anterior interosseous nerve** branch of **median nerve** supplies **NO** intrinsic muscles of hand.
- Similarly **radial nerve** and its branch **posterior interosseous nerve** provide **NO** nerve supply to any intrinsic muscles of hand.

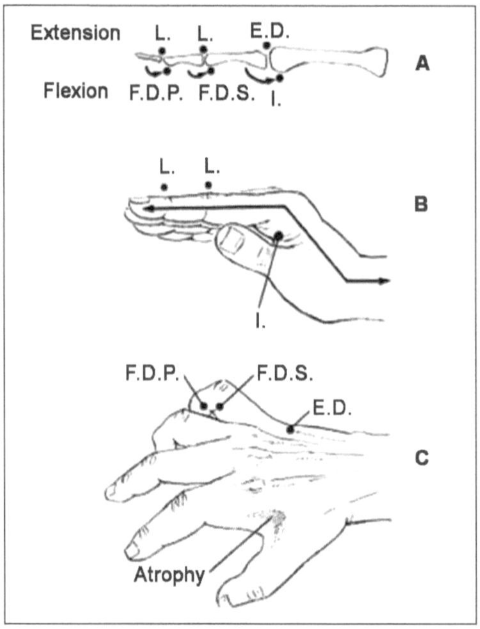

Ulnar Claw Hand

- The interossei and lumbricals produce the **"Z-position"** of hand acting through dorsal digital expansions.
- It produces:
  - **Flexion at the metacarpophalangeal joints** by the **interossei;** and
  - **Extension at the interphalangeal joints** by the **lumbricals.**
- In **distal section** of the ulnar nerve (at wrist), the **interossei and medial two lumbricals** are paralysed.
- The **proximal phalanges** are **hyperextended** by the **unopposed long extensors.**
- The **middle** and **distal phalanges** are **hyperflexed** by the **unopposed long flexors.**
- The result is a **"claw hand"**, which is the **opposite** of the **Z-position.**

Ulnar Paradox

- In **high ulnar nerve palsy, flexor carpi ulnaris** and **medial half of flexor digitorum profundus** is also paralysed producing **less clawing** of **medial two fingers.**

Complete Claw Hand

- A combined **median and ulnar nerve palsy** at the wrist results in **a full claw hand** with **thenar** and **hypothenar** flattening and **thumb adduction and flexion (a simian hand).**

Ulnar nerve in hand

Superficial branch
Palmaris brevis

Deep branch
1. All hypothenar muscles
   - Abductor digiti minimi
   - Flexor digiti minimi
   - Opponens digiti minimi
2. Adductor pollicis
3. 3rd and 4th lumbricals
4. All dorsal interosseous
5. All palmar interosseous
6. Deep head of flexor pollicis brevis

Median nerve in hand

Recurrent branch
All thenar muscles
i. Abductor pollicis brevis
ii. Flexor pollicis brevis–Superficial head
iii. Opponens pollicis
Except deep head of flexor pollicis brevis

Lateral branch
1st lumbrical

Medial branch
2nd lumbrical

Note:

- Acting alone palmar interosseous causes **adduction** of fingers **(PAD).**
- Acting alone dorsal interosseous causes **abduction** of fingers **(DAB).**

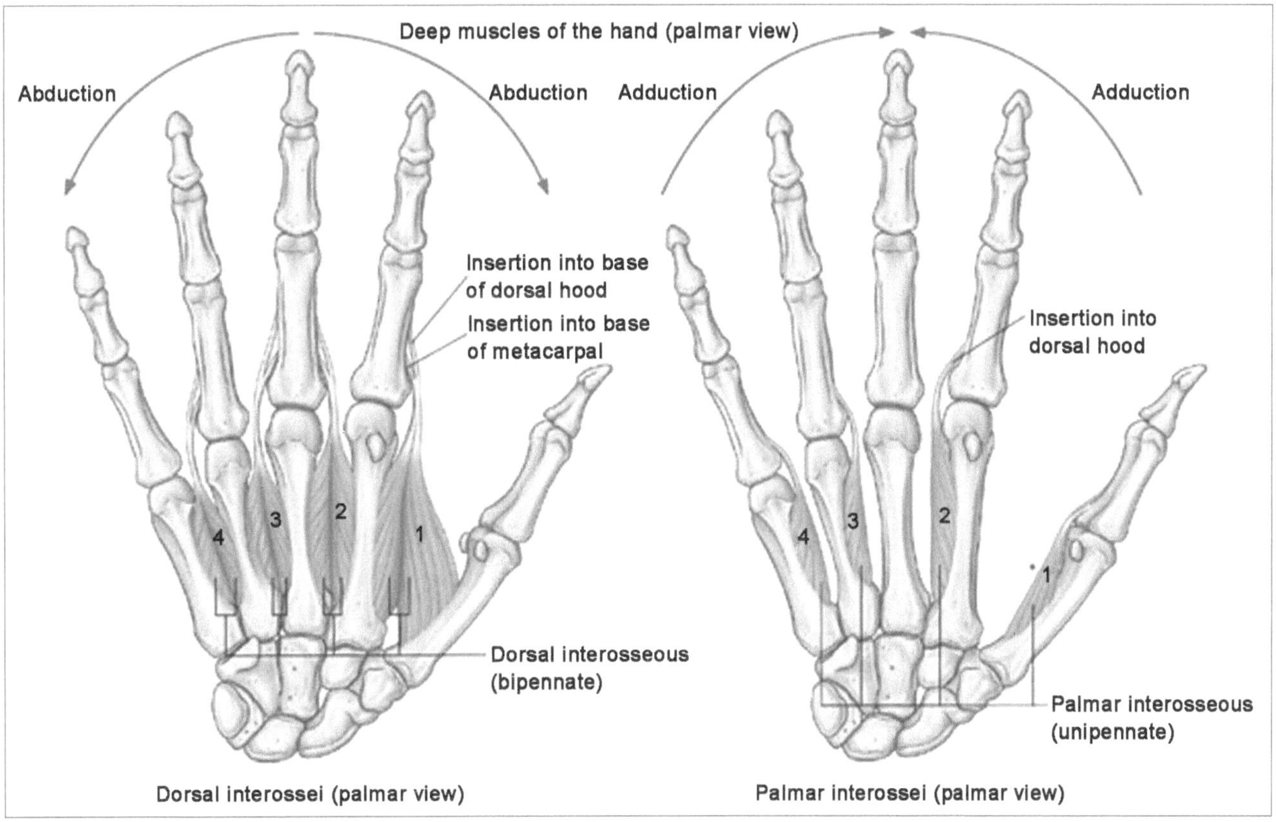

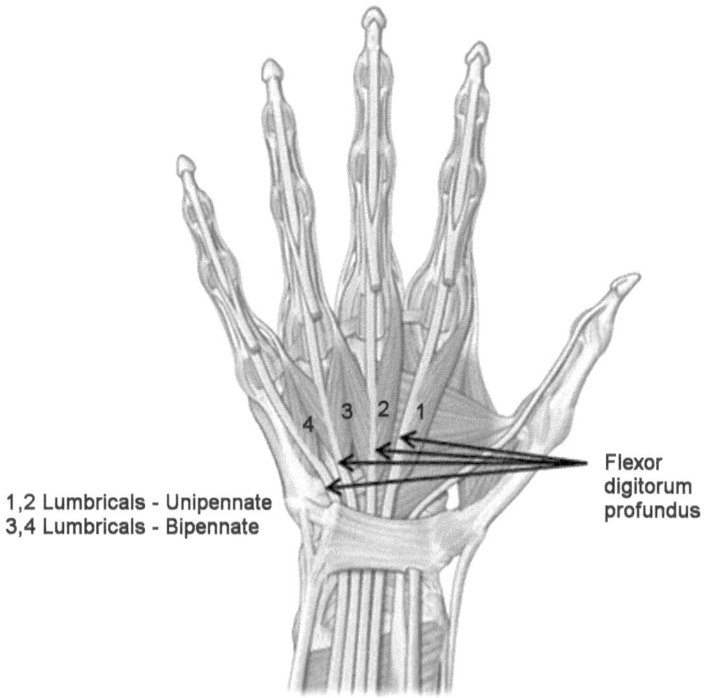

Lumbricals – Palmar view

- **Extensor digitorum and abductor pollicis longus** are supplied by **posterior interosseous nerve.**
- **Abductor pollicis brevis** is supplied by **recurrent branch** of **median nerve.**

Ans: (a) Interossei and lumbricals

Ref: *Keith L Moore, Clinically Oriented Anatomy, 7th Edition, Page 1227, 1238, 1239; Gray's Anatomy, 41st Edition, Page 893e; Vishram Singh, Textbook of Anatomy, Volume 1, 2nd Edition, Page 180,181; Gray's Atlas of Anatomy, Page 445, 447*

3. Ligation of the common hepatic artery will impair blood supply in:

(a) Right gastric and left gastric artery
(b) Right gastric and right gastroepiploic artery
(c) Right gastroepiploic and short gastric vessels
(d) Right gastric and short gastric vessels

Explanation:

- **Celiac trunk** is a ventral branch of **abdominal aorta.**
- It gives three branches:
  - Left gastric artery.
  - Splenic artery.
  - Common hepatic artery.
- **Common hepatic artery** – A segment of **hepatic artery** from its origin from **celiac trunk** to its **first branch, gastroduodenal artery.**
- **Proper hepatic artery** – From **gastroduodenal artery** to till its bifurcation into left and right hepatic artery.
- **Left gastric artery** is a direct branch of **celiac trunk.**
- **Right gastric artery** is a branch of **proper hepatic artery.**
- **Short gastric vessels** and **posterior gastric vessels** are branches of **splenic artery.**
- **Left gastroepiploic/gastro-omental artery** is a branch of **splenic artery.***

- **Right gastroepiploic/gastro-omental artery** is a branch of **gastroduodenal artery.***
- So ligation of common hepatic artery will impair blood supply in right gastric and right gastroepiploic artery.

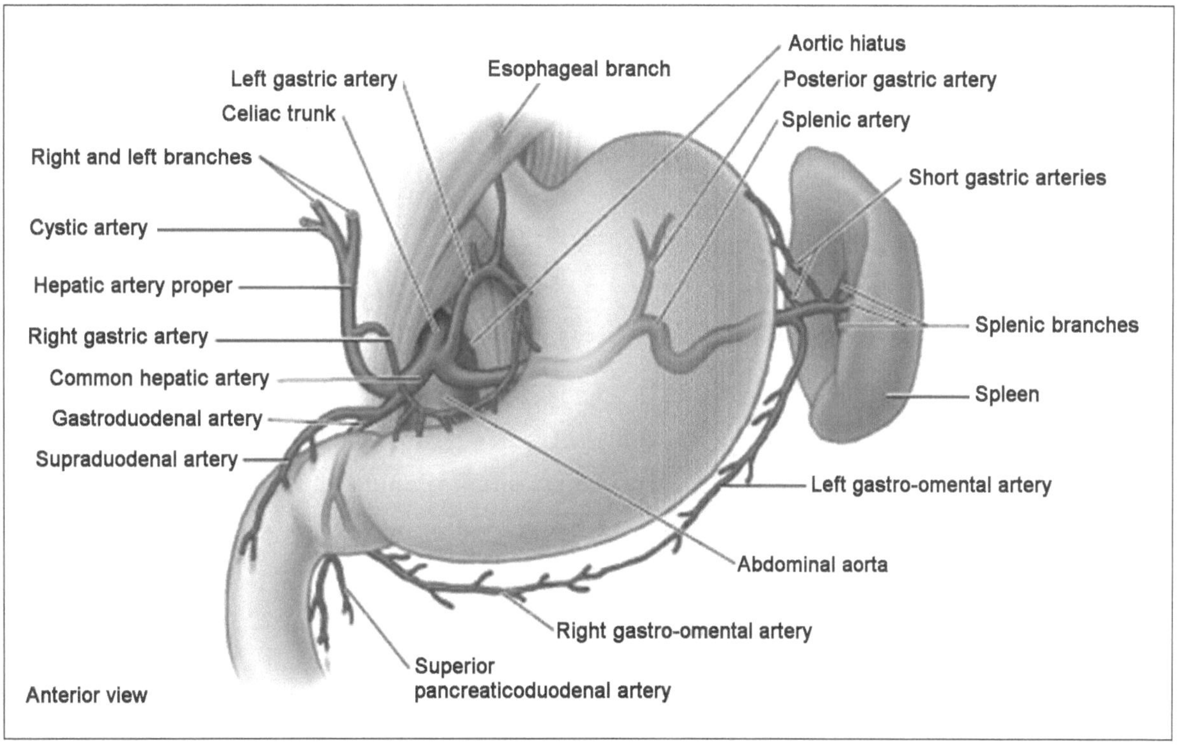

Ans: (b) Right gastric and right gastroepiploic artery

Ref: *Keith L Moore, Clinically Oriented Anatomy, 7th Edition, Page 420; Gray's Anatomy, 41st Edition, Page 1166*

4. Identify the cell marked in the histological image of the cerebellum shown below:

(a) Purkinje cells (b) Basket cells

(c) Golgi cells (d) Granular cells

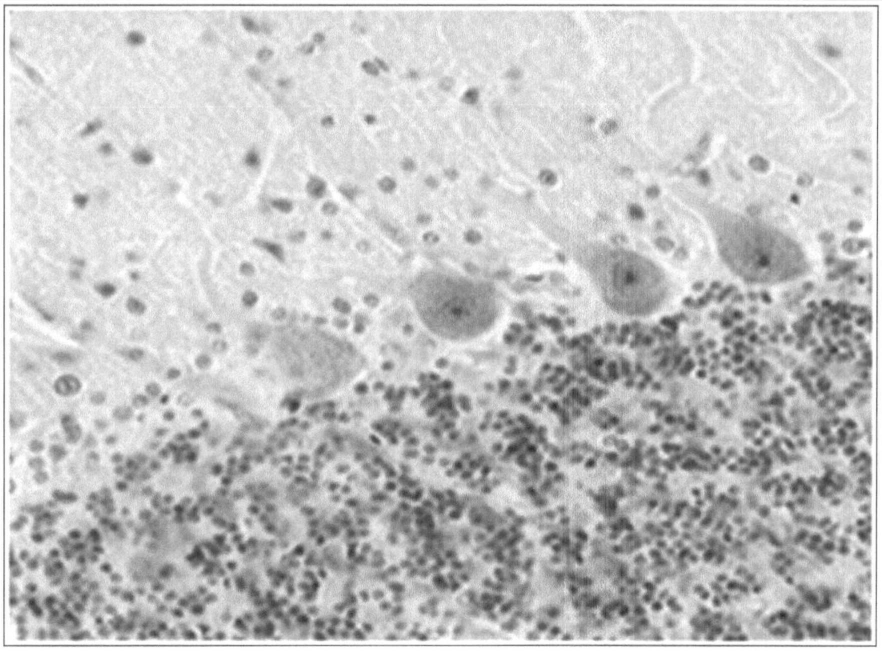

Explanation:

- The given image is a histological picture of **cerebellum** stained with **hematoxylin and eosin stain.**
- The histology of cerebellum and its **cortex** is same throughout **(Homotypical)** unlike the cerebral cortex.

CEREBELLUM

- **Grossly:**
  - Deep folds in cortex of cerebellum is called **folia** and is separated by **sulci.**
- **Histology:**
  - **Outer grey mater and inner white mater.**
  - **Grey mater – Three layer (Pneumonic : M-P-G)**
    - **Outer molecular layer (ML)** contains small neurons – **Stellate cells*, Basket cells*** and its **fibers.**
    - **Middle Purkinje layer (PL)** contains single layer of large **Purkinje cells* (Flask-shaped)** whose **dendrites** branch in **molecular layer.**
    - **Inner granule cell layer (GL)** contains **small granule cells, large Golgi type II cells*,** and empty spaces called **glomeruli.***

Note:

- The **sole efferent** from **cerebellar cortex** is through **Purkinje** cell axon which is **inhibitory** to **deep cerebellar nuclei**
- **Climbing fibres*** - Afferent to cerebellum from **contralateral inferior olivary nucleus** from **medulla.**
- **Mossy fibres*** - All afferent fibres to cerebellum except climbing fibres
- All **intrinsic neurons** in the cerebellar cortex are **inhibitory***
- **Granule cell*** is the only **intrinsic excitatory neuron** in **cerebellar cortex**

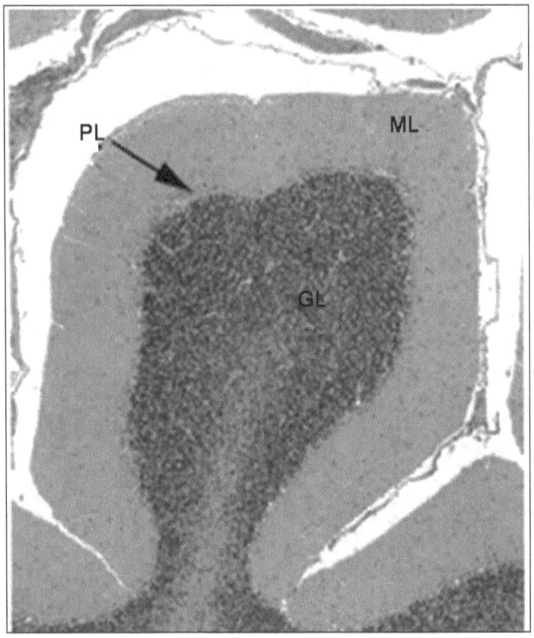

H and E (Low power)

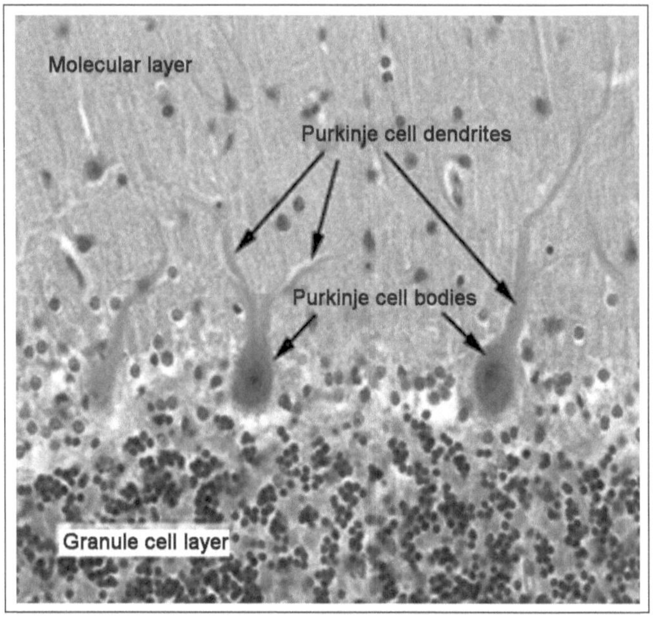

H and E (High power)

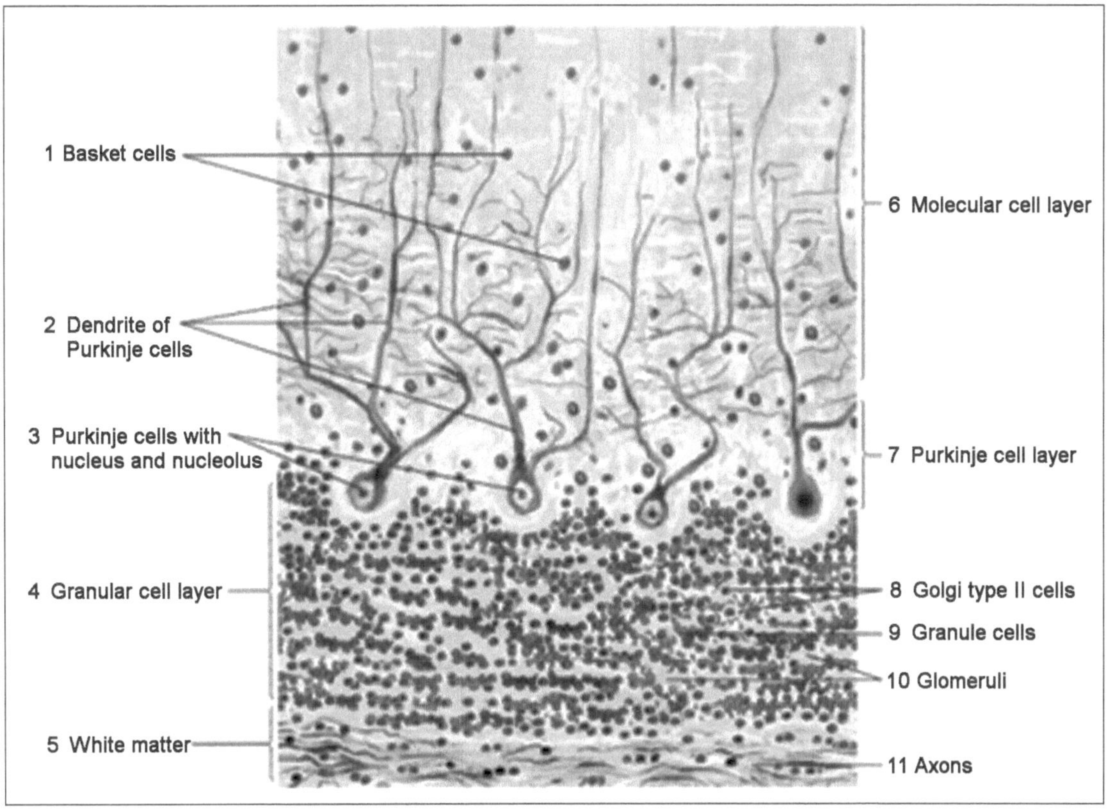

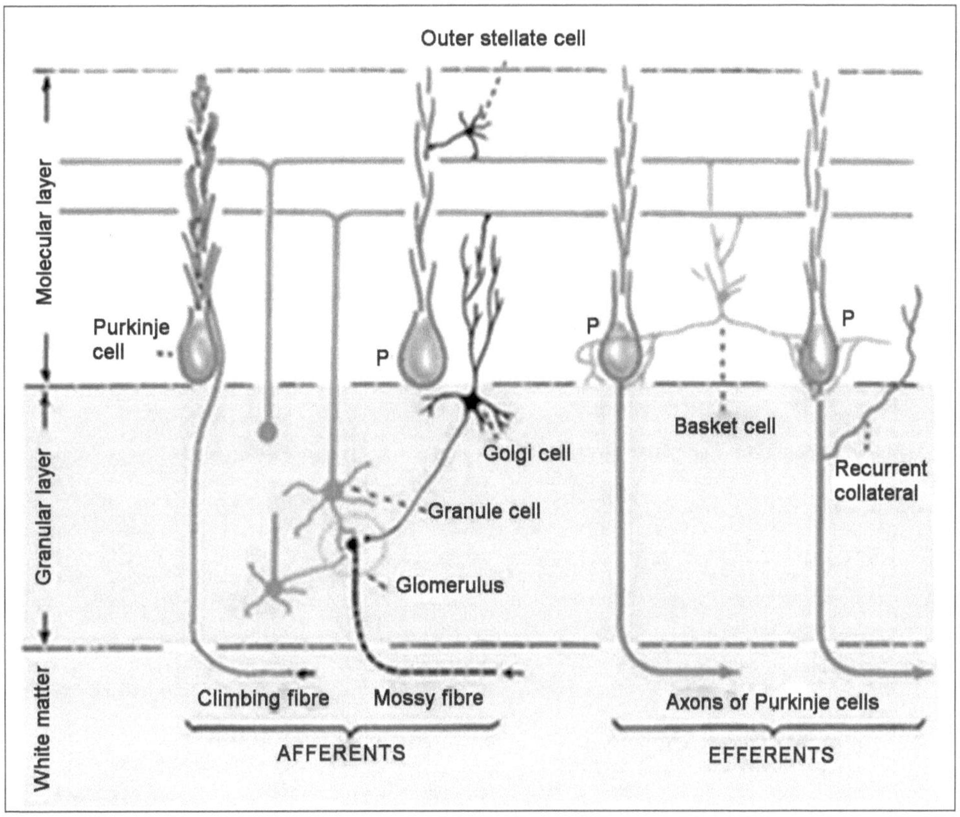

Ans: (a) Purkinje cells

Ref: *Wheater's Functional Histology, 6th Edition, Page 396; IB Singh, Human Histology, 6th Edition, Page 370, 371; di Fiore's Atlas of Histology, 11th Edition, Page 148; Vishram Singh, Clinical Neuroanatomy, 2nd Edition, Page 205-208*

5. Tumor of the uncinate process of pancreas affects which of the following vessel?

(a) Superior mesenteric artery (b) Portal vein

(c) Common hepatic artery (d) Inferior mesenteric artery

Explanation:

- The uncinate process is a hook-shaped continuation of the inferomedial part of the head of the pancreas.
- The **superior mesenteric vessels** descend **anterior to the uncinate process** of the pancreas and the third part of the duodenum, and posterior to the body of the pancreas.
- The uncinate process extends medially between superior mesenteric vessels anteriorly and the abdominal aorta posteriorly.
- On sagittal cross-sectional imaging, **the left renal vein, uncinate process, and third part of duodenum** can be seen lying between the superior mesenteric artery and the abdominal aorta.
- The **superior mesenteric vessels** may be compressed by a **tumor of uncinate process** at this site.

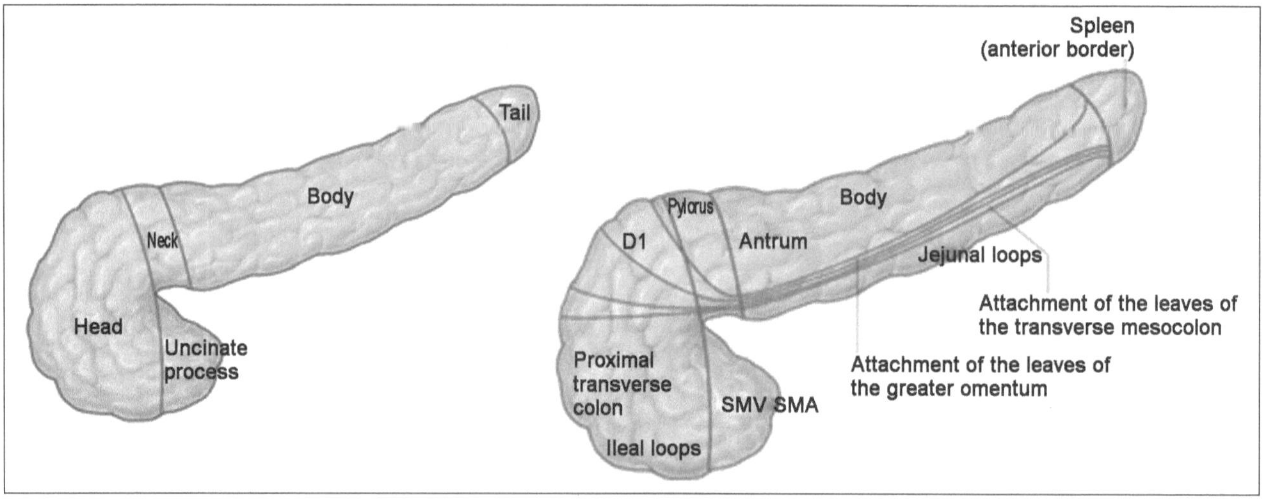

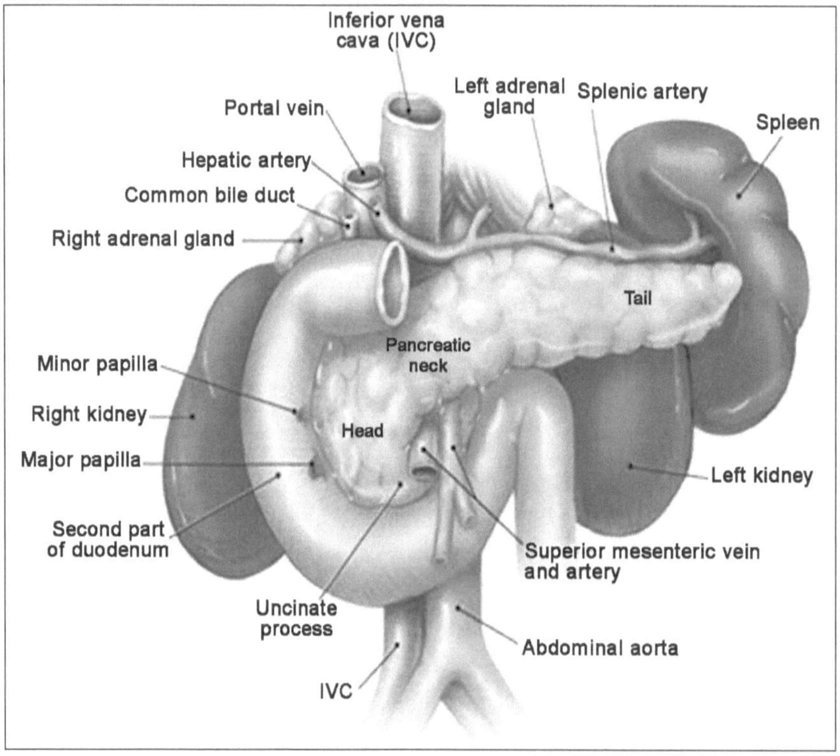

Note:

- **Portal vein** is related to **neck of pancreas** posteriorly.

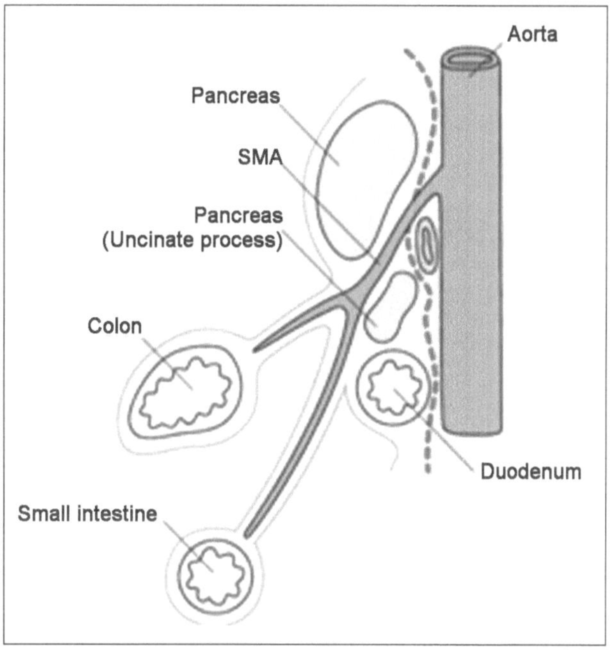

Ans: (a) Superior mesenteric artery

Ref: *Gray's Anatomy, 41st Edition, Page 1181*

6. Illustration showing histology of cartilage. Identify the type of cartilage:

(a) Hyaline cartilage
(b) Articular cartilage
(c) Elastic cartilage
(d) Fibrocartilage

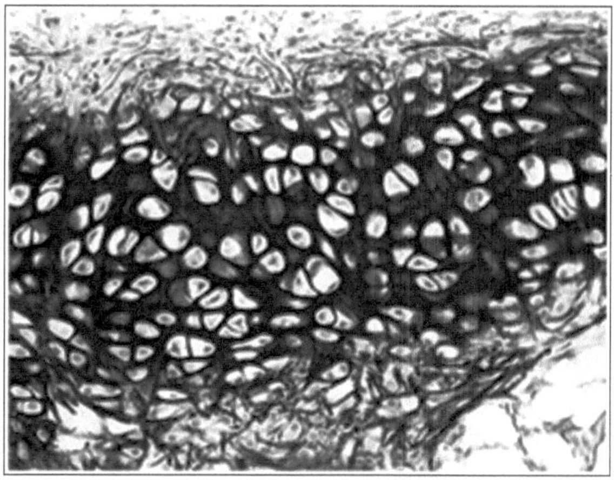

Explanation:

- Elastic cartilage (or yellow fibrocartilage) is similar in many ways to hyaline cartilage.
- The main difference is that instead of collagen fibres, the matrix contains numerous elastic fibres that form a network.
- The fibres are difficult to see in hematoxylin and eosin stained section.
- The elastic fibres can be clearly visualised if special methods for staining elastic fibres is used like resorcin, fusion and orcein.

- Elastic cartilage possesses greater flexibility than hyaline cartilage, and readily recovers its shape after being deformed.

	Hyaline cartilage	Elastic cartilage	Fibrocartilage
	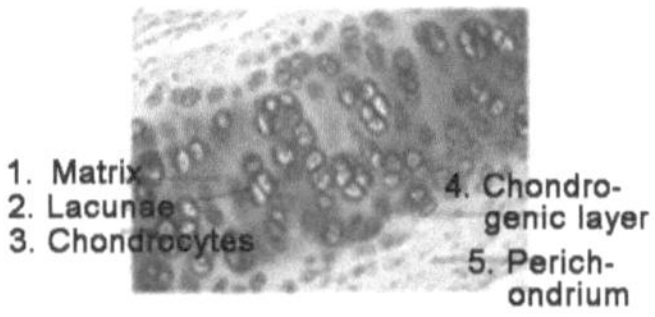	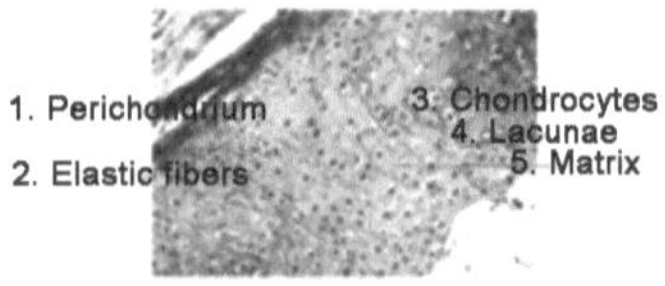	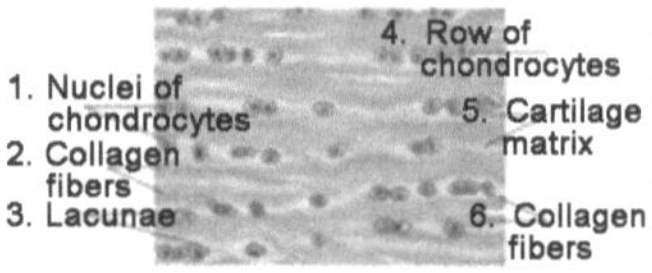
Color	**Glossy bluish and transparent**	**Yellowish**	**White, opaque**
Chondrocytes	Present inside lacunae as single or as isogenous cell clusters	Larger, more numerous and packed more closely inside lacunae as compared to hyaline cartilage	Few in numbers, scattered singly or arranged in rows
Matrix	**Homogenous, Basophilic,** collagen fibres delicate and not visible	Rich in elastic fibres	Thick bundles of collagen fibres run parallel within matrix
Perichondrium	Present (except articular cartilage and epiphyseal plates)	Present	**Absent**
Cell types	Chondroblasts and chondrocytes	Chondroblasts and chondrocytes	Chondrocytes and fibroblasts
Fibres	Type II collagen	Type II collagen and elastic fibres	Types I and II collagen
Ground substance	Proteoglycan – Aggrecan secreted by chondrocytes	Proteoglycan – Aggrecan	Proteoglycan – **versican** (secreted by fibroblasts
Calcification	Yes (i.e., during endochondral bone formation, during aging process)	**No calcification**	Yes (i.e., calcification of fibrocartilaginous callus during bone repair)
Site	Fetal skeletal tissue, epiphyseal plates, articular surface of synovial joints, costal cartilages of rib cage, cartilages of nasal, cavity, larynx (thyroid, cricoid, and arytenoids), rings of trachea and plates in bronchi	Pinna of external ear, external acoustic meatus, auditory (Eustachian) tube, cartilages of larynx (epiglottis, corniculate and cuneiform cartilages)	Intervertebral discs, symphysis publis, articular discs (sternoclavicular and temporomandibular joints) menisci (knee joint), triangular fibrocartilage complex (wrist joint), insertion of tendons

Ans: (c) Elastic cartilage

Ref: *Ross and Pawlina, Histology A Text and Atlas, 6th Edition, Page 206; Wheater's Functional Histology, 6th Edition, Page 182*

7. Remnants of Wolffian ducts in a female are in:

(a) Pouch of Douglas
(b) Broad ligament
(c) Uterovesical pouch
(d) Iliac fossa

Explanation:

- Parts of the mesonephric duct, may persist as Gartner duct cysts between the layers of the **broad ligament** along the lateral wall of the uterus and in the wall of the vagina.

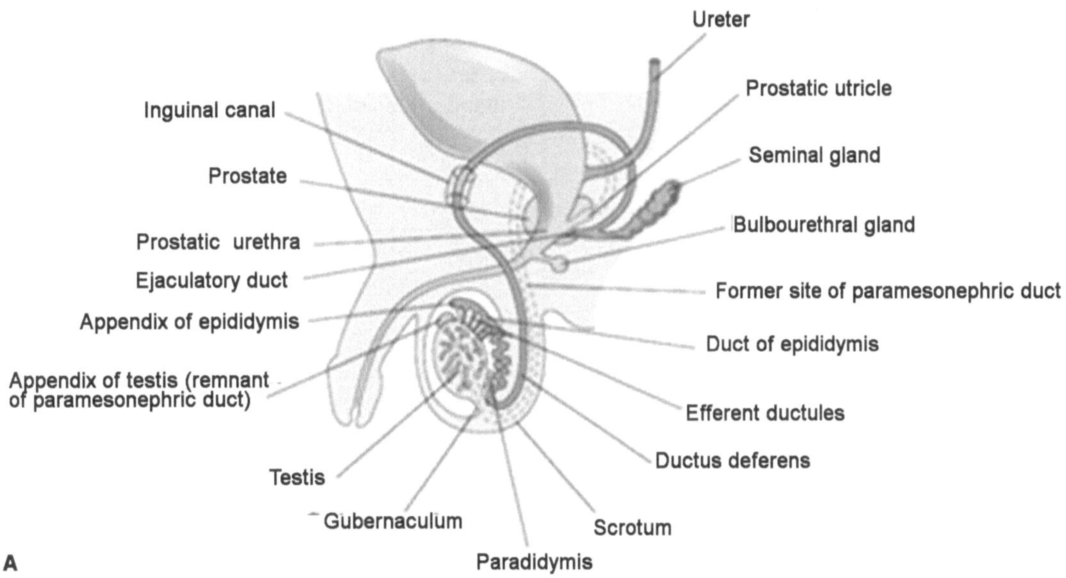
Ureter
Prostatic utricle
Inguinal canal
Seminal gland
Prostate
Bulbourethral gland
Prostatic urethra
Ejaculatory duct
Former site of paramesonephric duct
Appendix of epididymis
Duct of epididymis
Appendix of testis (remnant of paramesonephric duct)
Efferent ductules
Ductus deferens
Testis
Gubernaculum
Scrotum
Paradidymis

A

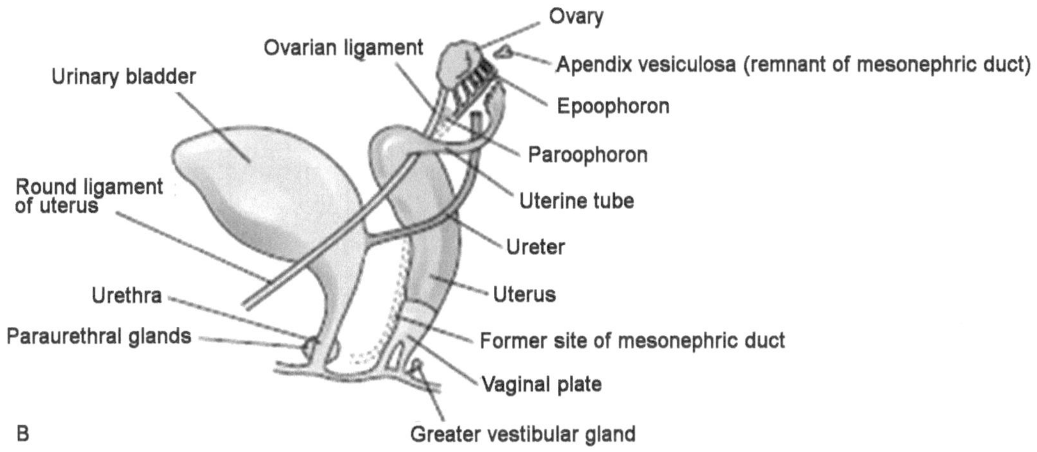
Ovary
Ovarian ligament
Apendix vesiculosa (remnant of mesonephric duct)
Urinary bladder
Epoophoron
Paroophoron
Round ligament of uterus
Uterine tube
Ureter
Urethra
Uterus
Paraurethral glands
Former site of mesonephric duct
Vaginal plate
Greater vestibular gland

B

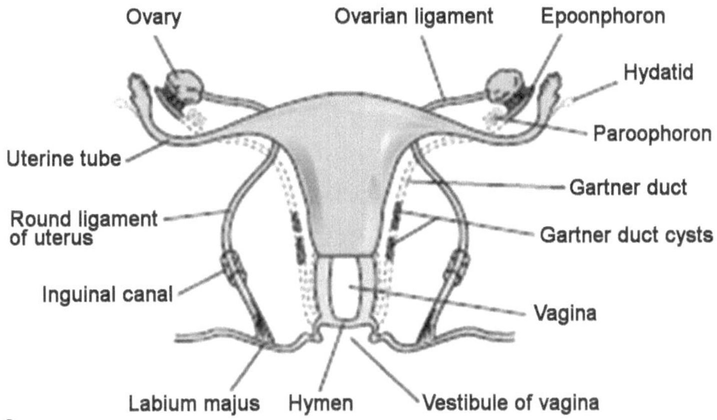
Ovary
Ovarian ligament
Epoonphoron
Hydatid
Paroophoron
Uterine tube
Gartner duct
Round ligament of uterus
Gartner duct cysts
Inguinal canal
Vagina
Labium majus
Hymen
Vestibule of vagina

C

Remnants of parts of the urogenital duct system in adult male and female

Male	
Mesonephric duct – Cranial end	Appendix of epididymis – Head of epididymis
Few mesonephric tubules	Paradidymis – Caudal to efferent ductules in testis
Paramesonephric duct – Cranial end	Appendix of testis – Head of testis
Paramesonephric duct – Caudal end	Prostatic utricle – Opens into prostatic urethra
Female	
Mesonephric duct – Cranial end	Appendix vesiculosa
Mesonephric duct – Caudal end	Gardern duct cysts – In broad ligament along the lateral wall of uterus and vagina
Few cranial mesonephric tubules + Mesonephric duct	Epoophoron – In mesovarium
Few caudal mesonephric tubules alone	Paraoophoron – In mesovarium
Paramesonephric duct – Cranial end (Not involved in tube formation)	Hydatid of Morgagni – In Mesovarium

Ans: (b) Broad ligament

Ref: *Keith L Moore, Clinically Oriented Embryology, 10th Edition, Page 265, 267; Langman's Medical Embryology, 12th Edition, Page 250*

8. Episiotomy extended beyond perineal body injured the structure immediately posterior to it. Which structure is likely injured?

(a) External anal sphincter
(b) Ishchiocavernosus
(c) Bulbospongiosus
(d) Urethral sphincter

Explanation:

Episiotomy

- It is an incision given in the perineum to enlarge the vaginal orifice to facilitate childbirth.

Median Episiotomy

- This incision begins at the frenulum of labia minora and proceeds backward in the midline up to the external anal sphincter.
- It cuts through the skin, vaginal wall, perineal body, and superficial transverse perinei muscle.
- Inadvertently, it may cut the external anal sphincter.

Mediolateral Episiotomy

- This incision begins at the labia minora and proceeds laterally at an angle of 45°.
- It cuts through the skin, vaginal wall, and bulbospongiosus muscle.

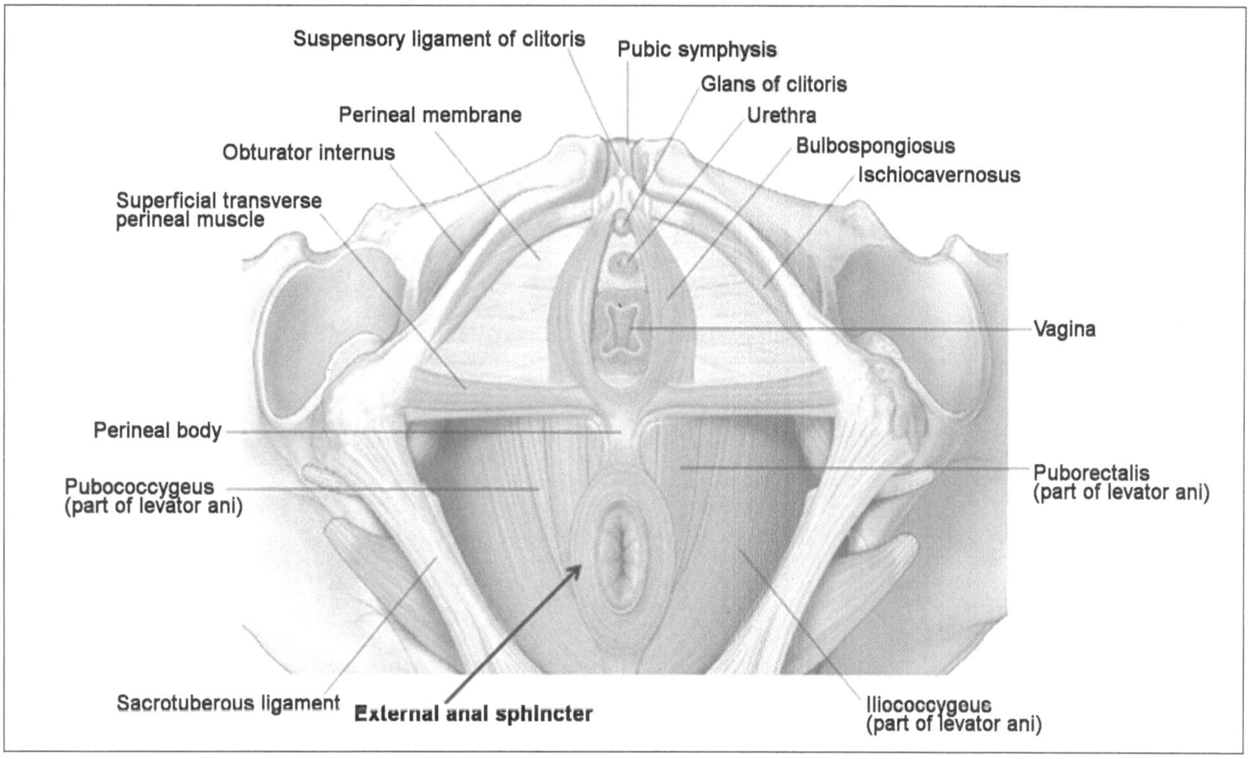

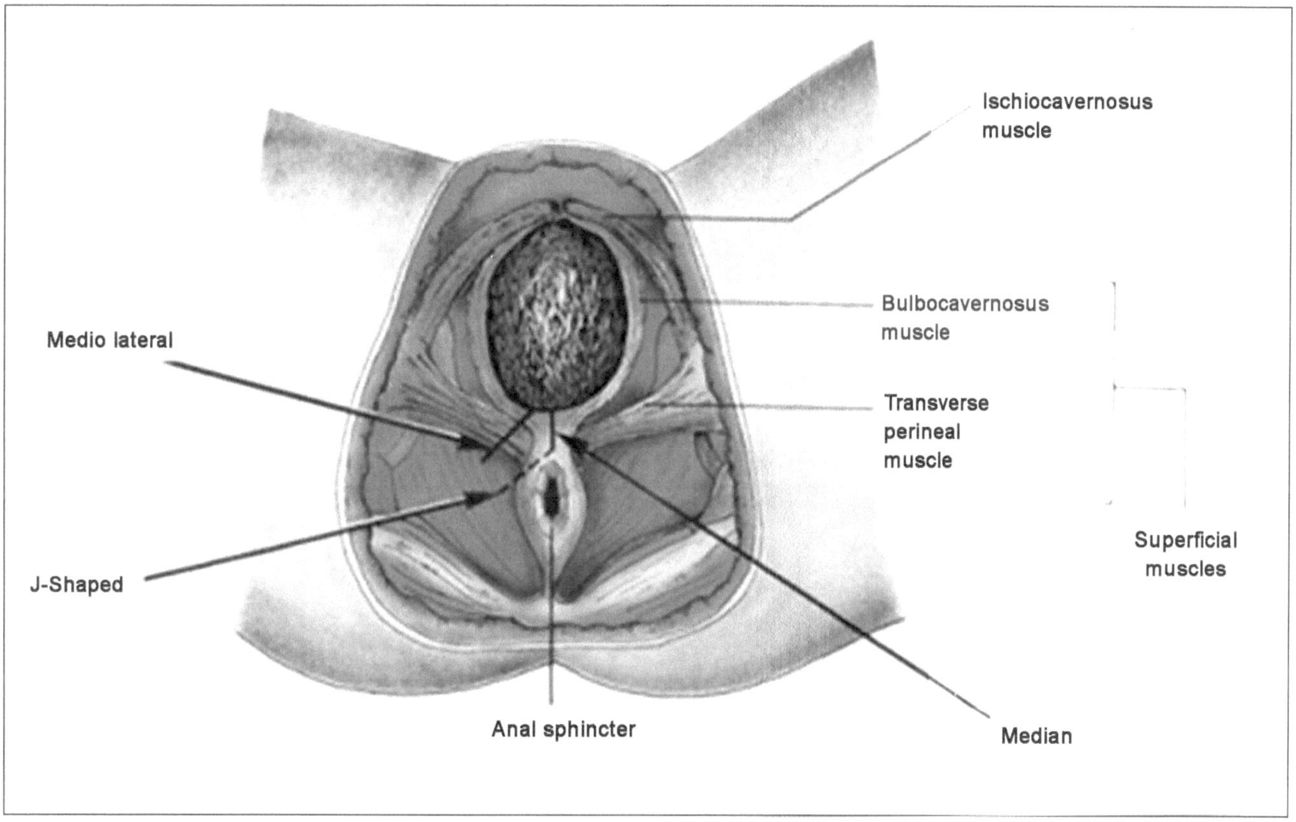

Ans: (a) External anal sphincter

Ref: *Keith L Moore, Clinically Oriented Anatomy, 7th Edition, Page 760; Gray's Atlas of Anatomy, 2nd Edition, Page 262; Vishram Singh, Page 232*

9. Saccule develops from:

(a) Saccus anterior
(b) Saccusmedius
(c) Pars inferior
(d) Pars superior

Explanation:

- All inner structures of ear develops from the **surface ectoderm*.**

Thickening of the surface ectoderm-
next to the hindbrain and dorsal to 2nd pharyngeal cleft

↓

Otic placode or otic disc

↓

Otic pit

↓

Otic vesicle or otocyst

→ Dorsomedial region of otocyst
↓
Endolymphatic appendage
↓
Endolymphatic duct and sac

→ Rest of the part of otocyst

→ Expanded pars superior
- Anterior, posterior and lateral semicircular canals ducts
- Utricle

→ Narrow pars inferior
- Cochlea
- Saccule
- Both connected by ductus reuniens

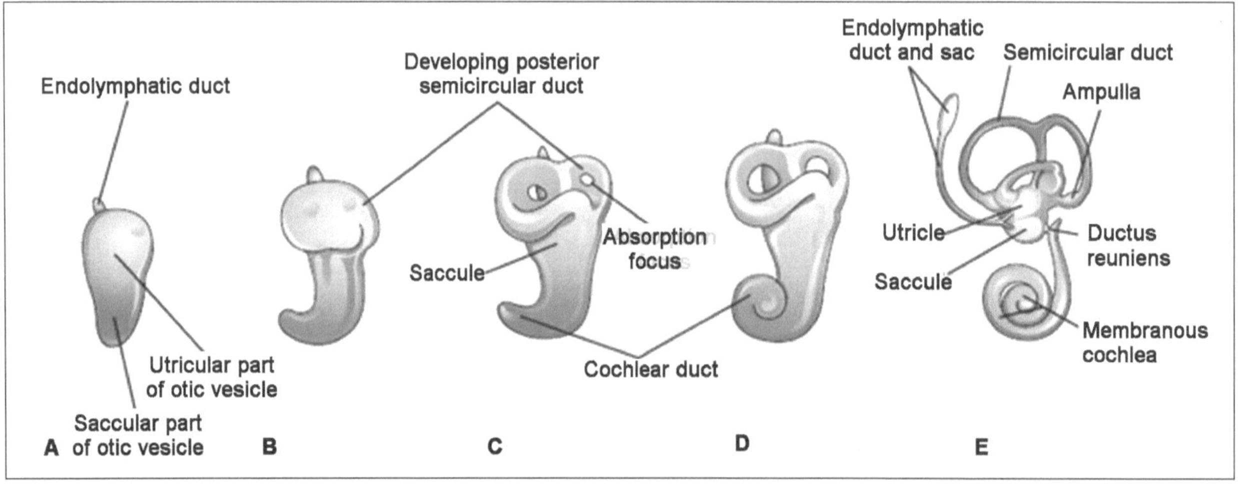

Development of inner ear

Ans: (c) Pars inferior

Ref: *Larsen's Human Embryology, 4th Edition, Page 583; Gray's Anatomy, 41st Edition, Page 658; Keith L Moore, Clinically Oriented Embryology, 10th Edition, Page 430*

10. Which of the following nerve supplies the marked structure?

(a) Dorsal scapular (b) Subscapular

(c) Suprascapular (d) From the dorsal rami of C1

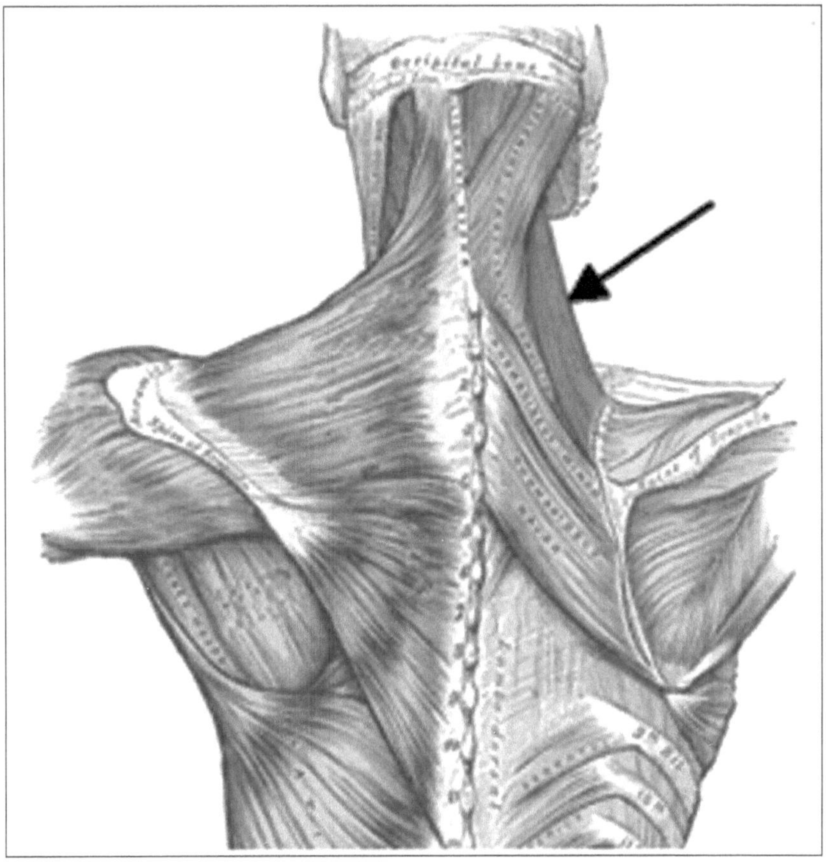

Explanation:

- Marked muscle is **Levator scapulae*.** It is supplied by **Dorsal scapular nerve* (C5).**

Name of the muscles	Motor innervation	Sensory innervation
Trapezius – Upper part	Solely by Accessory nerve	
Middle and Lower part	**Accessory nerve**	Proprioceptive branches from cervical plexus (C3, C4)
Rhomboid major and Rhomboid minor	**Dorsal scapular nerve** (C5 often C4)	
Levator scapulae	**Dorsal scapular nerve** (C5)	Proprioceptive branches from cervical plexus (C3, C4)
Supraspinatus	**Suprascapular nerve** (C5,6 often C4)	
Infraspinatus	**Suprascapular nerve** (C5,6)	
Subscapularis	Upper and lower **subscapular** nerves (via C5, 6)	
Teres major	Lower subscapular nerve (C5,6,7)	
Teres minor	**Axillary** nerve (C5,6)	
Latissimus dorsi	**Thoracodorsal** (C6,7,8)	

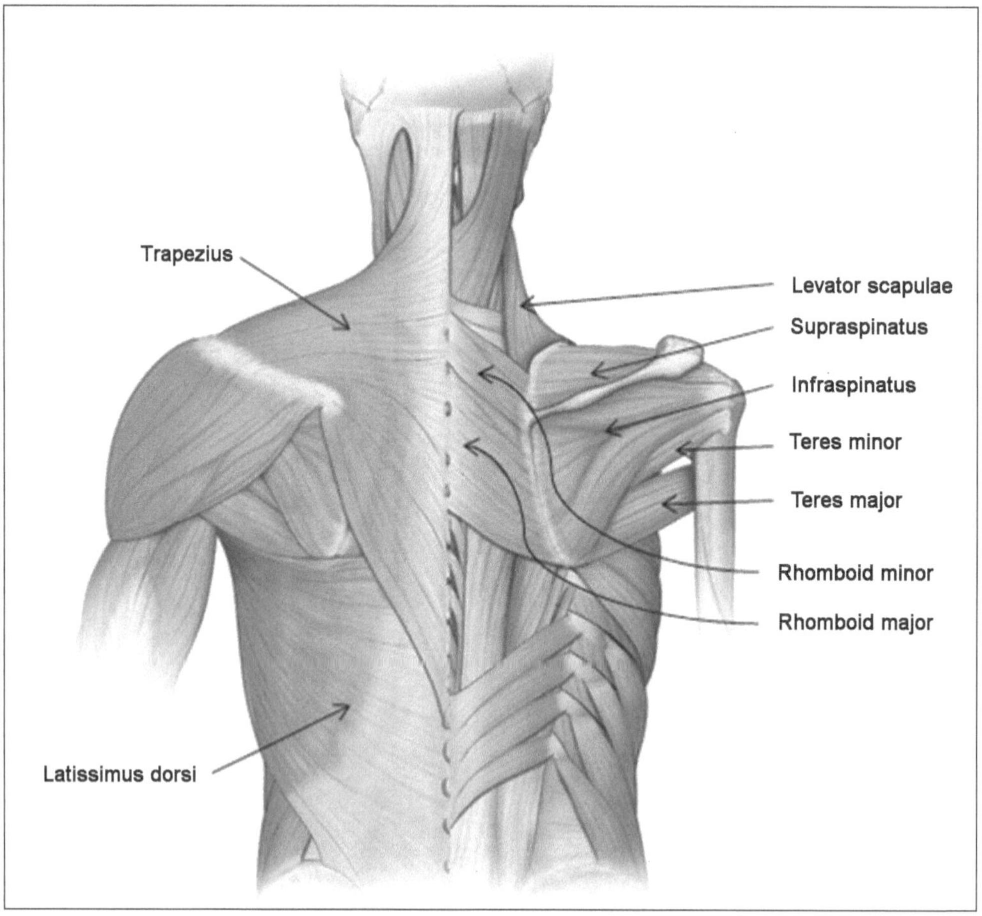

Dorsal muscles of scapula

First Cervical Nerve C1 (also called **Suboccipital nerve)**

- **Speciality:** It provides no cutaneous nerve hence **do not possess a dermatome.**
- **Divisions: (Supplies 5+5 muscles).**
- **Dorsal rami of C1:**
  - *Rectus capitis posterior major and minor.*
  - *Obliquus capitis superior and inferior.*
  - *Semispinalis capitis.*
- **Ventral rami of C1:**
  - *Rectus capitis anterior and lateralis.*
- The nerve joins with **hypoglossal nerve** and through **C1 fibres** supply
  - *Geniohyoid.*
  - *Thyrohyoid.*
  - *Superior belly of omohyoid.*

Note:

- Occasionally has a **cutaneous branch** that accompanies the **occipital artery** to the scalp, and connects with the **greater and lesser occipital nerves.**
- It may also **communicate** with the **accessory nerve.**
- Small sensory branches of dorsal rami of C1 to 3 supply the **dura mater of posterior cranial fossa around foramen magnum.**

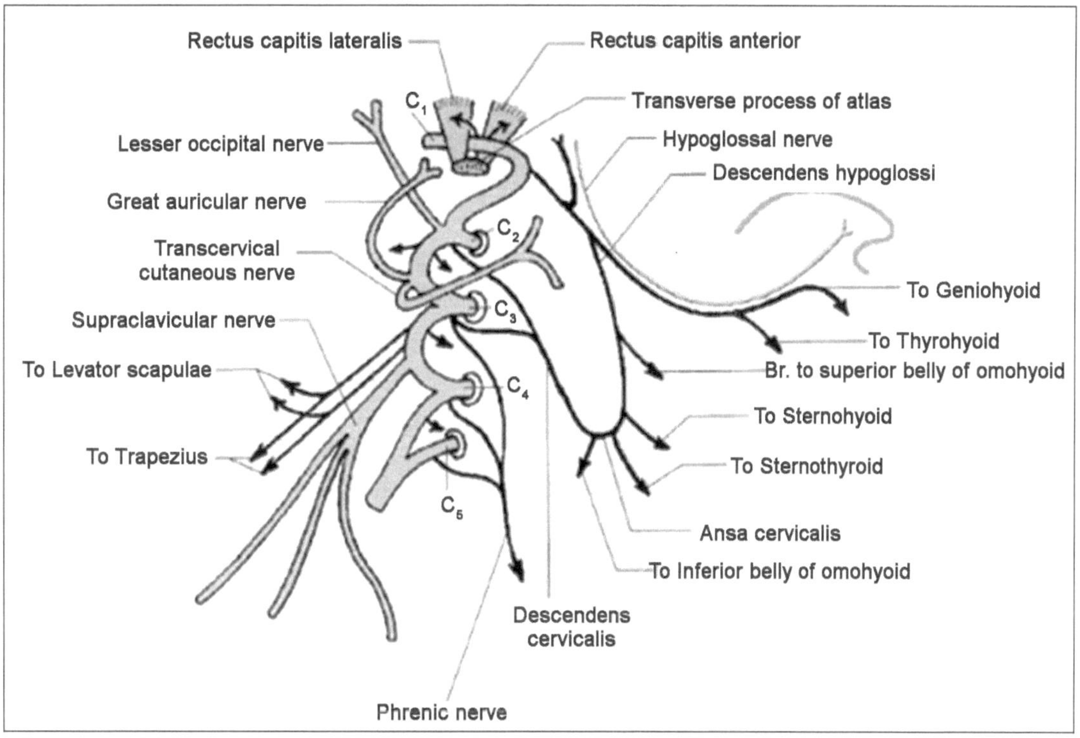

Cervical plexus

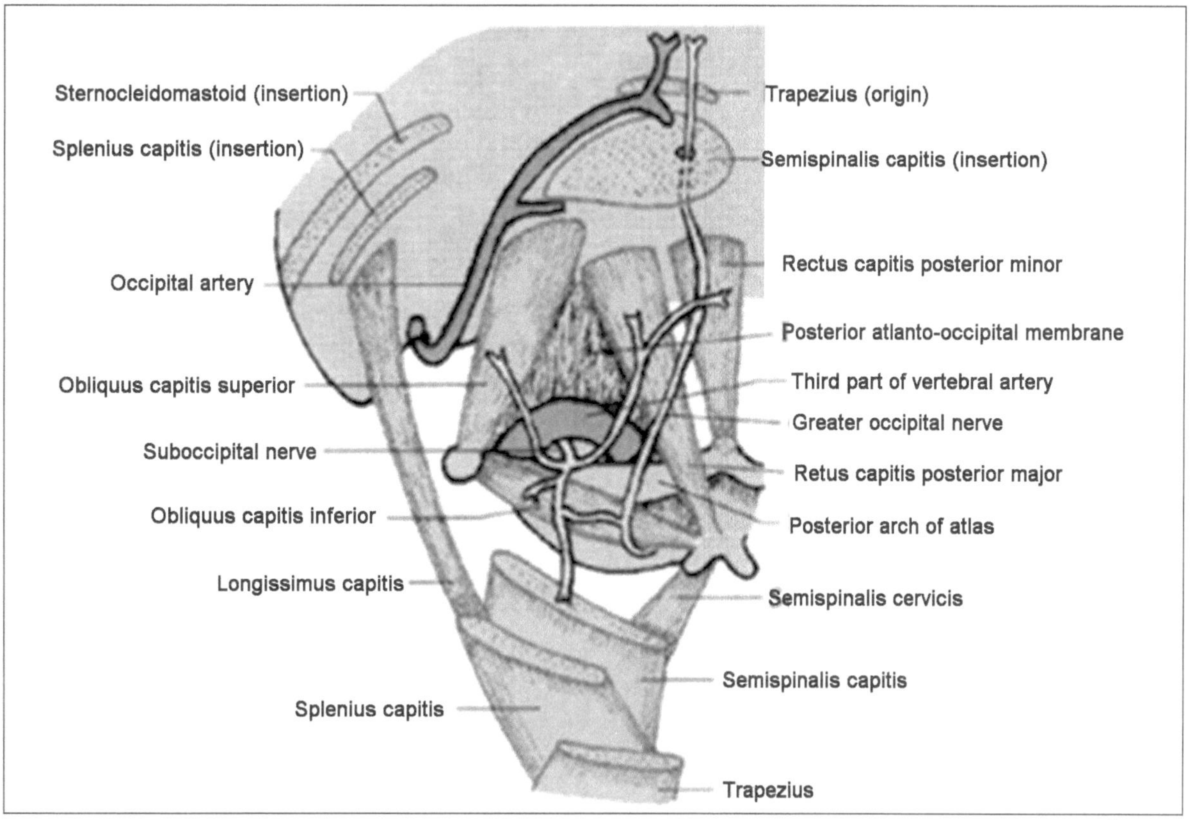

Suboccipital triangle – Left side

Ans: (a) Dorsal scapular

Ref: *Gray's Anatomy, 41st Edition, Page 768, 818, 823, 824; A.K.Datta, Essentials of Human Anatomy (Part II), 5th Edition, Page 103 and 104*

11. The upward extension of thyroid swelling is prevented by which of the following attached to thyroid cartilage?

(a) Thyrohyoid membrane
(b) Sternothyroid
(c) Pretracheal fascia
(d) Ligament of Berry

Explanation:

The convex lateral (superficial) surface of thyroid lobe is covered by **sternothyroid,** whose attachment to the oblique thyroid line prevents the upper pole of the gland from extending on to thyrohyoid.

- The **lateral lobe of thyroid** gland is **3 sided pyramid** in shape.
- The apex of the lateral lobe is sandwiched between **sternothyroid anterolaterally (Superficial)** and **inferior constrictor medially (Deep)**. Since the sternothyroid muscle is attached to the oblique line of thyroid cartilage above, thyroid enlargement cannot extend above.
- Sometimes the thyroid tumor extends backwards, as the false capsule is thin along the posterior borders of the lateral lobes.
- Posterior extension compresses the adjacent structures without forming a visible swelling on the front of the neck.

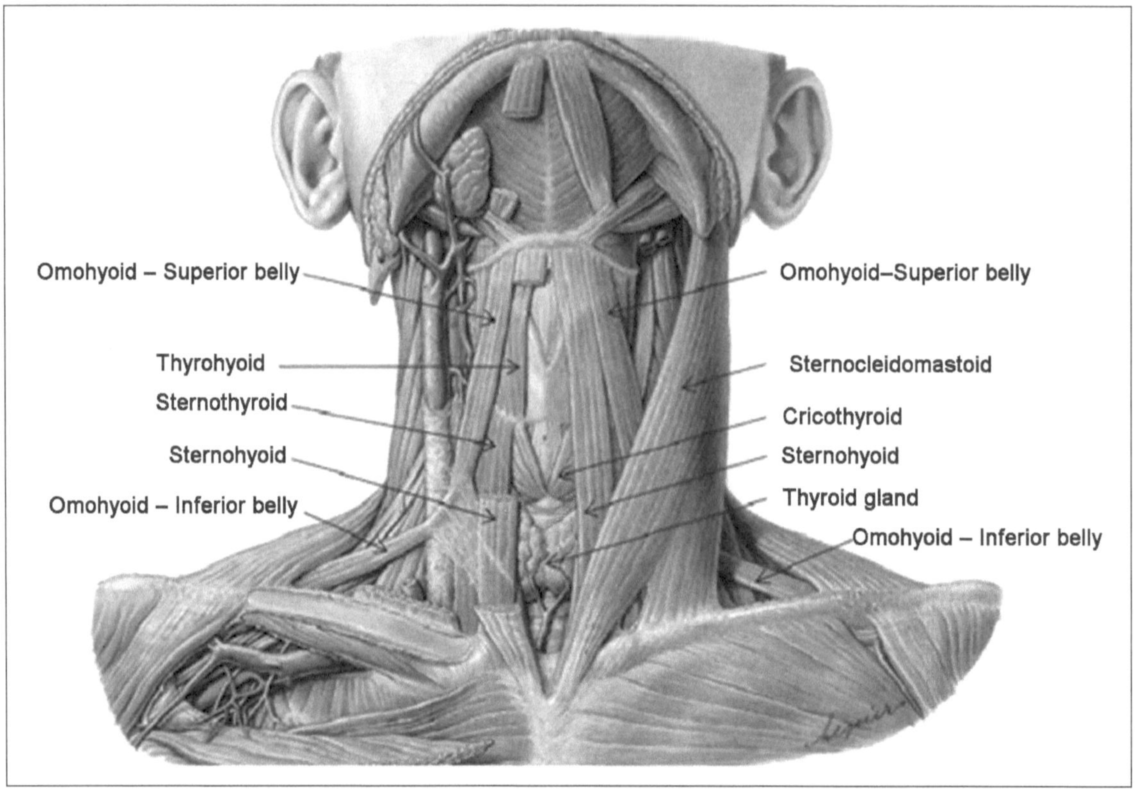

Suspensory Ligament of Berry

- It connects the **medial surface** of **thyroid lobe** to the **cricoid cartilage.**
- It is a thick ligament derived from **pretracheal fascia** forming **false capsule of thyroid.**
- Through this ligament **thyroid gland moves up and down during swallowing.**
- Thus thyroid swellings can be distinguished clinically from other swellings in the region of the neck.

Membranes and Ligaments of Larynx

	Extrinsic	Intrinsic
Membranes	Thyrohyoid	Cricovocal (Conus elasticus)
	Cricotracheal	Quadrate/Quadrangular
Ligaments	Median and lateral thyrohyoid	Vocal
	Cricothyroid	Vestibular
	Cricotracheal	

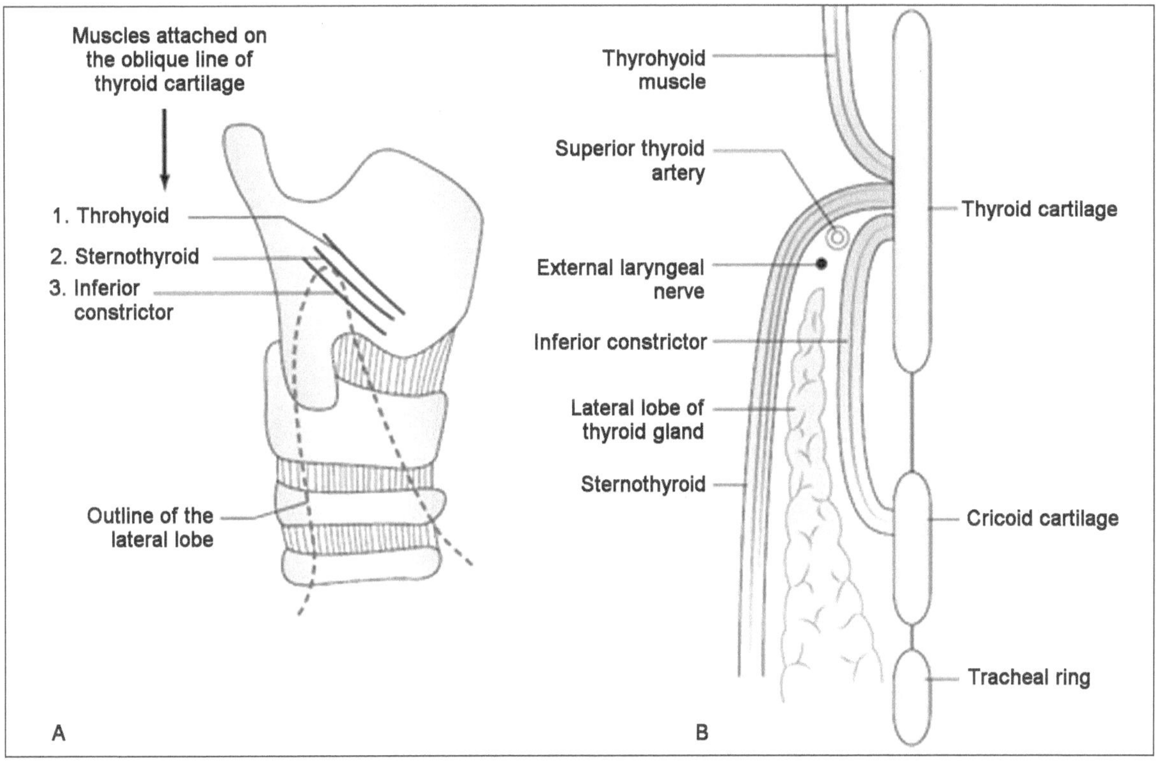

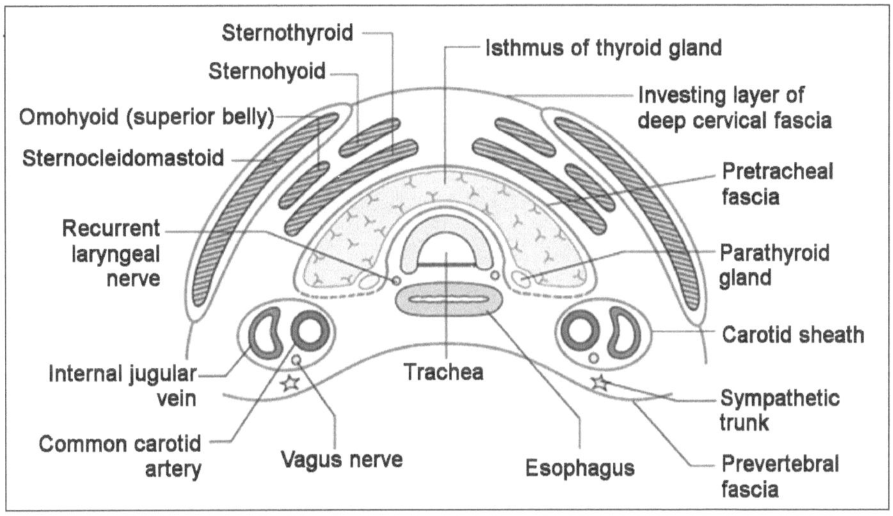

Ans: (b) Sternothyroid

Ref: *Gray's Anatomy, 41st Edition, Page 470; Keith L Moore, Clinically Oriented Anatomy, 7th Edition, Page 1631; Vishram Singh, Textbook of Anatomy, Volume III, 2nd Edition, Page 157, 158, 222, 223*

12. Identify the type of joint in the given picture:

(a) Syndesmosis
(b) Synarthrosis
(c) Symphysis
(d) Synovial joint

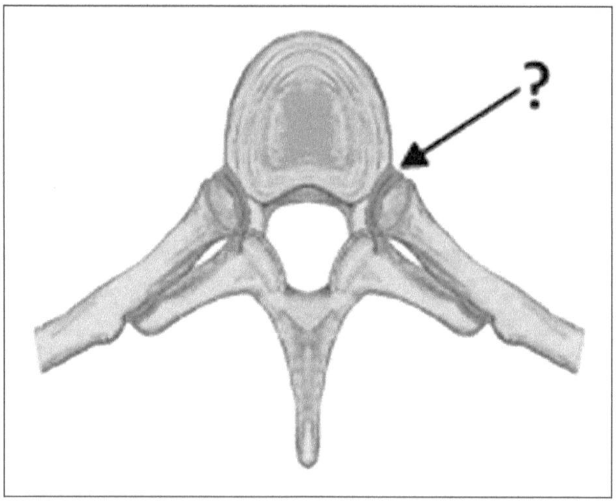

Explanation:

- **Costovertebral joints** – A **plane type of synovial joint** is formed by the articulation of articular facets on the head of ribs and costal facets on the bodies of thoracic vertebrae.
- The head of typical rib articulates with the body of numerically corresponding vertebra and also with the body of next higher vertebra.
- **1st, 10th, 11th and 12th ribs** articulate with the bodies of **corresponding vertebra.**

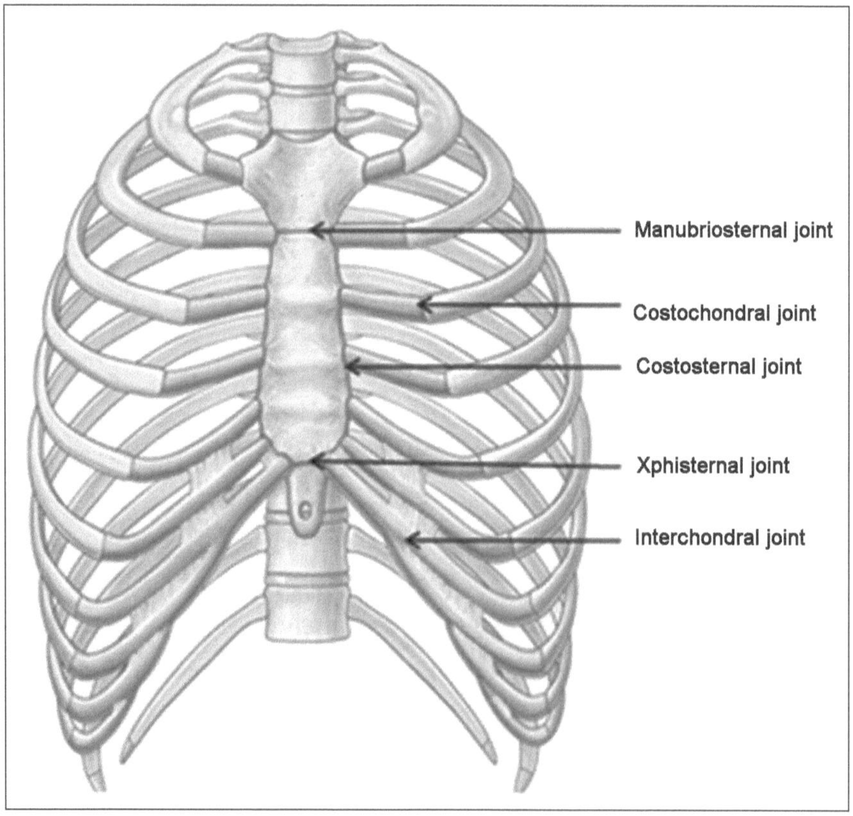

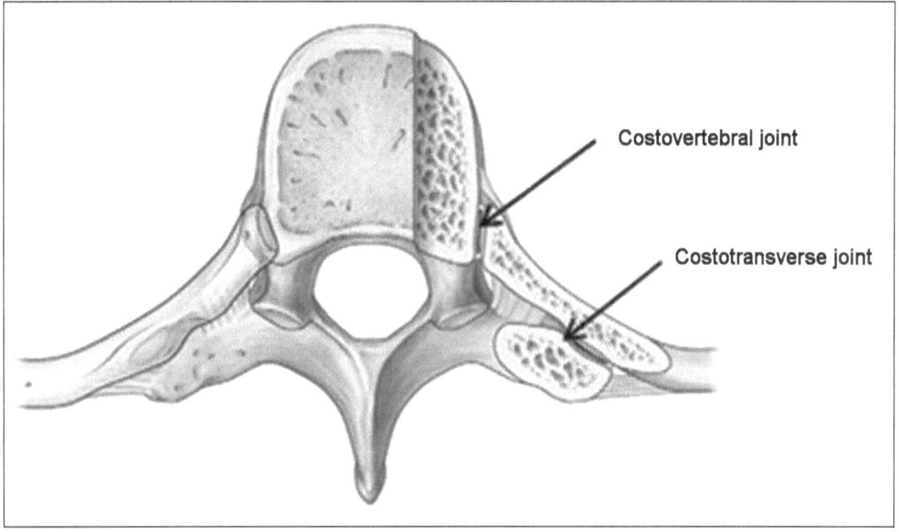

Joint Name	Articular ends	Type of joint
Costovertebral joint	• Head of rib with body of vertebra	Synovial joint
Costotransverse joint	• Tubercle of rib with transverse process of vertebra • Absent in 11th and 12th rib	Synovial joint
Costochondral joint	• Anterior end of rib with its costal cartilage	Primary cartilaginous joint (Synchondrosis)
Chondrosternal joint (Sternocostal joint)	• Medial end of 1st to 7th costal cartilages with lateral border of sternum	**1st chondrosternal joint – Primary cartilaginous joint (Synchondrosis)** **2nd to 7th chondrosternal joint –Synovial joint**
Interchondral joint	• Joint between 7th and 10th costal cartilages	Synovial joint
Manubriosternal joint	• Lower end of manubrium sterni with upper end of body of sternum	Secondary cartilaginous joint (Symphysis)
Xiphisternal joint	• Xiphoid process with the body of the sternum	Secondary cartilaginous joint (symphysis)

Functional Classification (Based on movement of joint):

Synarthrosis – Immovable joints, e.g., Sutural joints, primary cartilaginous joints.

Amphiarthrosis – Partly movable, e.g., Syndesmoses, Secondary cartilaginous joint.

Diarthrosis – Freely movable joints, e.g., Synovial joints.

Structural Classification (Based on type of connective tissue and presence or absence of joint cavity):

- Fibrous joints.
- Cartilaginous joints.
- Synovial joints.

Syndesmosis – It is a type of **fibrous joint** where two adjacent bones are connected by interosseous ligaments or membranes.

E.g. : Interosseous radioulnar and interosseous tibiofibular joints.

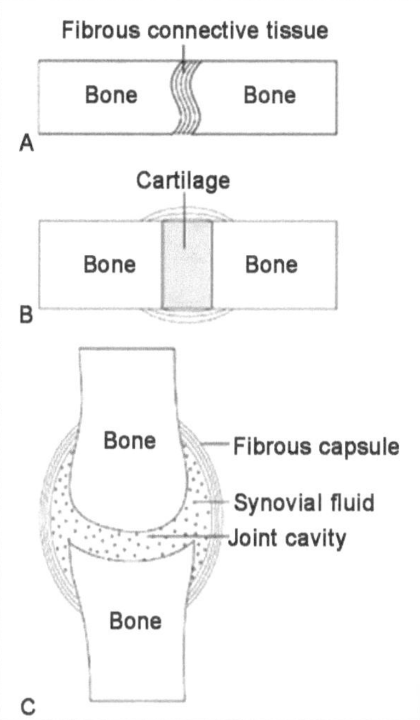

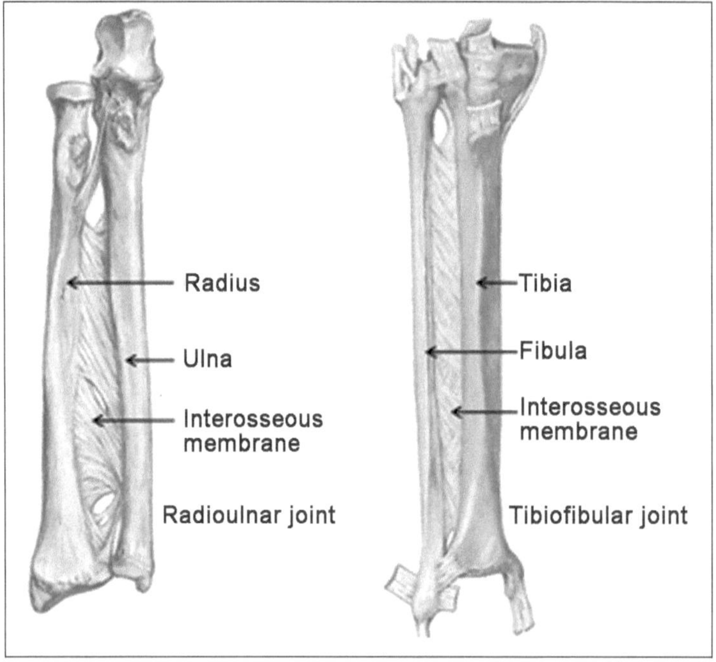

- **Symphysis** – It is type of **secondary cartilaginous joints** where articular surfaces of the bones are covered by hyaline cartilage which are connected by fibrocartilage, E.g.: Symphysis pubis, manubriosternal joint, Intervertebral joints.

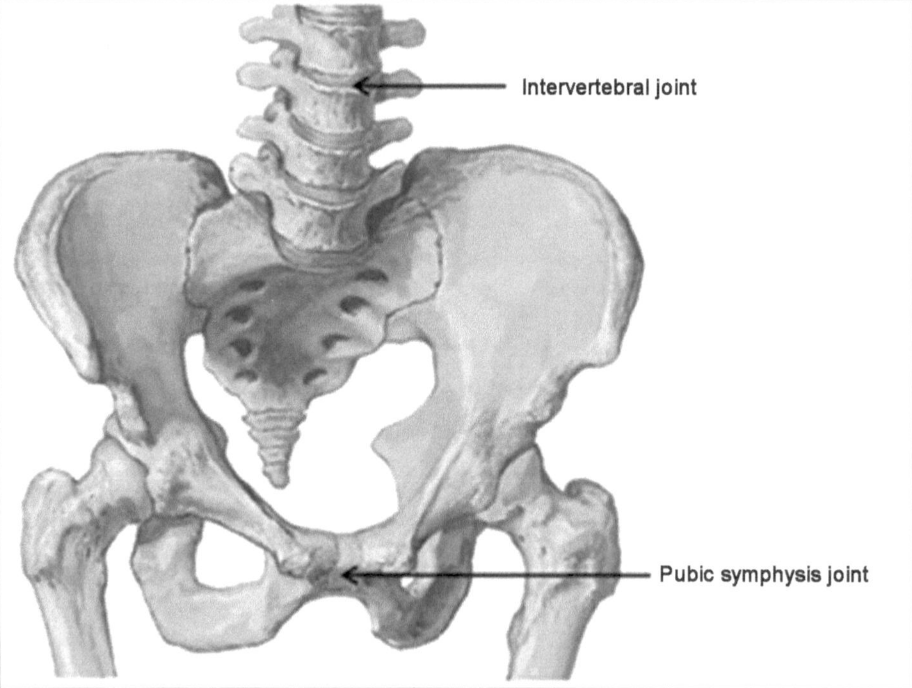

Note:

- Symphysis menti is not a true symphyseal joint.

Ans: (d) Synovial joint

Ref: *Gray's Anatomy, 41st Edition, Page 934; Keith L Moore, 7th Edition, Page 177; Vishram Singh, Textbook of Anatomy, Volume 1, 2nd Edition, Page 207; Vishram Singh, General Anatomy, 2nd Edition, Page 88-91; Netter Atlas of Human Anatomy, 6th Edition, Page 360, 460, 542*

13. In human cells, meiosis takes place at:

(a) Adrenal
(b) Adult ovary
(c) Prepubertal testis
(d) Hypothalamus

Explanation:

The meiosis is a special type of cell division that takes place only in the **reproductive organs** to produce **haploid gametes.**

Gametogenesis in Male (Spermatogenesis)

- In the male, primordial germ cells (PGCs) remain dormant from the **6th week** of embryonic development until puberty in the **seminiferous tubules** of testes.
- **At puberty,** seminiferous tubules mature and PGCs undergo a series of **mitotic divisions** to form spermatogonia.
- Throughout adulthood, spermatogonia produce **primary spermatocytes.**
- Each **primary spermatocytes** undergo **Meiosis I and Meiosis II** to produce **4 spermatids.**

- **Spermiogenesis**–The series of changes resulting in the transformation of spermatids into spermatozoa
- **Spermatogenesis**–Which begins at puberty, includes all of the events by which **spermatogonia** are transformed into **spermatozoa**

Note:

Meiosis does not occur in prepubertal testis.

Gametogenesis in Female (Oogenesis)

- In the female, PGCs differentiate into **oogonia,** which undergo **mitosis** to produce **more oogonia.**
- During **fetal life, oogonia** differentiates into **primary oocytes.**
- The primary oocytes enters into **meiosis I** since **fetal life** but remain **arrested** at **prophase I of first meiotic division** till **puberty*.**
- From puberty with every menstrual cycle, the arrested primary oocyte is stimulated to resume **meiosis.**
- If fertilization occurs, each primary oocyte yields one **definitive oocyte** and **three polar bodies.**

Note:

- **Meiosis II is completed only after fertilisation*.**
- Mitosis is a cell division that occurs in all somatic cells.

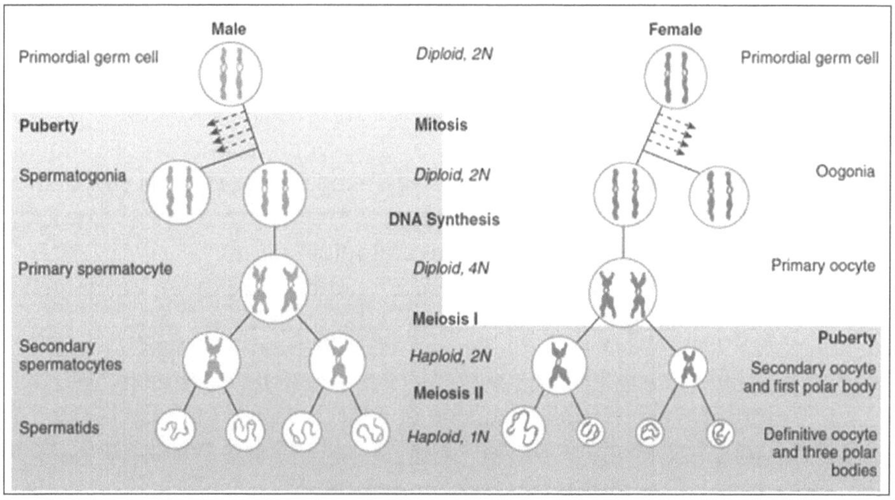

Gametogenesis in male and female

Ans: (b) Adult ovary

Ref: *Larsen's Human Embryology, 4th Edition, Page 20; Langman's Medical Embryology, 12th Edition, Page 24; Vishram Singh, Clinical Embryology, Page 26*

PHYSIOLOGY

1. VA/Q is infinity when:

(a) Pressure of oxygen in the alveolar air is less than dead space volume

(b) Partial pressure of oxygen and carbon dioxide are equal

(c) When PaO_2 is 159 mm Hg and $PaCO_2$ is 40 mm Hg

(d) No exchange of CO_2 and O_2 occur

Explanation:

VA/Q Ratio

- Alveolar ventilation-perfusion ratio (VA/Q) is the ratio of alveolar ventilation per minute to quantity of blood flow to alveoli per minute.
- Normally.
- Alveolar ventilation (VA) = **4.2 – 5.0 l/min.**
- Pulmonary blood flow (equal to cardiac output) (Q) = approx. 5 l/min.
- Hence **Normal VA/Q ratio = 0.84-0.9.**

Normal VA/Q Ratio

- When both alveolar ventilation (VA) and pulmonary blood flow (Q) is normal for the same alveolus, the ventilation-perfusion ratio (VA/Q) is also said to be normal. The exchange of gases is optimal and the alveolar pO_2 is about 104 mm Hg and pCO_2 is about 40 mm Hg.
- At the apex of the normal lung, there is more ventilation relative to blood flow, hence the VA/Q ratio is high.
- At the base, the blood flow is more than ventilation, hence VA/Q ratio is less than apex.

Alterations in VA/Q Ratio

- VA/Q ratio **increases** when the **alveolar ventilation increases**.
- Decrease in VA/Q ratio occurs when the blood flow is higher than the alveolar ventilation. Since the alveolar ventilation is not enough to provide oxygen, a fraction of venous blood passes through the pulmonary capillaries without becoming oxygenated. This fraction is called **shunted blood.** This shunted blood along with the additional deoxygenated blood from the bronchial veins to the pulmonary vein (about 2% of cardiac output) forms the so-called **physiological shunt**.
- When the ventilation (VA) is zero, yet there is still perfusion (Q) of the alveolus, the VA/Q is **zero.** So, alveolar air will have a pO_2 of 40 mm Hg and pCO_2 of 45 mm Hg.
- On the other extreme, when there is adequate ventilation (VA) but zero perfusion (Q), the ratio **VA/Q is infinity**. There is no exchange of gases through the respiratory membrane of the affected alveoli. In this case, **the alveolar air will have PO_2 of 149 mm Hg and a PCO_2 of 0 mm Hg.**

Ans: (d) No exchange of CO_2 and O_2 occur

Ref: *Guyton and Hall Textbook of Medical Physiology, 13th Edition, Page 525; Indu Khurana, Medical Physiology for Undergraduates, Page 319*

2. 'c' wave in JVP is due to:
(a) Right atrial contraction
(b) Bulging of tricuspid valve cusp into right atrium
(c) Passive filling of ventricle
(d) Right atrial relaxation

Explanation:

- The normal mean jugular venous pressure is 6 to 8 cm H_2O.
- **Jugular venous pulse.**
- The atrial pressure changes are transmitted to the great veins, producing three characteristic waves in the record of jugular pressure.

a wave	• Caused by **atrial contraction**, during which active filling of the right ventricle occurs
c wave	• Caused by the by the impact of the adjacent common carotid artery (or) • **Bulging of the tricuspid valve** into the atria during isovolumetric ventricular contraction
v wave	• Due to **increase in volume of blood in the right atrium** during ventricular systole when the tricuspid valve is closed
x descent and x' descent	• Reflects **atrial relaxation** and movement of the lower portion of the right atrium toward the right ventricle during final phases of ventricular systole
y decent	• Represents abrupt termination of the down stroke of the v wave during early diastole after the tricuspid valve opens and the right ventricle begins to fill passively

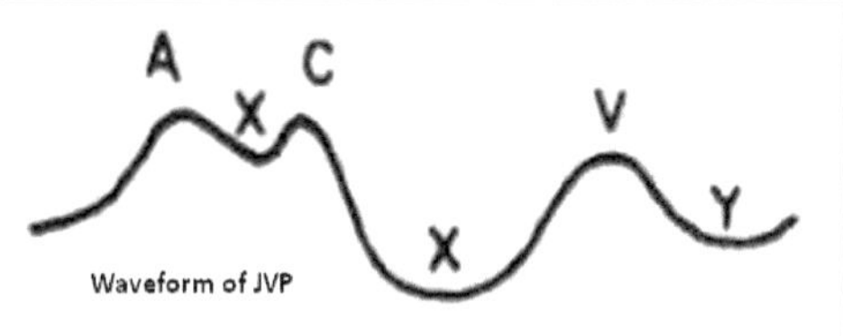

Ans: (b) Bulging of tricuspid valve cusp into right atrium

Ref: *BN Vijay Raghawa Rao, Clinical Examinations in Cardiology, Page 272; Ganong's Review of Medical Physiology, 25th Edition, Page 542*

3. Impaired function of aquaporin causes which of the following?
(a) Nephrogenic diabetes insipidus
(b) Liddle syndrome
(c) Cystic fibrosis
(d) Bartter's syndrome

Explanation:

- **Aquaporins** are the water channels made up of proteins. Diffusion of water across cell membranes depends on these integral membrane proteins.
- Out of 13 aquaporins identified, **4 aquaporins** have been found to play key role in kidney functions.

Types of aquaporin	Location in the nephrons
Aquaporin 1	Both basolateral and apical membrane of the proximal convoluted tubule Both basolateral and apical membrane of descending limb of loop of Henle
Aquaporin 2	Luminal membrane of collecting duct
Aquaporin 3	Basolateral membrane of collecting duct
Aquaporin 4	Basolateral membrane of medullary collecting duct

- **Aquaporin 2** is the key to action of vasopressin (ADH) on the collecting duct. Vasopressin increases the permeability of the collecting ducts, so that water enters the hypertonic interstitium of the renal pyramids. As a result, the volume of urine is decreased and concentrated.
- Vasopressin exerts its antidiuretic effect by activation of **V2 receptors** and insertion of **aquaporin 2** into the apical (luminal) membranes of the **principal cells of the collecting ducts**.
- There are two types of diabetes insipidus, central diabetes insipidus (vasopressin deficiency) or nephrogenic diabetes insipidus (kidneys fail to respond to ADH).
- In nephrogenic diabetes, there is either mutation of V2 receptor making it unresponsive to ADH or decreased expression of AQP 2.
- **Bartter syndrome** is characterized by chronic Na^+ loss in the urine, with resultant hypovolemia causing stimulation of renin and aldosterone secretion. Hyperkalemia and alkalosis is present and there is no hypertension in this condition. This condition occurs due to defective transport in the thick ascending limb. There is decreased sodium, chloride and potassium reabsorption. It is caused by mutations in the gene of any of the key proteins located in the thick ascending limb such as **Na–K–2Cl cotransporter (NKCC2), the potassium secreting channel (ROMK1), basolateral chloride channel the ClC–Kb Cl– channel (barttin).**
- Liddle's syndrome is characterised by mutations in the **amiloride-sensitive epithelial sodium channel (ENaC)** in the distal and collecting tubules. These mutations cause excessive activity of ENaC, resulting in increased reabsorption of sodium and water, hypertension, and metabolic alkalosis. This condition can be treated with amiloride, which blocks the excessive ENaC activity.

Ans: (a) Nephrogenic diabetes insipidus

Ref: *Ganong's Review of Medical Physiology, 25th Edition, Page 698; Clinical Biochemistry: Metabolic and Clinical Aspects (2008). United Kingdom: Churchill Livingstone/Elsevier, Page 52; Guyton and Hall Textbook of Medical Physiology, 13th Edition, Page 439*

4. Highest prolactin is seen during:

(a) REM sleep (b) 24 hours after parturition

(c) 1 hour after wakeup (d) 1 hour after running

Explanation:

- **Prolactin** is secreted by lactotropes of the anterior pituitary. Prolactin is structurally similar to growth hormone and human chorionic somatomammotropin (hCS). The half-life of prolactin is **20 mins**. Similar to Growth hormone prolactin acts through **JAK STAT pathway**.
- Prolactin causes milk secretion from the breast. It causes increase in mRNA levels in the breast and subsequent production of casein and lactalbumin. It prevents ovulation in lactating women.
- The normal plasma prolactin concentration is approximately **5 ng/ml in men** and **8 ng/ml in women**.
- The plasma prolactin level rises during sleep, the rise starting after the onset of sleep and persisting throughout the sleep period. Secretion is increased during pregnancy, reaching a peak at the time of parturition. Bromocriptine, L Dopa inhibits prolactin secretion.

Factors that affect prolactin levels

Parturition	Very marked increase
Nursing	
Pregnancy	
Sleep	Marked increase
Stress	
TRH	
Phenothiazines, butyrophenones	

Contd.

Contd.

Breast stimulation in non lactating women	Moderate increase
Hypoglycemia	
Strenuous exercise	
Sexual intercourse in women	
Estrogens	
Hypothyroidism	
Opioids	

Ans: (b) 24 hours after parturition

Ref: *Ganong's Review of Medical Physiology, 25th Edition, Page 333*

5. At a high altitude of 3000 m, a person complains of breathlessness. All of the following can be used for management of this person *except*:

(a) Oxygen supplementation
(b) Immediate rapid descent
(c) Acetazolamide
(d) Intravenous digoxin

Explanation:

ACUTE MOUNTAIN SICKNESS (AMS)

- Individuals who rapidly ascend to high altitude may experience sudden decrease in arterial oxygen and the rapid onset of signs and symptoms of hypoxia with altered CNS function. Some individuals who ascend quickly to moderate altitudes develop a syndrome called **acute mountain sickness (AMS).** Symptoms such as headache, sleeplessness, nausea, vision and hearing diminution, weakness, breathlessness, and dyspnoea on exertion. In most individuals, symptoms disappear 1 to 3 days after descent.
- Some of them develop **acute cerebral edema or high altitude pulmonary edema (HAPE).**
- **HAPE** is a life-threatening illness in which the person develops symptoms such as severe dyspnoea, orthopnoea, cough and copious crackles, sometimes cough with pink, frothy sputum.
- **High-altitude cerebral edema is** associated with the CNS symptoms such as confusion, ataxia, hallucinations, and loss of consciousness, can also occur and requires immediate descent.

Treatment

- In patients with AMS with complications such as HAPE or cerebral edema, **administration of oxygen** and **descent to lower altitude** are the immediate measures to be taken.
- For people with mild AMS, rest, hydration and symptomatic treatment will resolve the symptoms as acclimatization takes place.
- **Acetazolamide (carbonic anhydrase inhibitor):** Recommended as a prophylactic treatment to reduce symptoms of AMS and also can be used in established AMS.
- **Dexamethasone (glucocorticoid):** Used for prevention and treatment of AMS. This also increases exercise capacity at high altitude.
- **Nifedipine (calcium channel blocker):** This drug is used as a prophylactic measure to prevent HAPE and also in treating established HAPE.
- **Sildenafil and tadalafil (phosphodiesterase 5 inhibitors):** These are pulmonary vasodilators.

Ans: (d) Intravenous digoxin

Ref: *Cloutier, MM (2018), Respiratory Physiology, 2nd Edition, Page 170; Lumb, AB (2012), Nunn's Applied Respiratory Physiology, 8th Edition, Page 254*

6. Which is not seen in ACTH deficiency?

(a) Nausea (b) Fatigue
(c) Hyperpigmentation (d) Anorexia

Explanation:

ACTH Deficiency

- Lack of ACTH can lead to secondary adrenal insufficiency.
- Causes of secondary adrenocortical deficiency includes panhypopituitarism, isolated failure of ACTH production or exogenous glucocorticoid administration.
- When ACTH output is too low, cortisol and aldosterone production decrease, and eventually the adrenal glands may atrophy because of a lack of ACTH stimulation.
- Signs and symptoms of ACTH deficiency includes fatigue, weakness, weight loss, nausea, vomiting, and diarrhoea. These signs and symptoms are similar to Addison's disease but Hyperpigmentation is absent, serum sodium and potassium levels are relatively normal in secondary adrenal insufficiency.

Addison's Disease

- The condition used to be a relatively common complication of tuberculosis, but now it is usually due to autoimmune inflammation of the adrenal.
- Addison's disease occurs due to chronic deficiency of glucocorticoids and mineralocorticoids secreted by adrenal cortex.
- Glucocorticoid deficiency produces weight loss, malaise, anorexia, nausea, vomiting, weakness and diarrhoea. Any exposure to stress including mild infection is fatal since glucocorticoids are essential for adaptation to stress. Patients undergoing surgery are administered with glucocorticoids to cope with the stress. This critical need for extra glucocorticoids and the associated difficulties in times of stress is called an **Addisonian Crisis.**
- Mineralocorticoid deficiency produces hyponatremia, hyperkalemia, acidosis and decreased ECF volume with hypotension.
- Increased ACTH secretion occurs due to feedback mechanism causing hyperpigmentation in skin and mucous membrane. Pigmentation of skin creases of the hand and gum are common.

Ans: (c) Hyperpigmentation

Ref: *Guyton and Hall Textbook of Medical Physiology, 13th Edition, Page 979*

7. Identify the sleep wave marked in the EEG during sleep wake cycle:

(a) Sleep stage 1 (b) Sleep stage 2
(c) Sleep stage 3 (d) REM sleep

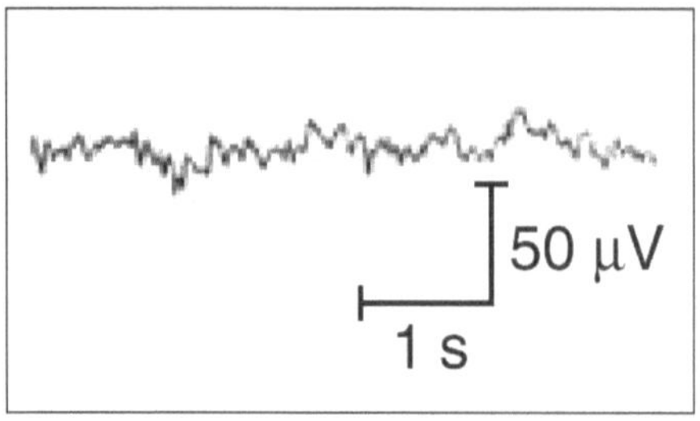

Explanation:

- The term EEG was introduced by **Hans Berger**, a German psychiatrist.

- EEG is used to record the electrical activity of the brain usually by surface electrodes placed on the scalp.
- The EEG waves are classified based on their **frequency** and **amplitude**. The frequency and amplitude differ based on different stages of **mental alertness**.

Types of EEG waves	Frequency (Hz)	Amplitude (μV)	Conditions and location
Delta (δ)	1-4	20-200	• **Very deep sleep, infancy** • Persons with **serious organic brain disease**
Theta (θ)	4-7	10	• Seen in **hippocampus** • **Parietal and temporal** regions in **children** • **Emotional stress** in some adults
Alpha (α)	8-13	50	• **Awake, quiet and resting state** with **eyes closed** • Recorded from **parieto occipital** region
Beta (β)	14-30	5-10	• During mental activity alpha waves are replaced by **asynchronous, high frequency** and **low voltage beta** waves • Recorded from **parietal** and **frontal region** of the scalp

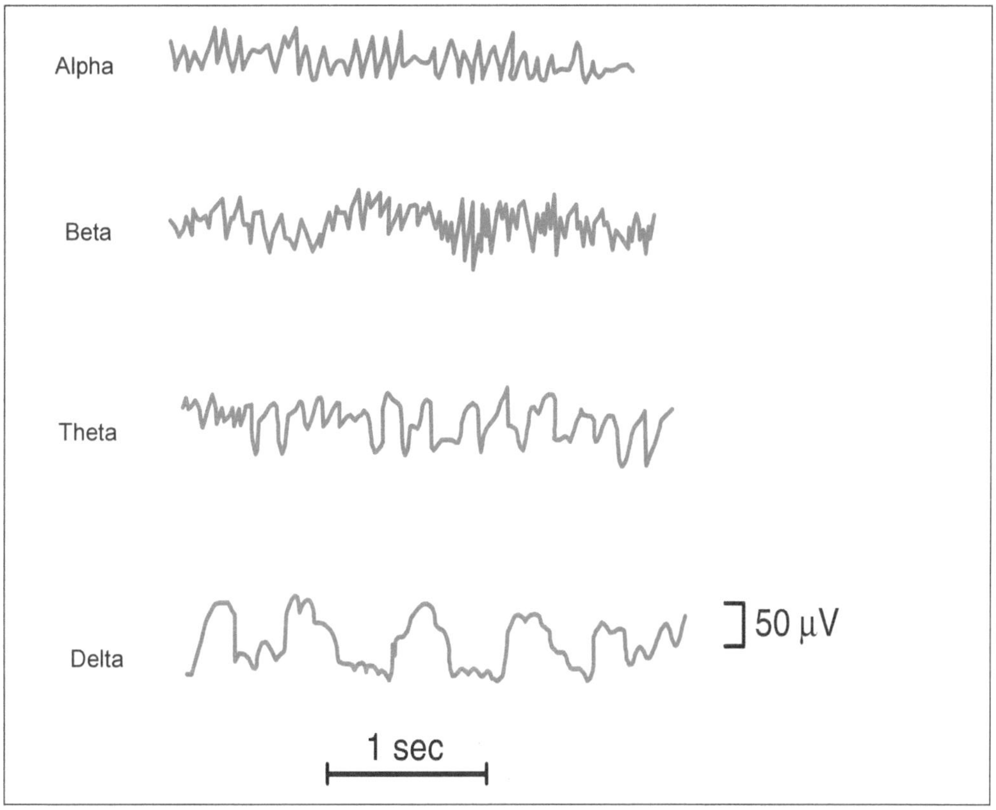

Sleep and EEG

- **Non-rapid eye movement sleep (NREM)** and **Rapid eye movement (REM)** sleep alternate in a sleep wake cycle.

Non-REM Sleep

- Also known as **slow wave sleep or orthodox sleep**.
- **Stage 1 (Very light sleep):** Low amplitude and mixed frequency activity is seen in EEG. Predominantly theta wave is seen during this stage.

- **Stage 2 (Light sleep):** Characterized by appearance of sinusoidal waves called as **sleep spindles* (12-14 Hz)** and high voltage biphasic waves called **K complexes*** (evoked by auditory stimulus).
- **Stage 3:** Moderate deep sleep characterized by delta waves.
- **Stage 4:** Deep sleep with **predominant delta activity.** Rhythmic slow waves with marked synchronization.

REM Sleep

- **REM sleep** also called as **fast wave sleep or desynchronized sleep or paradoxical sleep or dream sleep or deepest sleep**. During REM sleep, high frequency and low amplitude waves are seen. Arousal by environmental stimuli is difficult during this stage. Since the EEG pattern is of wakefulness and the person is asleep, this is called as **paradoxical sleep.**

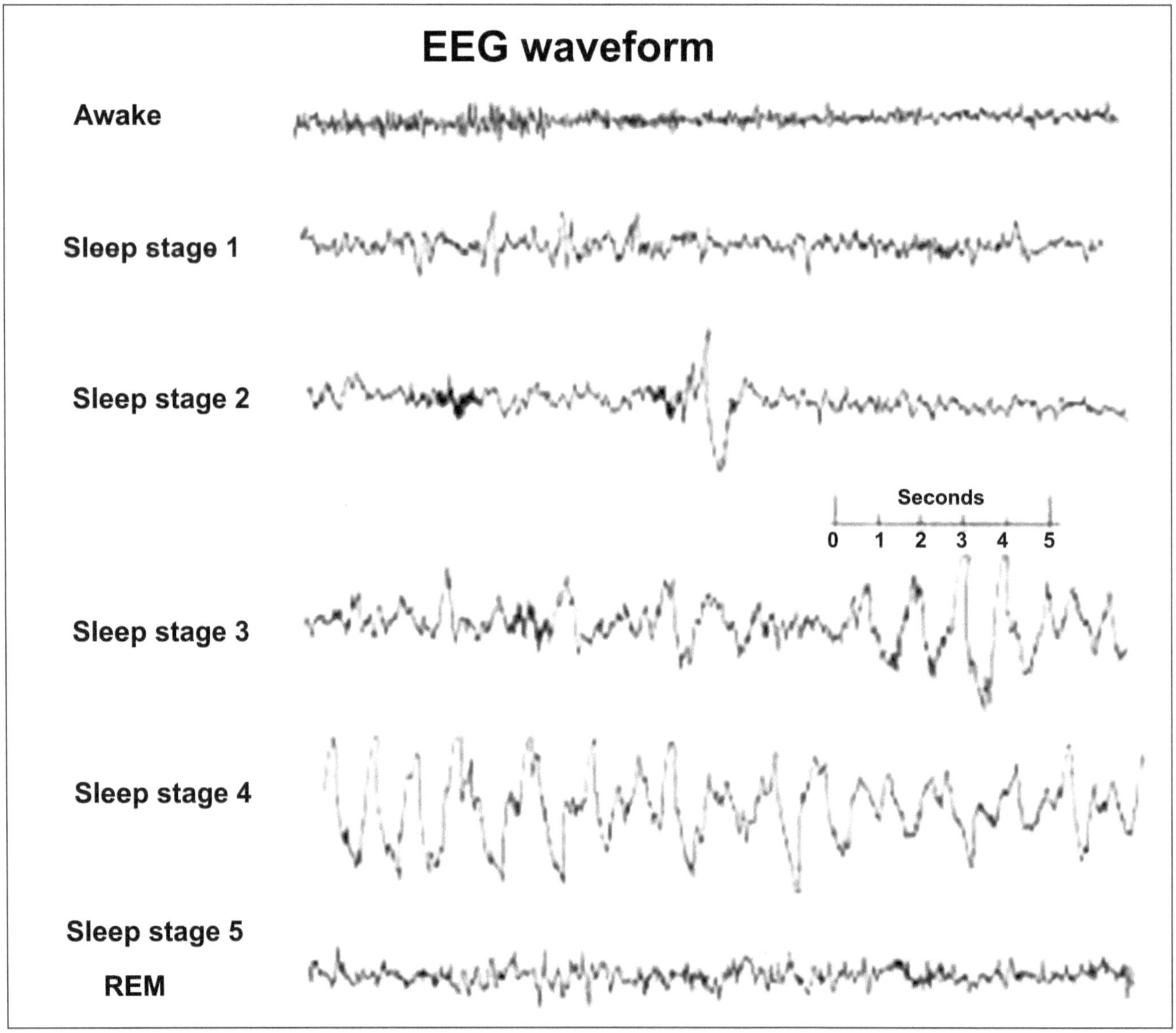

Ans: (d) REM sleep

Ref: *Barret et al., Ganong's Review of Medical Physiology, 25th Edition, Page 274; Indu Khurana Medical Physiology for Undergraduates, Page 866*

8. A patient slept keeping his arm by side, now he developed tingling and numbness sensation over the arm. Which of the following fibre is affected?

(a) C fibre
(b) Aβ fibre
(c) B fibre
(d) Sympathetic fibre

Explanation:

Saturday Night Palsy

- Compression of **radial nerve** occurs to individuals who sleep with their arms under their heads for long periods.
- Prolonged direct pressure on the upper medial arm or axilla causes compressive neuropathy of the radial nerve. This leads to numbness and tingling sensation of the arm. Usually occurs after **alcohol intoxication** since the reflex activity is diminished and hence this condition is called as **Saturday night palsy or Sunday morning palsy.**
- The radial nerve is composed of the **C5 to T1 nerve roots**, which arise from the posterior segment of the brachial nerve plexus.
- Large diameter motor, touch and pressure fibres (**Aβ fibres**) are affected. Pain fibres are relatively intact. Conversely, pressure on a nerve can cause loss of conduction in **large-diameter motor, touch and pressure** fibres while pain sensation remains relatively intact.

Erlanger and Gasser's Classification of Nerve Fibres

- Nerve fibres are classified into **A, B and C** based on their **diameter, electrical characteristics and functions.**
- The large axons are concerned primarily with **proprioceptive sensation, somatic motor function, conscious touch and pressure.**
- Small axons conduct **pain, temperature and autonomic functions.**

Fibre type	Function	Fibre diameter	Conduction velocity
Aα	Proprioception; somatic motor	12-20	70-120
Aβ	Touch, pressure	5-12	30-70
Aγ	Motor to muscle spindles	3-6	15-30
Aδ	Pain, temperature	2-5	12-30
B	Preganglionic autonomic	<3	3-15
C, Dorsal root	Pain, temperature	0.4-1.2	0.5-2
C, sympathetic	Postganglionic sympathetic	0.3-1.3	0.7-2.3

- Susceptibility of nerve fibres to various agents such as hypoxia, pressure and local anesthetics differs based on the type of nerve fibres.

	Most Susceptible	Intermediate	Least susceptible
Hypoxia	B	A	C
Pressure	A	B	C
Local anaesthetics	C	B	A

Ans: (b) Aβ fibre

Ref: *Barrett et al., Ganong's Review of Medical Physiology, 25th Edition, Page 84; Ansari FH, Juergens AL, Saturday Night Palsy [Updated 2020 May 13]. In: StatPearls*

9. Late emptying of gastric content due to presence of hypertonic and acidic content in the duodenum is due to:

(a) Gastrocolic reflex
(b) Gastroileal reflex
(c) Enterogastric reflex
(d) Myenteric reflex

Explanation:

- Gastrointestinal reflexes are essential to control **gastrointestinal motility and secretion.**
- **Enterogastric reflex, gastrocolic and colonoileal reflex** are the reflexes that involve **sympathetic innervation**. These reflexes transmit signals long distances to other areas of the gastrointestinal tract through sympathetic chain.

Enterogastric Reflex

- Enterogastric reflex is a neural mediated reflex that **inhibits gastric emptying**.
- This reflex is initiated by the stimulation of receptors in the **duodenal mucosa** and passes to the **stomach** through the **myenteric plexus**.
- Distension of the stomach or presence of acid in the upper part of intestines causes **enterogastric reflex**.
- **Stimuli of enterogastric reflex**
  - Distension of duodenum.
  - Acidity of the contents ($pH < 4$).
  - High or low osmolarity of chyme.
  - Presence of fat.
  - Protein digestion products in the chyme.

Gastrocolic Reflex

- **Contraction of colon** induced by **entry** of food into the **stomach**.
- Immediately after ingestion of food there is increase in motility of large intestines which causes defecation. This is usually seen in **children** and this reflex is **suppressed in adults**.
  - The **early phase** (**initial 10 mins**) of the gastrocolic reflex is initiated by **distension** of **stomach** and is conducted through the **extrinsic nerves** of the autonomic nervous system.
  - Later, **gastrin and cholecystokinin** are secreted into the blood stream in significant amounts which causes **late phase** of **gastrocolic reflex**.

Colonoileal Reflex

Reflexes from the colon to inhibit emptying of ileal contents into the colon.

Peristalsis

- Peristalsis is defined as a motor pattern of the gut organ musculature that can propel content into the **anal** (**antegrade peristalsis**) or **oral** (**retrograde peristalsis**) direction.
- Bolus present in the intestine stretches the intestinal musculature which stimulates the inhibitory neurons present in front of the bolus to cause relaxation and stimulatory neurons at the oral end of the bolus to propel the bolus in anal direction. This occurs due to myenteric plexus. This is called as **myenteric reflex or peristaltic reflex.**
- The peristaltic reflex plus the anal direction of movement of the peristalsis is called the **"law of the gut".**
- Apart from nervous signals, several hormonal factors also affect peristalsis.
  - **Gastrin, CCK, insulin, motilin and serotonin** enhance intestinal motility.
  - **Secretin and Glucagon** inhibit small intestinal motility.

Ans: (c) Enterogastric reflex

Ref: *Guyton and Hall Textbook of Medical Physiology, 13th Edition, Page 803-13; Barret et al., Ganong's Review of Medical Physiology, 25th Edition, Page 500*

10. Which of the following glycoprotein is found in glomerular basement membrane?

(a) Chondroitin sulfate
(b) Keratan sulfate I
(c) Heparan sulfate
(d) Keratan sulfate II

Explanation:

The glomerular capillary membrane makes the filtration barrier which consists of three major layers:

- **Capillary endothelium:** The endothelium of the capillary is fenestrated with pores (70-90 nm Diameter). This layer is freely permeable to everything in the blood except for RBCs and platelets.
- **Capillary basement membrane:**
  - Consists of gel like meshwork of glycoproteins and proteoglycans.
  - Effectively prevents filtration of plasma proteins due to the strong negative electrical charges associated with the proteoglycans.
  - The GBM contains laminin, type IV collagen, nidogen, and **heparan sulfate proteoglycan (HSPG).**
- **Layer of epithelial cells surrounding the outer surface of the capillary basement membrane (podocytes)**
  - These cells have long foot like processes (pedicels) that encircle the outer surface of the capillaries.
  - The foot processes are separated by gaps called **slit pores** or **filtration slits** that are **25 nm wide** through which the glomerular filtrate moves.
  - Slit pores are composed of several proteins, including nephrin (NPHS1), NEPH-1, podocin (NPHS2), α-actinin 4 (ACTN4) and CD2-AP.
- The glomerular membrane permits the free passage of neutral substances up to 4 nm in diameter. Substances above 8 nm size are totally excluded.
- Apart from the size of the molecules charge of the molecules also affects its filtration through glomerular capillary membrane.
- The total area of glomerular capillary endothelium across which filtration occurs in humans is about **0.8 m^2**.

Ans: (c) Heparan sulfate

Ref: *Miner JH, Glomerular Basement Membrane Composition and the Filtration Barrier, Pediatric Nephrology, 2011 Sep 1;26(9):1413-17; Guyton and Hall Textbook of Medical Physiology, 13th Edition, Page 335 and Vander's Renal Physiology, 7th Edition, Page 8*

11. In comparison to normal healthy person in the evening time, which among the following have elevated both ACTH and cortisol?

(a) Just after awakening in the morning
(b) Cushing's disease
(b) Addison's disease
(d) After exercise

Explanation:

- **Corticotropin releasing hormone (CRH)** from the **hypothalamus** under higher CNS control is responsible for **ACTH secretion**.
- **Circadian** and **pulsatile nature** of **ACTH** and **cortisol secretion** is one of the important features of **hypothalamo pituitary adrenocortical axis**.
- ACTH is secreted from **pituitary** in **irregular bursts** throughout the day. **Plasma cortisol** tends to **rise** and **fall** in response to these bursts.
- The **suprachiasmatic nucleus*** of the hypothalamus controls **the circadian rhythms of the body.**
- The greatest ACTH secretory activity occurs before waking up in the morning and diminishes late in the afternoon and early evening.

- The plasma cortisol level ranges between a high of about **20 μg/dl an hour before arising in the morning** and a low of about 5 μg/dl around midnight.
- Stressors such as physical trauma, exercise, mental stress, etc increases the ACTH and cortisol secretion.
- In **Addison's disease** there is **deficiency** of **mineralocorticoids** and **glucocorticoids**.
- **Cushing's syndrome** is characterised by **hypersecretion of cortisol**. Excess ACTH secretion is the most common cause of Cushing's syndrome and is characterized by high plasma levels of ACTH and cortisol.

Ans: (d) After exercise

Ref: *Barrett et al., Ganong's Review of Medical Physiology, 25th Edition, Page 366; Guyton and Hall Textbook of Medical Physiology, 13th Edition, Page 977*

BIOCHEMISTRY

1. If the percentage of thymine residues in DNA is 28%, what is the percentage of cytosine?

(a) 28% (b) 44%

(c) 36% (d) 22%

Explanation:

Nucleic acids are polymers of nucleotides.

DNA

Primary Structure

- DNA is a polymer of **10^{10}deoxyribonucleotides.**
- Made up of four different types of **deoxyribonucleotides:**
  - Adenine deoxyribonucleotide (dA).
  - Thymine deoxyribonucleotide (dT).
  - Guanine deoxyribonucleotide (dG).
  - Cytosine deoxyribonucleotide (dC).
- Consists of two helical strands which runanti parallel to each other.
- Nucleotides of each strand are bound to each other by covalent 3'- 5' phosphodiester linkage.
- Strand end with free 5' phosphate group at 5' end. Opposite end bears a free 3' OH or phosphate group at 3' end.
- Primary structure is the number and sequence of different deoxyribonucleotides in its strands joined together by phosphodiester linkages.
- Backbone of primary structure – linear strand of interconnected sugar phosphate residues while the purine and pyrimidine projects laterally from the backbone.

Secondary Structure of DNA

- This consists of a double stranded helix formed by the two polydeoxyribonucleotide strands around a central axis.
- DNA is a **double helix**. Each of its two strands is coiled about a central axis, usually a right handed helix. The two sugar phosphate backbones wind around the outside of the bases like the banisters of a spiral staircase and are exposed to the aqueous solution.
- The phosphodiester bonds in the two interwoven strands run in opposite directions.
- Therefore the strands are called antiparallel.
- Thus the polarity of the two strands will be 3' – 5' and 5' – 3'. The 3' – 5' strand is called coding or "**template strand**" and 5' – 3' strand is called **noncoding 'strand'.**
- The aromatic rings of bases are hydrophobic and they are stacked in the interior, nearly perpendicular to the long axis of the helix.
- Adenine base of one strand of DNA is hydrogen bonded to a thymine in the opposite strand (two hydrogen bonds); while the guanine is hydrogen bonded to a cytosine (three hydrogen bonds).
- The ratio of purine to pyrimidine bases in the DNA molecule is always around 1 i.e. $(G + A)/(T+ C) \approx 1$. This is known as Chargaff's rule.

- Bases are hydrogen bonded to each other. Complementary base pairing is there.

  A=T (The content of adenine equals to that of thymine).

  GEC (The content of guanine equals to that of cytosine).

  Applying this rule, if **thymine is 28%, adenine is also 28%.**

Therefore concentration of guanine and cytosine together = 100 – (2 × 28) = 44.

Since, guanine and cytosine concentrations are equal, G=C= 44/2 = 22%.

- In DNA, the glycosidic bonds between sugar and bases are not directly opposite each other and two grooves of unequal width form around the double helix.
- The edge of the helix that measures more than 180° from glycosidic bond to glycosidic bond is called the major groove and if it is less than 180° it is called minor groove.

Ans: (d) 22%

Ref: *Textbook of Biochemistry for Medical Students, DM Vasudevan, 9th Edition, Chapter 34, Page 593*

2. A patient complains of knee pain. Routine investigations are unremarkable and still, the patient is unsatisfied. Urine turns black on standing. Which of the following enzyme is deficient?

(a) Homogentisate oxidase (b) Xanthine oxidase

(c) Phenyl alanine hydroxylase (d) Dihydroorotate dehydrogenase

Explanation:

Alkaptonuria

- Autosomal recessive disorder.
- Metabolic defect of **phenyl alanine** and **tyrosine** metabolism due to **deficiency of homogentisic acidoxidase*.**
- **Homogentisic acid** accumulates in the tissues and blood and appears in urine.
- **Urine** turns **black*** on standing (immediately, if **alkali** is added).
- In long-standing cases, deposition of homogentisic acid derivatives in cartilages of ears and other exposed parts leads to generalised pigmentation of connective tissues and deposition in joints leads to **arthritis**, a condition called **Ochronosis***.
- It is due to oxidation of homogentisic acid followed by polymerisation to form blue-black pigments.

Biochemical Abnormalities

Homogentisic acid
↓
Benzoquinone acetate
Polyphenol oxidase ↓
Alkaptone bodies

- Pigmentation of the **sclera of eyes** (usually at an advanced age) leading to dark blots on the white area of the eyes.
- **Skin darkening**, especially in around the sweat glands and in the sun-exposed areas.
- **Brown colored sweat.**
- **Arthritis** (especially of the spine).
- **Brown or black coloration of urine** if left exposed in air after collecting it.
- Darkening of ears.
- **Kidney stone** formation.
- **Stone** in the **prostate.**

- **Ochronosis** leads to degenerative arthritis in later life.
- **Cardiac valves** may also be affected leading to high incidence of heart diseases.
- No mental retardation.

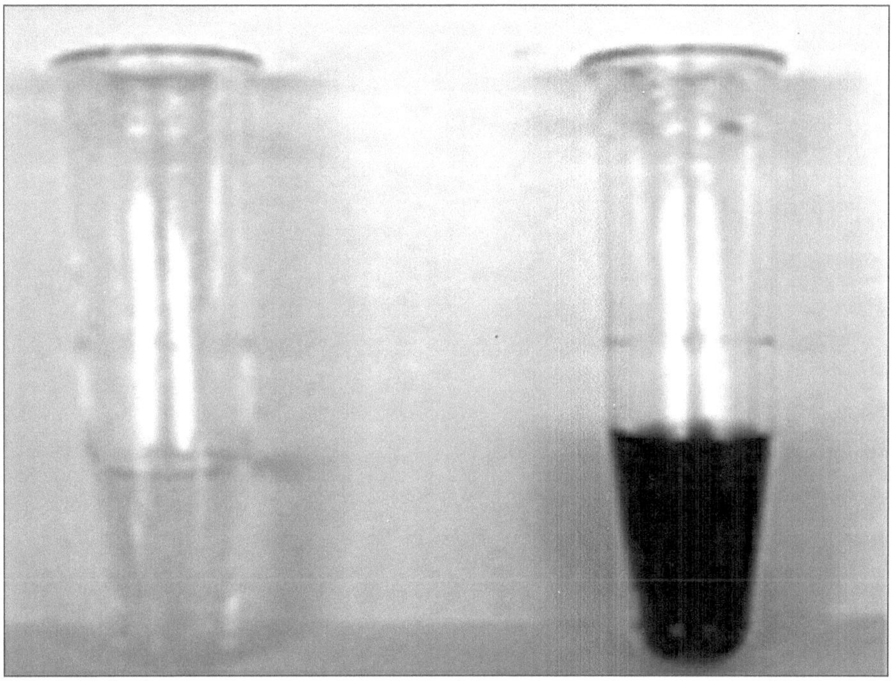

Diagnosis

- Blackening of urine on standing.
- Positive **ferric chloride test–bluish green color** on addition of ferric chloride.
- Positive **Benedict's test.**
- Glucose oxidase negative.

Ans: (a) Homogentisate oxidase

Ref: *Textbook of Biochemistry for Medical Students, DM Vasudevan, 9th Edition, Chapter 17, Page 310*

3. A female is on maize as a staple diet. History of diarrhea and lesion in the neck region is found. It is due to the deficiency of:

(a) Zinc (b) Niacin
(c) Thiamine (d) Riboflavin

Explanation:

Niacin (B3)/Nicotinic Acid/Nicotinamide

- **Sources** – Yeast, Rice polishings, Peanuts, Cereals, Legumes, Meat fish etc.
- RDA –Adults ~ 15 mg , Pregnancy and lactation ~ 22-25 mg.
- Depends on tryptophan content in the diet (60 mg Tryptophan E 1 mg NAD+).

Requirement Increases in:

- Increased calorie intake or expenditure.
- Acute illness or early convalescence.
- After severe injury, infection and burns.

- High corn or Maize diet.
- Pregnancy and lactation.

Causes for Niacin Deficiency

- Malnutrition.
- Consumption of Maize (Corn) as staple diet.
- Sorghum (Jowar / Guinea corn) as staple diet.
- Nutritional deficiency of pyridoxine.
- Isoniazid (INH) therapy.
- Hartnup's disease.
- Malignant carcinoid syndrome.

Deficiency Manifestations

- Nicotinic acid deficiency produces a disease called pellagra (Pelle = skin; agra = rough).
- Cardinal features described as **"3 D's"** are:
  - Dermatitis.
  - Diarrhea; and
  - Dementia.
- **Precipitating Factors are:**
  - High-corn diet; and
  - Alcoholism.

CLINICAL FEATURES

- **Skin Lesions:**
  - Typically involves areas of **skin exposed to sunlight** and subjected to pressure, heat or other types of trauma or/irritation.
  - These include face, neck (**Casal Necklace**), dorsal surfaces of the wrist, forearms, elbows, breasts and perineum.
  - The skin becomes reddened, later brown, thickened and scaly.
- **GI Manifestations:**
  - Anorexia, nausea, vomiting, abdominal pain, with alternating constipation/diarrhea.
  - Diarrhea becomes intractable later.
  - Gingivitis and stomatitis with reddening of the tip and margin of the tongue, which become swollen and cracked.
  - **Achlorhydria** present in about 40% cases.
  - Thickening and inflammation of the colon, with cystic lesions of the mucosa, which later becomes atrophic and ulcerated.
- **Cerebral Manifestations:**
  - Headache, insomnia, depression and other mental symptoms ranging from mild psychoneuroses to severe psychosis.

- **General Effects:**
  - Inadequate growth, loss of weight and strength, anemia which may be due to associated deficiency of other vitamins, dehydration and its consequences resulting from diarrhoea.
- **Additional Factors:**
  - Simultaneous deficiency of riboflavin (Vit B2) or pyridoxine (B6) can contribute to the etiology of pellagra. Both of these are required for synthesis of niacin from tryptophan.
  - Incidence of pellagra is more in **women** than men, reason is oestrogen metabolites can inhibit tryptophan metabolism and prevents synthesis of niacin from aminoacid tryptophan.
- **Association of Pellagra in Other Diseases:**
  - In carcinoid syndrome: Pellagra can occur. There is overproduction of 5-OH tryptamine (5-HT) which may use more than 60 per cent of tryptophan producing deficiency of Niacin synthesis.
  - In Hartnup disease: Pellagra may be associated.

Ans: (b) Niacin

Ref: *Textbook of Biochemistry for Medical Students, DM Vasudevan, 9th Edition, Chapter 29, Page 505*

4. Replacement of alanine by which of the following amino acid will increase UV absorbance of protein at 280 nm wavelength?

(a) Arginine (b) Guanine
(c) Tryptophan (d) Lysine

Explanation:

- Proteins absorb light at specific wavelength.The amino acids **tyrosine** and **tryptophan** have a very specific absorption at **280 nm**, allowing direct measurement of **protein concentration**.
- UV absorbance at **280 nm** is routinely used to estimate protein concentration in laboratories.
- Amino acids with aromatic rings are the reason for the absorbance peak at 280 nm.

Ans: (c) Tryptophan

Ref: *Textbook of Biochemistry for Medical Students, DM Vasudevan, 9th Edition, Chapter 3, Page 31*

5. NO is synthesized from:

(a) L citrulline (b) L arginine
(c) Glycine (d) Lysine

Explanation:

- Nitric oxide (NO) is formed in the body from amino acid arginine.

Formation of NO

- **Arginine** is acted upon by an enzyme called nitrogen oxide synthase, a cytosolic enzyme and converts arginine to citrulline and nitric oxide (NO).
- Nitric oxide synthase (NOS) is a very complex cytosolic enzyme which requires five redox cofactors: NADPH, FAD, FMN, heme and tetrahydrobiopterin (FH4).
- NO is a wonder molecule having diverse biological functions like PGs. Endothelium derived relaxing factor (EDRF) which produces vasodilatation.

Synthesis of Nitric oxide

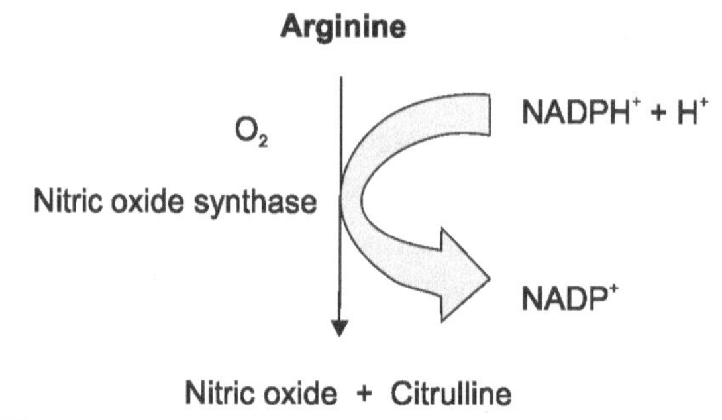

Nitric Oxide Synthase (NOS)

- Dioxygenase.
- Contains heme, FAD, FMN and tetrahydrobiopterine.
- It utilizes NADPH and molecular oxygen.

Mechanism of Action

Through c GMP, activates protein kinase C in smooth muscle.

Isozymes of NOS

- Neuronal NOS (nNOS or NOS-I): "Ca^2+ activated.
- Macrophage NOS (induced NOS, iNOS, or NOS II): Ca^2+ independent.
- Endothelial NOS (eNOS or NOS III): Ca^2+ activated.

Functions of NO

- It acts as a **vasodilator** and causes **relaxation of smooth muscles.**
- It has important role in the regulation of **blood flow** and maintaining **blood pressure.**
- It is involved in **penile erection**.
- Acts as a neurotransmitter in the brain and peripheral autonomic nervous system.
- May have also role in relaxation of skeletal muscles.
- Inhibits adhesion, activation and aggregation of platelets.
- May constitute part of a primitive immune system and may mediate bactericidal actions of macrophages.
- Low level of nitric oxide may be involved in causation of pylorospasm of infantile hypertrophic pyloric stenosis.

NO in Disease and Treatment

- **Nitroglycerine:** The important coronary artery vasodilator used in Angina Pectoris acts to increase intracellular release of NO and cGMP↑.
- **In septic shock:** Bacterial lipopolysaccharide present in blood causes uncontrolled production of NO leading to dilatation of blood vessels and lowering of BP.
- **In eclampsia and pre-eclampsia:** The hypertension is due to decreased production of nitric oxide (NO) due to probably formation of ADMA (asymmetric dimethyl arginine).
- **Iron supplements:** Iron supplements can dramatically reduce dry cough symptoms in heart patients. Cardiac patients using ACE inhibitors, widely prescribed for hypertension, heart failure and other cardiac conditions often suffer from a dry cough. It is the biggest reason for people stopping taking their medication.

Iron supplements act by decreasing the production of nitric oxide, which is linked to inflammation of the bronchial cells in the lungs.

Ans: (b) L arginine

Ref: *Textbook of Biochemistry for Medical Students, DM Vasudevan, 9th Edition, Chapter 16, Page 297*

6. Apolipoprotein B 48 is a remnant of:

(a) RNA editing
(b) RNA alternate splicing
(c) DNA editing
(d) RNA interference

Explanation:

- Apolipoprotein (apo) B is a large **glycoprotein** that serves an indispensable role in the **assembly** and **secretion of lipids**, including **triglyceride** and **cholesterol** of both dietary and endogenous origin, and also in the intravascular transport and receptor-mediated uptake and delivery of distinct classes of lipoproteins.
- Mammalian lipoprotein metabolism has evolved a complex partitioning of transport processes for lipid of dietary and endogenous origin, a phenomenon reflected in the existence of two forms of the apo B protein. Referred to as apo B100 and apo B48, each is encoded by a single APOB gene. The molecular mechanism responsible for the production of apo B48 in mammals involves a site-specific RNA modification, referred to as C-to-U RNA editing.
- Human liver secretes **apo B100**, the product of a **large mRNA** encoding 4536 residues.
- The small intestine of all mammals secretes apo B48, which arises following C-to-U deamination of a single cytidine base in the nuclear apo B transcript, introducing a translational stop codon,UAA.
- This process, referred to as apo B **RNA editing**, operates through a multicomponent enzyme complex.
- Due to RNA editing leading to introduction of stop codon,UAA during translation, premature termination of synthesis of apo B100 occurs.This results in the synthesis of apo B48, in small intestine of all mammals, a protein that is colinear with the amino terminal 2152 residues of the full-length form.
- **Apo B100 is** the major protein component of **LDL** and contains the domain required for interaction of this lipoprotein with the LDL receptor.
- **Apo B48** circulates in association with **chylomicrons** and **chylomicron remnants**, and these particles, by virtue of their content of apo E, are cleared by a distinct receptor referred to as the LDL-receptor related protein.

Ans: (a) RNA editing

Ref: *Textbook of Biochemistry for Medical Students, DM Vasudevan, 9th Edition, Chapter 12, Page 227*

7. Which of the following dietary fiber absorbs maximum water?

(a) Mucilage
(b) Hemicellulose
(c) Gums
(d) Pectin

Explanation:

- The unavailable or **indigestible** carbohydrate in diet is called dietary fiber.
- Dietary fiber is necessary to maintain the **normal motility** of gastrointestinal tract.
- Diet rich in fiber improves bowel motility, prevents constipation, decreases reabsorption of bile acids thus lowering cholesterol level and improves glucose tolerance.
- Has **hypoglycemic** and **hypolipidemic** effect.
- The beneficial effect is more with soluble fiber present in vegetables and only a diet having plenty of vegetables and green leaves will have the desired effect.

- Fiber requirement is about 30 g/day.
- The inclusion of fiber rich food in weight reducing diets is found to be helpful, since it provides a feeling of fullness without consumption of excess calories.
- **Disadvantage of dietary fiber:** Reduces absorption of minerals like calcium and iron.

Table showing properties of some dietary fibers		
Fiber	**Chemical nature**	**Physiological effect**
Cellulose	Polymer of glucose	Retains water in feces; promotes peristalsis, increases bowel action
Hemicellulose	Pentoses, hexoses and uronic acid	Retains water in feces, increases bile acid excretion
Lignin	Aromatic alcohols hypocholesterolemic	Antioxidant, increases bile acid excretion
Pectins	Partially esterified Rhamno galacturonan	Absorbs water, slows gastric emptying, binds bile acids, increases their excretion

Ans: (d) Pectin

Ref: *Textbook of Biochemistry for Medical Students, DM Vasudevan, 9th Edition, Chapter 31, Page 550-55*

8. Vitamin B_{12} is found maximum in:

(a) Green leafy vegetables (b) Roots and tubers
(c) Vegetarian diet (d) Animal products

Explanation:

Sources of Vitamin B_{12}

- It is present in foods of animal origin only and is not present in foods of vegetable sources.
- In nature it is obtained via synthesis by bacteria in soil, water and animal intestine.
- Good and rich animal sources are: liver, eggs, fish, meat, kidney. Fair sources are: milk and dairy products.
- Pure vegetarians should take enough milk/and milk products and one egg twice a week so that they do not develop B_{12} deficiency in the long run.

Daily Requirements

- In normal adults: 3 μg/day.
- Infants: 0.3 μg/day.
- Children: 1 to 2 μg/day.
- In pregnancy and lactation: Requirement is increased approx. 4 μg/day.

Absorption and Excretion

Vitamin B_{12} is absorbed from Ileum.

Requirements:

- Presence of HCl; and
- Intrinsic factor (IF) of Castle, a constituent of normal gastric juice.

Intrinsic Factor (IF):

- A glycoprotein secreted by parietal cells, a constituent of gastric mucoproteins. In addition to amino acids, contain hexoses, hexosamines and sialic acid.

  Note: Atrophy of fundus of stomach and a lack of free HCl (achlorhydria) is usually associated with pernicious anemia, caused by B_{12} deficiency.

MECHANISM OF ABSORPTION

- Vitamin B_{12} is absorbed from the **distal third of the ileum** via specific binding site (receptors) that binds the "**B_{12}.IF complex**". The removal of B_{12} from 'intrinsic factor' (IF) in presence of Ca^{++} ions and a releasing factor (RF) secreted by duodenum take place and B_{12} enters the ileal mucosal cells for absorption into the circulation.
- **Transport in the blood:** Vitamin B_{12} is transported in blood in association with specific proteins named Transcobalamine I and Transcobalamine II and III.
- Physiologically Transcobalamine II is more important.
- **Normal serum level of B_{12}:** Normal serum level varies from 0.008 to 0.42 µg/dl. (Average = 0.02 µg/dl).
- **Excretion:** Normally there is practically no urinary excretion. But following parenteral administration there is urinary excretion upto 0.3 µg/day.
- **Storage:** Stored in Liver. A man on normal nonvegetarian diet may store several mg (= 4 mg). As storage is high, development of deficiency state takes long time

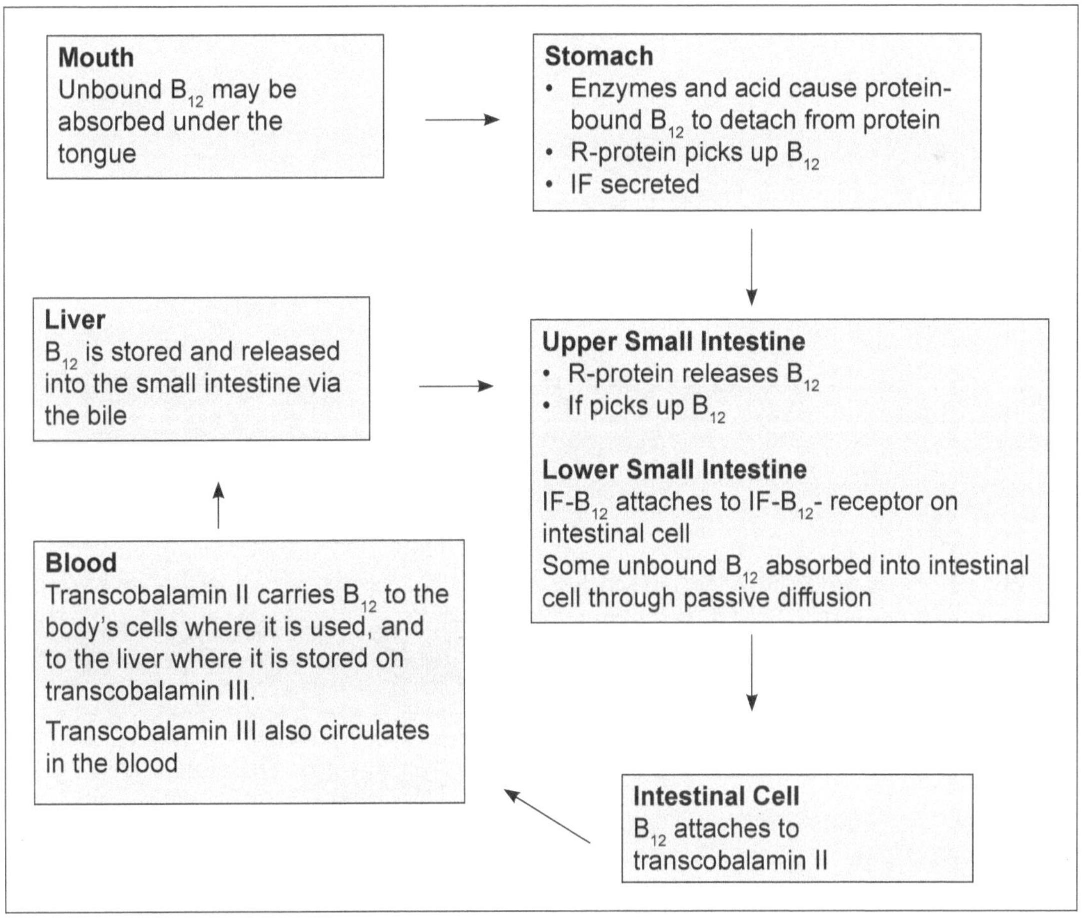

BIOROLE OF VITAMIN B_{12}

- **Methyl malonyl-CoA to succinyl-CoA conversion:**

  Vitamin B_{12} is required as a coenzyme for the conversion of L-methyl malonyl CoA to succinyl-CoA. The reaction is catalyzed by the enzyme isomerase.

  L-Methyl Malonyl-CoA _____ B_{12} ___________ Succinyl-CoA.

  Isomerase.

  Normal healthy individuals excrete less than <2 mg/day which is not detectable.

  Note: In B_{12} deficiency: Methyl malonic acid accumulates and excretion of methyl malonic acid in urine is increased. Methyl malonic aciduria is a sensitive index for B_{12} deficiency.

- **Methylation of Homocysteine to Methionine:** This requires tetrahydrofolate (FH4) as a $-CH_3$ carrier.
- Methylation of pyrimidine ring to form thymine.
- **Conversion of Ribonucleotides to deoxyribonucleotides:** It is of importance in DNA synthesis.

  Ribonucleotides ______ B_{12} ____________ Deoxyribonucleotides.

  Reductase.

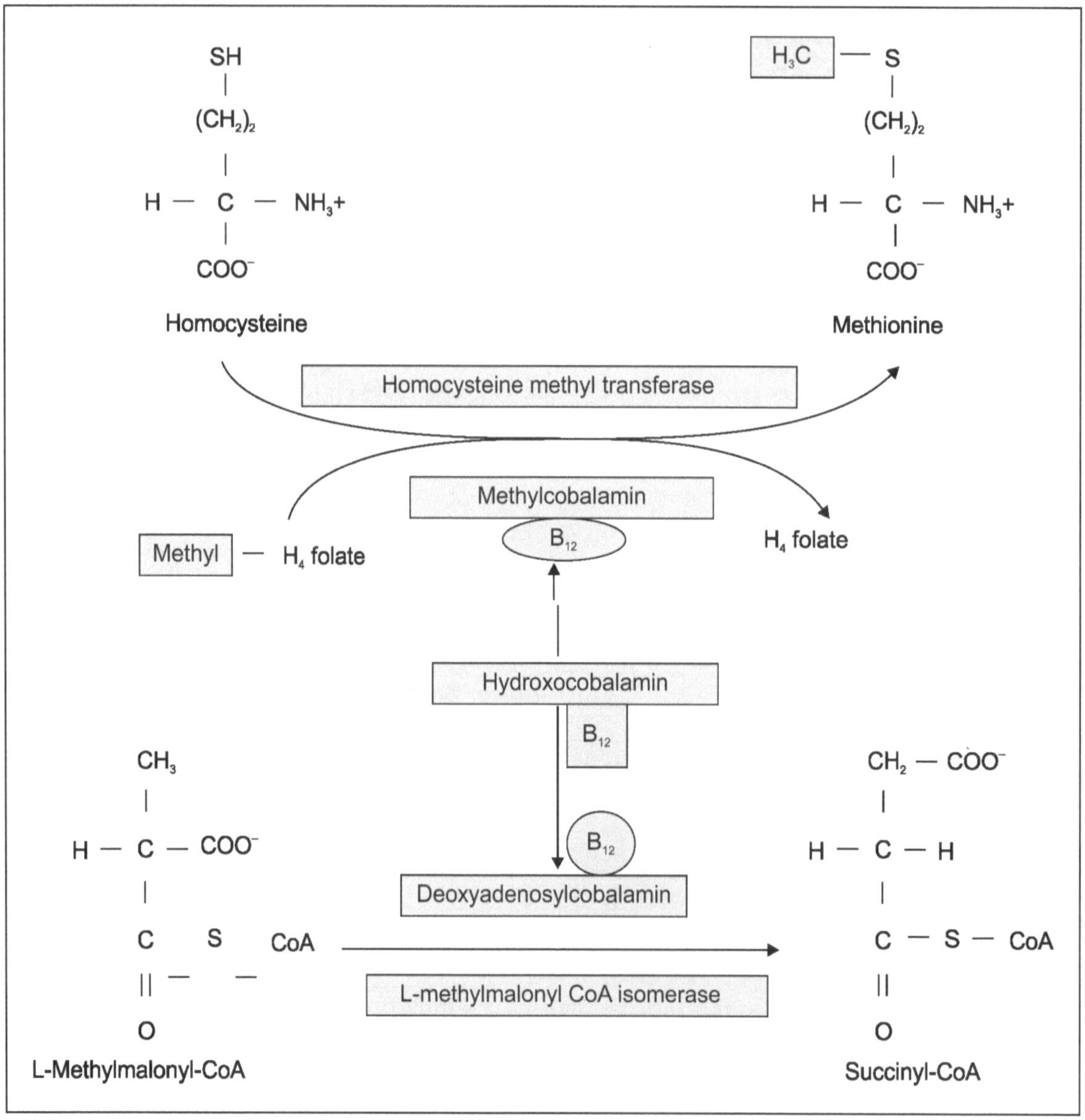

VITAMIN B_{12} DEFICIENCY

- **Causes**
  - Malnutrition.
  - Malabsorption.
  - Congenital failure to secrete IF/HCl.
  - Parietal cell destruction/damage.
  - Autoimmune disease.
  - Lack of B_{12}–IF complex receptors.
  - Partial/Total gastrectomy.
  - Pancreatic disorders/pancreatectomy.
  - Pregnancy.
  - Old age.

FOLATE TRAP (METHYL TRAP HYPOTHESIS)

- B_{12} is necessary as coenzyme for conversion of N5–methyl FH4 to form methyl-B_{12} which is required for conversion of homocysteine to methionine.
- In B_{12} deficiency, the above reactions cannot take place and folate is permanently trapped as N5–methyl. FH4 and is therefore not available for C1-transfer. It is called as folate trap. This results in diminished synthesis of thymidylate and DNA. Increased folate levels are observed in plasma and the activity of the enzyme homocysteine methyl transferase is low.

DEFICIENCY MANIFESTATIONS

I. Adult Pernicious Anemia:

- Vitamin B_{12} deficiency produces macrocytic anemia. In addition to hematological manifestation, it is combined with neurological features (subacute combined degeneration of the cord). It is an autoimmune disease, antibodies to IF and parietal cells found.

In addition to hematological changes, the following changes are seen:

- Mucosal atrophy of stomach and inflammation of tongue (glossitis), inflammation of mouth (stomatitis), and pharynx (pharyngitis), Absence of HCl (Achlorhydria).
- Degenerative changes of posterior and lateral columns of the spinal cord, resulting in peripheral sensory disturbances, hyperactive reflexes, ataxia, paralysis.

Cause: Increased concentration of methyl malonic acid, which competes with malonyl-CoA leading to impairment of FA synthesis.

Hematological Changes:

Peripheral blood picture shows:

- Macrocytic type of anemia with megaloblasts, erythroblasts and normoblasts.
- Granulocytopenia with occasional myelocytes.
- Thrombocytopenia.
- Reduction in RB cells count and Hb content.

Other **biochemical changes** are:

- Serum B_{12} level is decreased.
- Urinary B_{12} level is decreased.
- Rise in fecal B_{12} excretion.
- Schilling test shows decrease in labelled B_{12} absorption.

- Urinary excretion of methyl malonic acid is increased.
- Auto-antibodies to IF (intrinsic factor) and parietal cells (canalicular lipoproteins).

Bone Marrow:

- **Shows evidences of arrested development of all elements:** Erythroid, myeloid and thrombocytes.
- Megaloblasts and myeloblasts accumulate at the expense of more mature cells, viz., erythroblasts, normoblasts and myelocytes.
- Number of megakaryocytes decrease.
- **DNA synthesis:** In pernicious anemia, DNA synthesis in maturing red blood cells is depressed, due to:
  - Failure in conversion of ribonucleotides to deoxyribonucleotides; and
  - Partly owing to the failure in forming the thymidylic acid by the methylation of deoxyuridylic acid.

  The fall in DNA synthesis results in prolongation of resting phases between successive mitoses of maturing RB cells as also a rise in the RNA levels ↑ in those cells so that the resulting macrocytic RB cells has a much higher RNA: DNA ratio ↑ than the normal RB cells. The lengthening of resting phase may be the ultimate reason for the formation of Megaloblasts in pernicious anemia.

II. Congenital Pernicious Anemia:

Occurs in postnatal period, before 2½ years of age:

- Due to lack of intrinsic factor (IF).
- It is not accompanied by gastric acid secretion/or abnormalities of gastric mucosa.

III. Juvenile Pernicious Anemia:

- Failure to secrete intrinsic factor (IF).
- Associated achlorhydria and atrophic gastritis.
- Antibodies to IF/and/or parietal cells have been demonstrated (autoimmune in nature).

IV. Following Surgical Operations:

Pernicious anemia may occur in the following:

- Total gastrectomy
- Extensive resections of small intestine.

V. Tapeworm Infection of GI Tract:

A megaloblastic anemia, responsive to vitamin B_{12} therapy occurs with infestation with "Fish tapeworm", Diphyllobothrium latum, which eats up unusually large amounts of vitamin B_{12} from the gut, creating B_{12} deficiency to the host.

B_{12} Deficiency Symptoms:

- Macrocytic hypochromic Anemia–'folate trap'.
- Neurological manifestations.
- Mild – Paresthesia.
- Advanced – Confusion, Loss of memory, Psychosis.
- Homocysteinuria / Methylmalonyl aciduria.

Neurological Problems may be due to:

- Methyl malonyl CoA ↑ – Inhibits acetyl CoA carboxylase.
- Substitutes malonyl CoA in fatty acid synthesis–Branched FA – Affects membrane integrity.
- Propionyl CoA ↑– Inhibits acetyl CoA carboxylase.
- **Cobalamin Deficiency Assessment**

  Serum Cobalamin (ELISA).

  Schilling test – Radio labelled Cobalamin (1μG) given orally.

- In Gastric atrophy – radioactivity in feces.
- In Nutritional deficiency – enhanced absorption – radioactivity in liver region – very little in feces.
- Methyl malonic acid in urine.
- Homocysteinuria.
- Peripheral smear – Megaloblasts are seen.

Methyl Malonic Aciduria: This is of two types:

- **Due to vitamin B_{12} deficiency:** Vitamin B_{12} is required as a coenzyme for "isomerase" which converts methyl malonyl CoA to succinyl CoA. In vitamin B_{12} deficiency, this conversion cannot take place, as a result methyl malonic acid ↑accumulates in blood and tissues and excreted in urine. Excretion of methyl malonic acid in urine is a sensitive index for vitamin B_{12} deficiency.
- **Inherited deficiency of the enzyme isomerase:** In this vitamin B_{12} deficiency is not there. It is observed as inherited disorder in infants and young children, with severe metabolic acidosis.
- **In pernicious anemia:** 0.5 to 1.0 μgm/day given parenterally will maintain in complete hematological and neurological remissions.

Ans: (d) Animal products

Ref: *Textbook of Biochemistry for Medical Students, DM Vasudevan, 9th edition, Chapter 29, Page 514*

9. Enzyme activated by decrease in insulin : glucagon ratio:

(a) Glucokinase
(b) Hexokinase
(c) Glucose 6 phosphatase
(d) PFK

Explanation:

Insulin—Secreted from **pancreatic islet ß cells**, released in response to elevated glucose.

ACTIONS OF INSULIN

(A) **Net decrease of delivery of glucose** to systemic blood by liver.

(B) **Increase in the rate of utilisation** of glucose by tissue cells.

MECHANISMS

(A) **Diminished glucose levels** in blood is due to:

- Decreased hepatic glycogenolysis.
- Increased hepatic glycogenesis by its direct action on Protein phosphatase-1, thus converting glycogen synthase 'b' (inactive) to glycogen synthase 'a' (active).
- Decreased gluconeogenesis.

(B) **Increase in the rate of utilisation of glucose by tissue cells:**

Glucose is removed from the blood more readily and is utilised more actively for:

- Oxidation for energy production.
- Increases lipogenesis; and
- For glycogenesis.

The overall effect of insulin is antagonistic to that of adrenal glucocorticoids and growth hormone. Its primary action in extrahepatic tissues is to facilitate entrance of glucose into the cells. In the liver, which is freely permeable to glucose, insulin exerts a regulatory influence upon the activity of glucokinase.

Effects of insulin on blood glucose: Uptake of glucose by cells and storage as triacylglycerols and glycogen	
Metabolic effect	**Target enzyme**
↑Glucose uptake (muscle, adipose)	↑Glucose transporter (GLUT4)
↑Glucose uptake (liver)	↑Glucokinased (increased expression)
↑Glycogen synthesis (liver, muscle)	↑Glycogen synthase
↓Glycogen breakdown (liver, muscle)	↓Glycogen phosphorylase
↑Glycolysis, acetyl-CoA production (liver, muscle)	↑PFK-1 (by ↑ PFK-2)
	↑Pyruvate dehydrogenase complex
↑Fatty acid synthesis (liver)	↑Acetyl-CoA carboxylase
↑Triacylglycerol synthesis (adipose tissue)	↑Lipoprotein lipase

Actions of Insulin

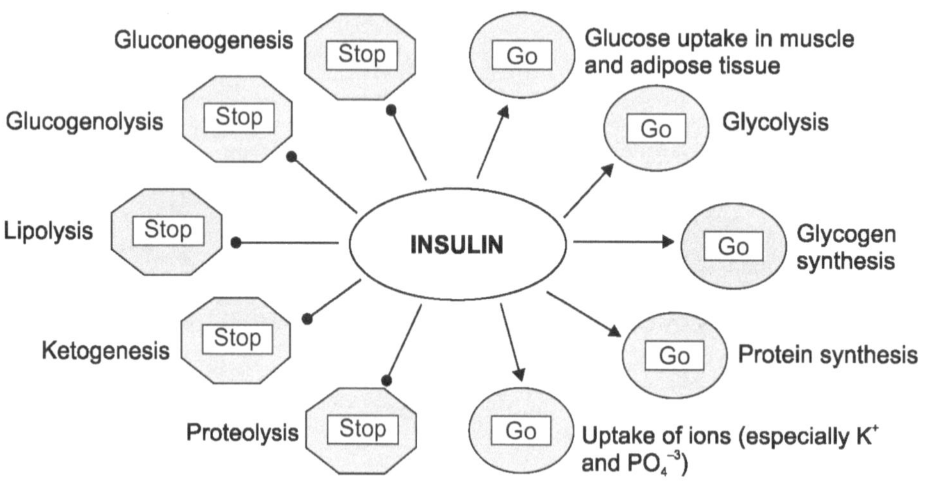

Glucagon—Secreted from pancreatic islet alpha cells, it acts through stimulating cAMP.

- In response to hypoglycemia, α-cells produce glucagon which produces rapid glycogenolysis in liver. It activates phosphorylase enzyme, by increasing cyclic AMP level, which mediates its action through cyclic AMP mediated protein kinase. Active protein kinase, activates phosphorylase kinase which in turn activates the enzyme glycogen phosphorylase.

Note: Glucagon cannot produce glycogenolysis in muscle as it lacks the receptor.

- Glucagon also enhances "gluconeogenesis" from amino acids, pyruvates and lactates.

Effects of glucagon on blood glucose: Production and release of glucose by the liver		
Metabolic effect	**Effect on glucose metabolism**	**Target enzyme**
↑ Glycogen breakdown (liver)	Glycogen→glucose	↑ Glycogen phosphorylase
↓ Glycogen synthesis (liver)	Less glucose stored as glycogen	↓ Glycogen synthase
↓ Glycolysis (liver)	Less glucose used as fuel in liver	↓ PFK-1
↑ Gluconeogenesis (liver)	Amino acids, Glycerol, Oxaloacetate } → glucose	↑ FBPase-2 ↓ Pyruvate kinase ↑ PEP carboxykinase
↑ Fatty acid mobilization (adipose tissue)	Less glucose used as fuel by liver, muscle	↑ Triacylglycerol lipase Perilipin phosphorylation
↑ Ketogenesis	Provides alternative to glucose as energy source for brain	↑ Acetyl-CoA carboxylase

Blood glucose level is the balance between hyperglycemic and hypoglycemic hormones.

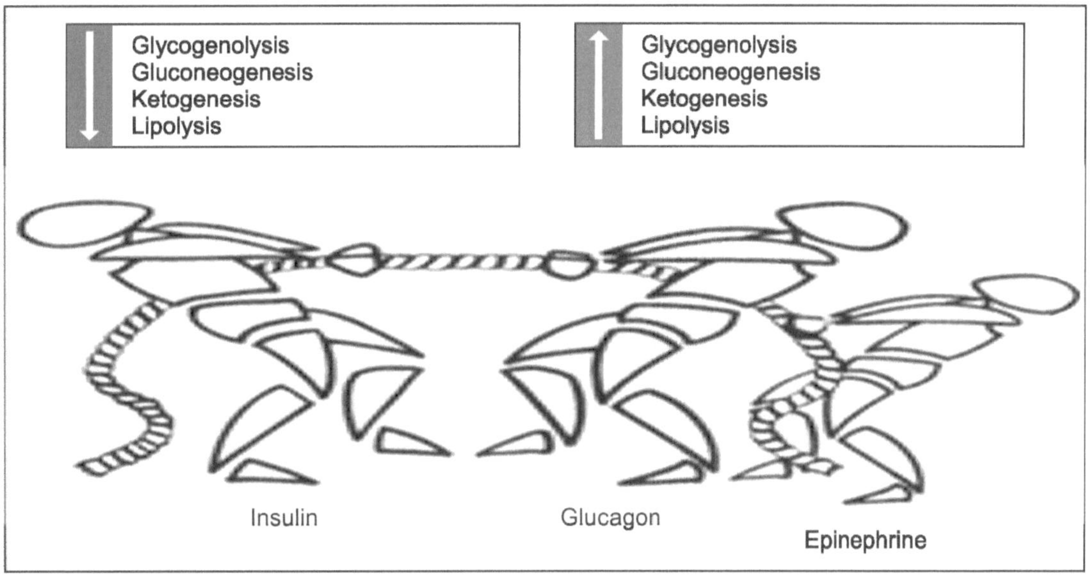

Ans: (c) Glucose 6 phosphatase

Ref: *Textbook of Biochemistry for Medical Students, DM Vasudevan, 9th Edition, Chapter 9, Page 167*

10. The given below clinical features occurs due to deficiency of:

(a) B_{12}
(b) B_1
(c) B_2
(d) B_3

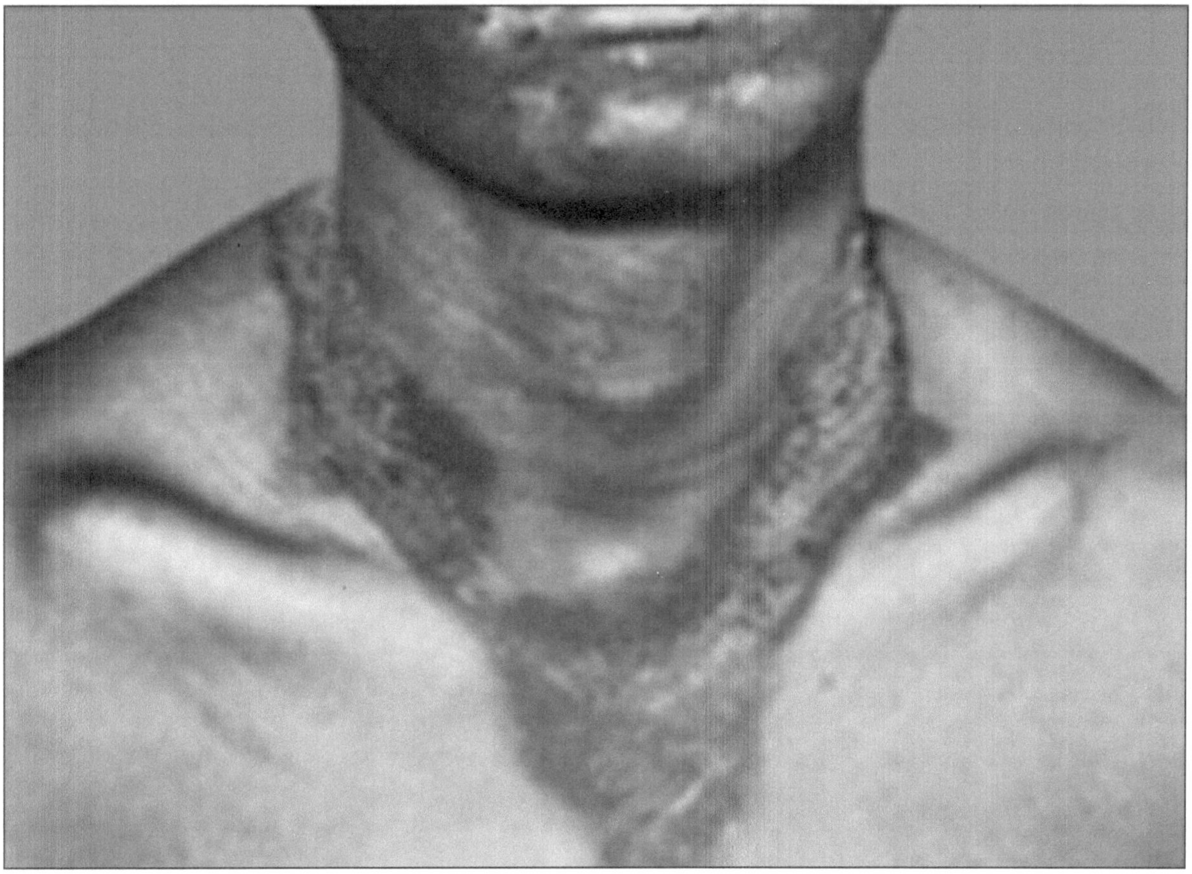

Explanation:

Niacin Deficiency (Vitamin B_3)

• Causes clinical syndrome called **Pellagra** **Risk factors** • Alcoholics • Prolonged antibiotic use • Congenital defects of intestinal and kidney absorption of tryptophan (**Hartnup disease**) • **Carcinoid syndrome** (↑conversion of tryptophan to serotonin) **Early symptoms** • Loss of appetite • Generalized weakness • Irritability • Abdominal pain • Vomiting	**Other features** • Bright red glossitis • Characteristic skin rash that is **pigmented** and **scaling**, particularly in skin areas exposed to sunlight • **Casal's necklace** – Rash forms a ring around the neck • Vaginitis • Esophagitis • Diarrhea (due to **proctitis** and **malabsorption**) • Depression • Seizures • Dementia • Pellagra syndrome—the **four Ds: dermatitis**, **diarrhea** and **dementia** leading to **death**

Ans: (d) B_3

Ref: *Textbook of Biochemistry for Medical Students, DM Vasudevan, 9th Edition, Chapter 29, Page 505*

11. A 45-year-old man presents with Paresthesia. His Hb is 6 g/dl. Peripheral smear shows macrocytes and neutrophils with hypersegmented nuclei. Endoscopy reveals atrophic gastritis. Which of the following deficiency is more likely?

(a) Vitamin B_{12} deficiency
(b) Niacin deficiency
(c) Riboflavin deficiency
(d) Folate deficiency

Explanation:

Pernicious Anemia (PA)

- Pernicious anemia (PA) is a macrocytic anemia that is caused by vitamin B_{12} deficiency, as a result of intrinsic factor deficiency.
- **Paresthesia** is one of the neurological manifestations of vitamin B_{12} deficiency. Hb value of 6 g% is suggestive of **anemia**.
- Peripheral smear showing **macrocytes** and neutrophils with **hypersegmented** nuclei are the characteristic features of **megaloblastic anemia**.
- Endoscopy findings reveal **atrophy of gastric mucosa** which might have resulted in the **deficiency of intrinsic factor** which in turn leads to deceased absorption of vitamin B_{12} and its deficiency.

Ans: (a) Vitamin B_{12} deficiency

Ref: *Textbook of Biochemistry for Medical Students, DM Vasudevan, 9th Edition, Chapter 29, Page 514*

12. True about structure of protein:

(a) 2° structure is 3D
(b) 2° structure stabilized by disulphide bond
(c) 3° structure is 3D
(d) 1°, 2° and 3° structure are destroyed by denaturation.

Explanation:

- As protein is a macromolecule and made of several 100 or 1000 of amino acids, the structure is more complex.

- Because proteins are very large molecules and because, their ultimate folded structure is important for their function, the structure of proteins is described into 4 levels of organization namely:
  - Primary.
  - Secondary.
  - Tertiary; and
  - Quaternary structures.

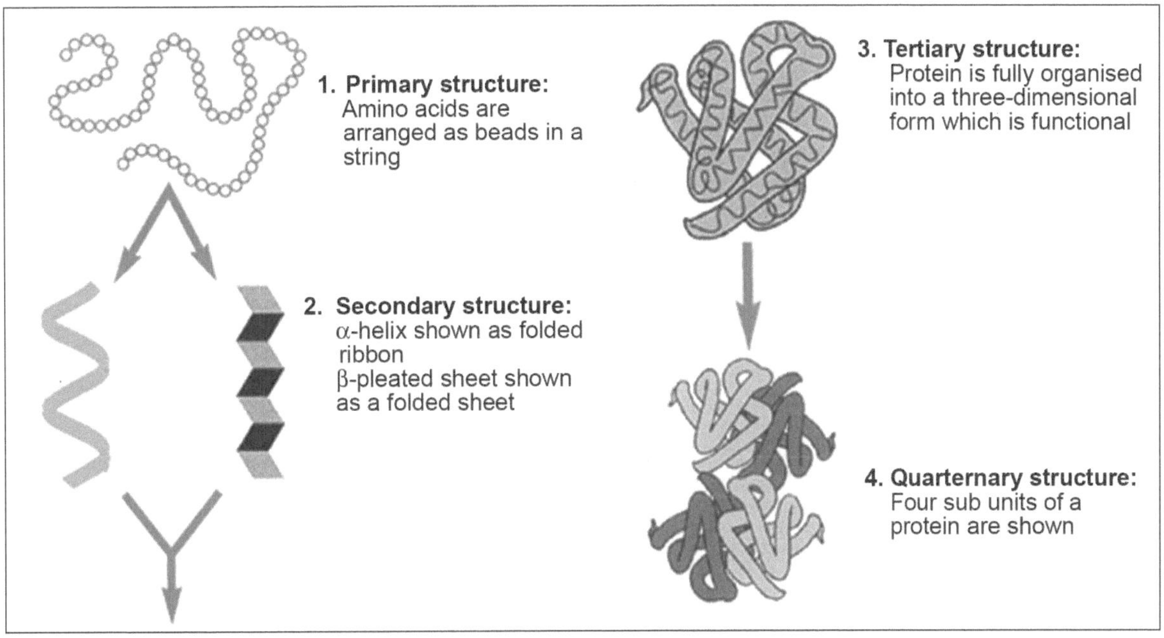

Primary Structure

- Total number of amino acids, types of amino acids, arrangement (sequence) of amino acids.
- It is the backbone of the peptide/protein.
- Linear and covalent (peptide) structure of peptide.
- Stabilized by the peptide bond.
- Genetically determined.
- Alterations in the primary structure occurs due to mutations.
- Less biologically active or totally non-functional proteins may occur due to mutations.

E.g.: HbA – Glutamate at the 6th position of beta–chain.

HbS (sickle cell) glu is replaced by valine at 6th position of beta chain.

Polypeptide backbone

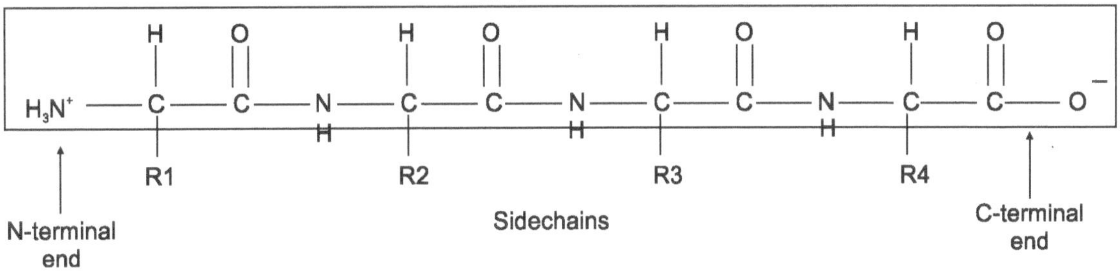

PROPERTIES OF PEPTIDE BOND

- Covalent bond; strong.
- Does not have any charge.

- Has a partial double bond character.
- Has no freedom of rotation around C—N bond.
- Limits the movement of peptide backbone.
- Rotation is possible between the N—C (phi) and the C—C bonds (psi angle) in the peptide backbone.
- Determine the path of the polypeptide.
- Extent of twists and turns – determine protein folding.
- Only limited, psi and phi combinations permitted.

Proteins, however, are not rigid; are flexible.

Planar.

The –C=O and –NH are trans with respect to each other.

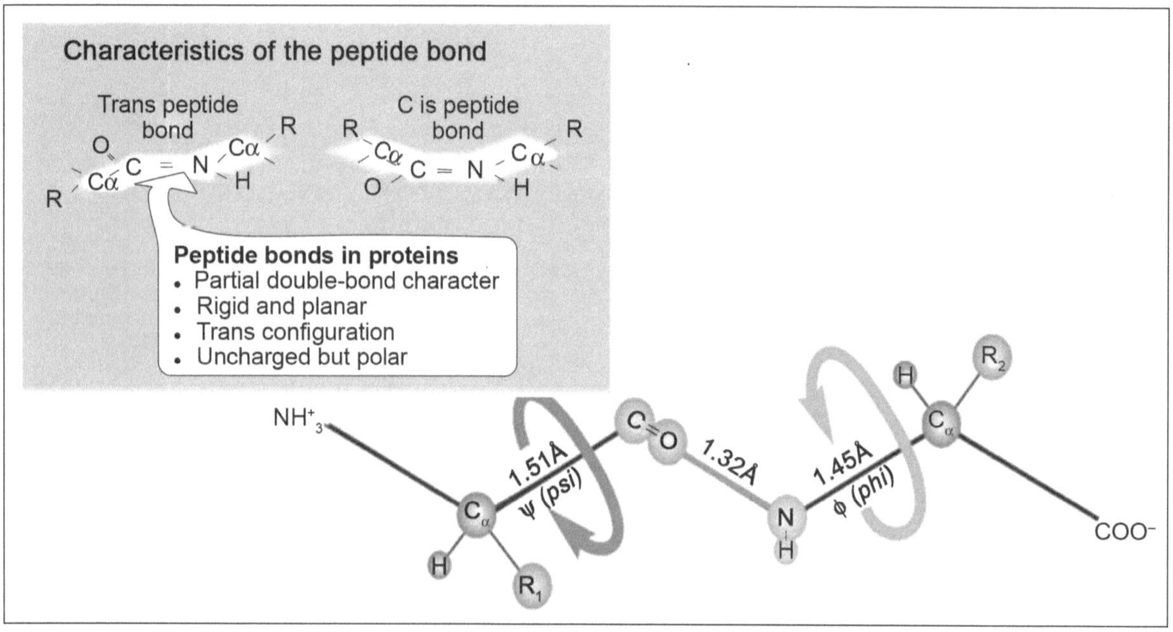

Secondary Structure

Folding of the peptide chain in to stable and specific coiling is the secondary structure of protein.

- **Repetitive**
  - α – Helical.
  - β – Pleated sheet.
- **Non-repetitive**
  - Bends.
  - Loops.

α-helix

- α-helix is the most stable conformation formed spontaneously with the lowest energy.
- Polypeptide backbone is coiling around an imaginary axis.
- The helix can be either right-handed or left-handed.
- The naturally occurring alpha helices found in proteins are all right-handed because of the less stearic clashes between side chains and the bakbone.
- There are 3.6 amino acid residues per turn of the helix.
- The vertical distance of each turn, pitch of 0.54 nm.

- Spacing of amino acids – 1.5 Å.
- Tightly coiled polypeptide backbone – inner part of the helix; side chains – extend outwards from the central axis.
- First amino and last carboxyl groups–not involved in H bonding.
- Each C=O is H-bonded to the NH of a peptide bond (4 residues).
- Amino acids spaced which are apart in sequence are spatially closer to one another.
- Large R groups donot favour alpha-helix formation.
- Glycine destabilizes the helix.
- Proline is a helix breaker.

  Examples: Both fibrous (keratin) and globular (Hb, Mb) proteins possess alpha-helix structure.

Beta-Pleated Sheet

- It is the second type of regular repetitive pattern (thus the name b) occuring in the secondary structure of a protein.
- The peptide backbone of a beta-sheet is partly extended with a 'pleated appearance'.
- The distance between adjacent amino acids along a b-strand is 3.5 Å.
- The side chains of adjacent amino acids orient in opposite directions to avoid steric clashes.
- Hydrogen bonds–formed between neighbouring polypeptide chains / within a single polypeptide chain folded into segments.
- Hydrogen bonds–formed between neighbouring polypeptide chains / within a single polypeptide chain folded into segments.
- Adjacent chains in a beta-sheet can run in opposite directions (antiparallel β sheet), in same direction (parallel β sheet) or both ways (mixed β sheets).
- Hence, 2 varieties of β - pleated forms.

  Parallel: Where H-bonded chains extend in the same direction.

  E.g.: Superoxide dismutase.

  Anti-parallel: H-bonded chains run in opposite directions.

  E.g.: Fibroin (silk).

Tertiary Structure

- The polypeptide chain with secondary structure mentioned above may be further folded, superfolded twisted about itself forming many sizes. Such a structural conformation is called tertiary structure.
- It is only one such conformation which is biologically active and protein in this conformation is called as native protein.
- Thus the tertiary structure is constituted by steric relationship between the amino acids located far apart but brought closer by folding (3 D structure).
- Folding not regular, non-repetitive.
- Stabilized mainly by hydrophobic bonds.
- Charged polar amino acids on outside.
- Non-polar amino acids inside, Uncharged polar amino acids (ser, thr, asn, gln, tyr, trp) inside / outside.
- Domains–Fundamental functional and 3D structural units of a polypeptide.
- Core of a domain is built of motifs.

- Folding inside a domain is usually independent of folding in other domains.

Quaternary Structure

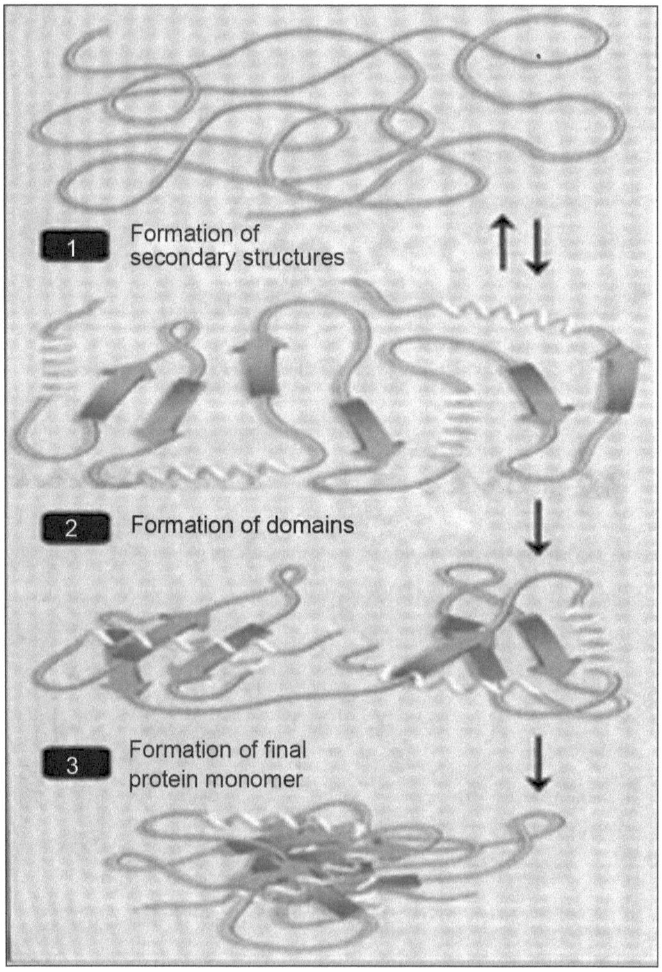

- Refers to the spatial relationships between individual polypeptide chains of an oligomeric protein.
- It is applicable only to the proteins with two or more polypeptide chains (subunits).
- Types of linkages involved in binding various subunits–Weak, non-covalent forces like ionic bonds, Van der Waal's forces.

  E.g.: Hemoglobin, Immunoglobulins.

The bonds responsible for interaction between groups of amino acids are as follows:

- **Hydrophobic interactions:** Normally occur between non polar side chains of amino acids such as alanine, leucine, methionine, isoleucine and phenylalanine.They constitute the major stabilising forces for tertiary structure forming a compact three-dimensional structure.
- **Hydrogen bonds:** Normally formed by the polar side chains of the amino acids.
- **Ionic or electrostatic interactions:** These are formed between oppositely charged polar side chains of amino acids, such as basic and acidic amino acids.
- **Van der Waal Forces:** Occur between nonpolar side chains.
- **Disulfide bonds:** These are the S–S bonds between –SH groups of distant cysteine residues.

Ans: (c) 3° structure is 3D

Ref: *Textbook of Biochemistry for Medical Students, DM Vasudevan, 9th Edition, Chapter 3, Page 34-39*

13. Van den Bergh test done for:

(a) Direct bilirubin
(b) Indirect bilirubin
(c) Both for direct and indirect bilirubin
(d) Total bilirubin

Explanation:

- The bilirubin can be detected by **van den Bergh reaction,** where diazotized sulfanilic acid (sulfanilic acid in HCl and sodium nitrite) reacts with bilirubin to form a purple colored complex, azobilirubin. Normal serum gives a positive van den Bergh reaction.
- When bilirubin is **conjugated**, the purple color is produced immediately on mixing with the reagent, the response is said to be van den Bergh **direct positive.**
- When the bilirubin is **unconjugated**, the color is obtained only when alcohol is added, and this response is known as **indirect positive**.
- If both conjugated and unconjugated bilirubin is present in increased amounts, a purple color is produced immediately and the color is intensified on adding alcohol. Then the reaction is called **biphasic**.
- In **Hemolytic** jaundice, unconjugated bilirubin is increased. Hence van den Bergh test is indirect positive. In **obstructive** jaundice, conjugated bilirubin is elevated, and van den Bergh test is direct positive.
- In **hepatocellular** jaundice, a biphasic reaction is observed, because both conjugated and unconjugated bilirubins are increased.

Ans: (c) Both for direct and indirect bilirubin

Ref: *Textbook of Biochemistry for Medical Students, DM Vasudevan, 9th Edition, Chapter 21, Page 397*

14. Restriction endonuclease will act on which of the following:

(a) GAATTC
CTTAAG

(b) AAGAAG
AAGAAG

(c) TACGAG
TACGAG

(d) GAGAGG
GAGAGG

Explanation:

- **Restriction endonucleases:** (They are compared to chemical knife). Certain endonucleases, enzymes that cut DNA at specific DNA sequences within the molecule, are a key biological tool in recombinant DNA technology. These enzymes were originally called restriction enzymes because their presence in a given bacterium restricted the growth of certain bacterial viruses called bacteriophages.
- Specific endonucleases.
- Recognize specific short sequences of DNA and cleave the DNA at or near the recognition sequence.
- Recognition sequences are palindromes.
- **Palindrome:** Sequence of DNA that is the same when one strand is read from left to right or the other strand is read from right to left–consists of adjacent inverted repeats.

  Reads the same in 5' to 3'.
- Example of a palindrome:

  GAATTC

  CTTAAG.
- Restriction enzymes are isolated from bacteria.
- Derive names from the bacteria.

  Genus–first letter capitalized.

Species–Second and third letters (small case).

Additional letters from "strains".

Roman numeral designates different enzymes from the same bacterial strain, in numerical order of discovery.

- Example: EcoRI

E	Escherichia
Co	Coli
R	R strain
I	First enzyme discovered from Escherichia coli R.

- **Mechanism of action:** Each restriction endonuclease enzyme recognises and cleaves a specific double-stranded DNA sequence that is 4 to 7 bp long. These DNA cuts result in:
- **Blunt ends** (by Bam H I)

(a) Cut with *Sma* I

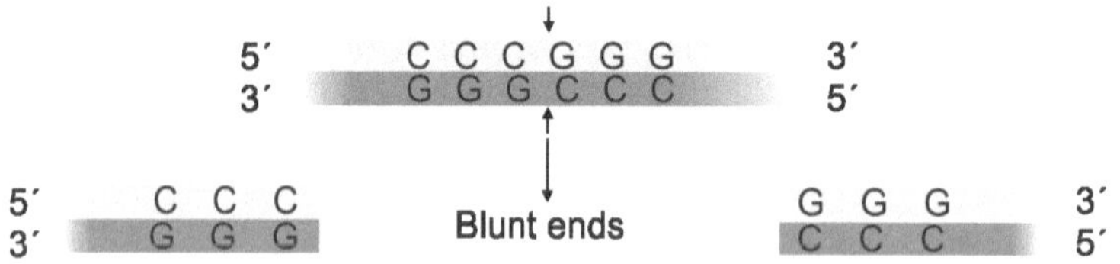

(b) Cut with *Bam* HI

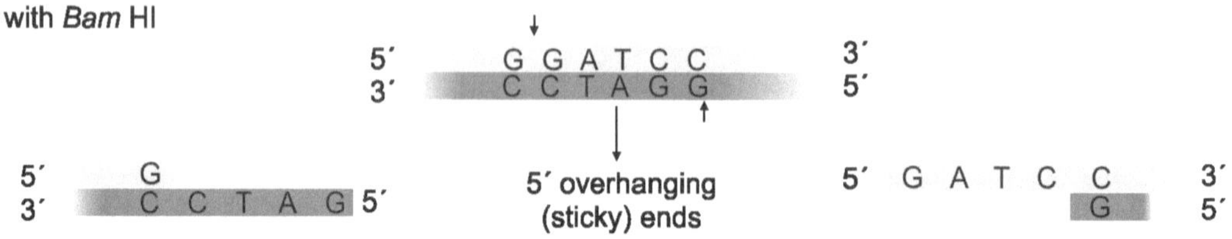

(c) Cut with *Pst* I

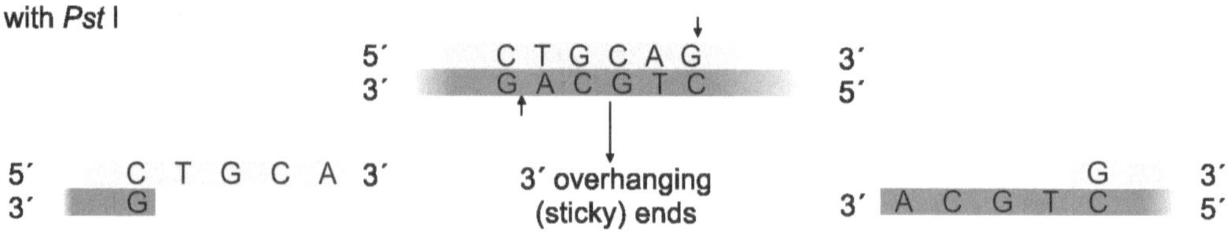

- **Sticky ends** (also called staggered or cohesive ends) by Bam HI or Eco R I.

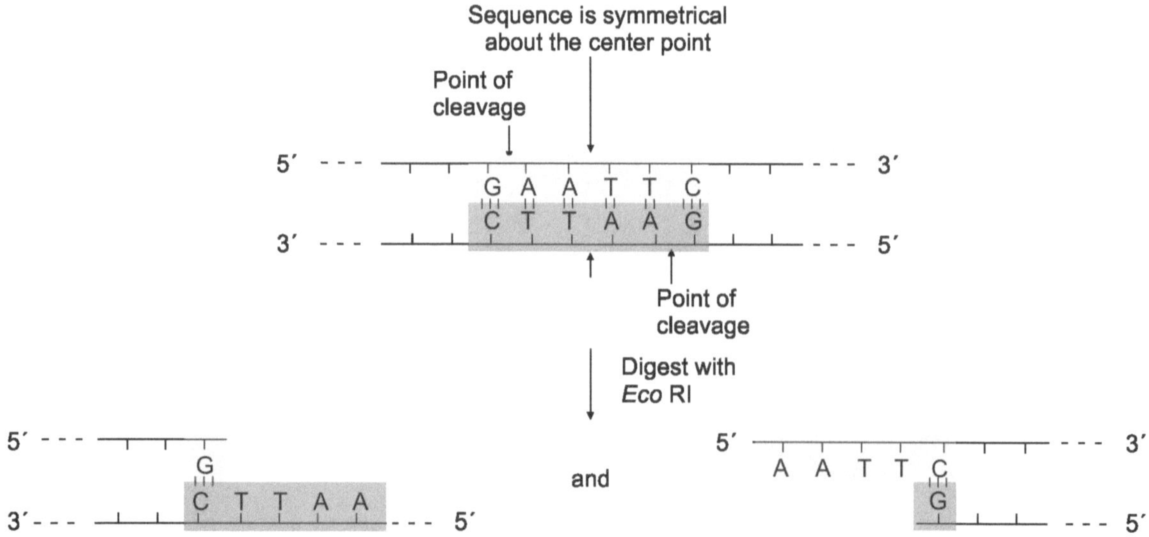

Sticky ends are particularly useful in preparation of chimeric or hybrid DNA molecule.

- By using different restriction endonucleases for the digestion of a particular DNA, a restriction map with characteristic sites of action can be prepared.
- When DNA is digested with a given enzyme, the ends of all the fragments would have the same DNA sequence. The fragments produced can be isolated by agarose electrophoresis or polyacrylamide gel electrophoresis. This is an essential step in cloning and a major use of these enzymes.

Ans: (a) GAATTC
CTTAAG

Ref: *Textbook of Biochemistry for Medical Students, DM Vasudevan, 9th Edition, Chapter 37, Page 544*

15. Hormone acting via tyrosine kinase receptor is:

(a) TRH (b) TSH

(c) Insulin (d) MSH

Explanation:

Mechanism of action of **insulin** along with actions.

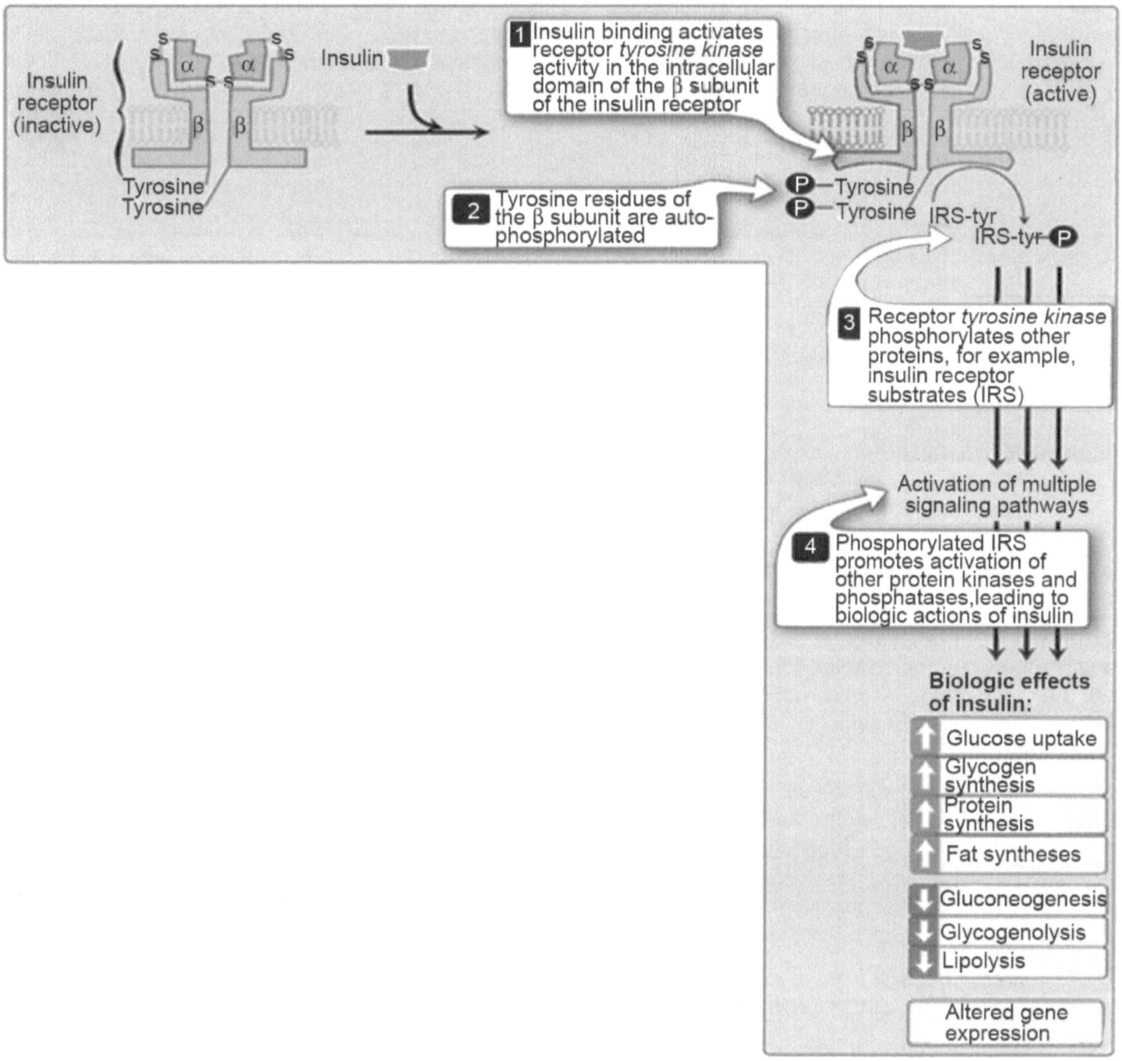

Ans: (c) Insulin

Ref: *Textbook of Biochemistry for Medical Students, DM Vasudevan, 9th Edition, Chapter 9, Page 167*

PHARMACOLOGY

1. A patient was recently started on fluphenazine. Few weeks later, he developed tremors, rigidity, bradykinesia and excessive salivation. First line of management for this patient is:

(a) Selegiline (b) Trihexyphenidyl

(c) Pramipexole (d) Amantadine

Explanation:

- **Fluphenazine:** It is an antipsychotic drug.
- The **neurological related adverse drug reactions (ADRs)** associated with chronic use of antipsychotic drugs are described in detail in the following table:

Neurological ADR	Clinical manifestations	Time of onset of ADR	Underlying mechanism	Management
Acute dystonia	Acute skeletal muscular spasm involving back, face, neck or tongue	1-5 days	Due to blockade of dopamine receptors	**Centrally acting anticholinergic drugs** (*Diphenhydramine, Benztropine*) are useful
Akathisia	Subjective experience of restlessness without anxiety	5-60 days	Not clearly understood	Decrease dose/change the offending drug; **Benzodiazepines** (*Clonazepam*) and **beta blockers** (*Propranolol*) are useful
Parkinsonism	Rigidity, tremors, bradykinesia, tremor, shuffling gait and mask like face	5-30 days	Due to blockade of dopamine receptors	Decrease dose/change the offending drug **Amantadine** (*Preferred due to absence of anticholinergic side effects*) over **Centrally acting anticholinergic drugs** (*Diphenhydramine, Benztropine*)
Neuroleptic malignant syndrome	Fatal complication associated with high degree fever, rigidity, myoglobinemia and unstable blood pressure	Weeks to months	Due to blockade of dopamine receptors	Stop the offending drug immediately Supportive care including **dantrolene** and **bromocriptine** are useful
Perioral tremor also called as 'Rabbit syndrome'	Delayed manifestation and extension of Parkinsonism	Months to years	Not clearly understood	The following medications may be useful: **Amantadine** (*Preferred due to absence of anticholinergic side effects*) over **Centrally acting anticholinergic drugs** (*Diphenhydramine, Benztropine*)
Tardive dyskinesia	Dyskinesia involving facial region; May also be associated with choreoathetosis or dystonia	Months to years	Upregulation/ supersensitivity of postsynaptic dopamine receptors	Decrease dose/change the offending drug; **VMAT2 inhibitors** (*Valbenazine and Deutetrabenazine*) may be useful

Ans: (d) Amantadine

Ref: *Roberson ED, Treatment of Central Nervous System Degenerative Disorders, In: Brunton LL, Hilal-Dandan R, Knollmann BC, Editors, Goodman and Gilman's The Pharmacological Basis of Therapeutics, 13th Edition, New York: McGraw-Hill 2018, Page 327-38*

2. Drug of choice for invasive aspergillosis is:

(a) Liposomal amphotericin B
(b) Caspofungin
(c) Posaconazole
(d) Voriconazole

Explanation:

- **Aspergillosis:** A fungal disease caused by a fungus *Aspergillus.*
- It has been established that **more than 50 species** of *Aspergillus* can cause Aspergillosis.
- Most common cause of invasive Aspergillosis is ***A. fumigatus.***
- The treatment of various clinical conditions associated with *Aspergillus* species infection are tabulated as follows:

Clinical condition associated with aspergillus species infection	First line drugs/Other options	Second line drugs	Remarks
Prophylaxis	Posaconazole Itraconazole	Micafungin Amphotericin B	Therapeutic Drug Monitoring (TDM) of first line drugs may be required
Invasive aspergillosis	Voriconazole Isavuconazole	Amphotericin B Caspofungin Posaconazole Micafungin	First line drugs are superior in efficacy when compared to second line drugs; Therapeutic Drug Monitoring (TDM) of Voriconazole is recommended
Single aspergilloma	Surgery	Itraconazole Voriconazole Amphotericin B	Surgery is the best option in single large cavity aspergilloma
Aspergillosis involving chronic pulmonary disease	Itraconazole voriconazole	Posaconazole Amphotericin B Micafungin	Therapeutic Drug Monitoring (TDM) of drug(s) is recommended
ABPA [*Allergic Bronchopulmonary Aspergillosis*]/**SAFS** [*Severe Asthma with Fungal Sensitization*]	Itraconazole	Voriconazole Posaconazole	Requires chronic therapy

Ans: (d) Voriconazole

Ref: *Denning DW. Aspergillosis, In: Jameson JL, Kasper DL, Longo DL, Fauci AS, Hauser SL, Loscalzo J, Editors, Harrison's Principles of Internal Medicine Vol II, 20th Edition, New York: McGraw-Hill 2018, Page 1532-37*

3. Which of the following is used as a first line drug in postmenopausal osteoporosis?

(a) Estrogen
(b) Raloxifene
(c) Biphosphonates
(d) Combined OCPs

Explanation:

- **Drugs Used for Treatment of Osteoporosis:**
  - Calcium and Vitamin D.
  - Biphosphonates.
  - Monoclonal antibody (Denosumab).
  - SERMs (Raloxifene).
  - Calcitonin.
  - PTH analogues (Teriparatide).

Important facts about drugs used for treatment of osteoporosis are tabulated as follows:

	Calcium and Vitamin D	Biphosphonates	Denosumab	SERMs (Raloxifene)	Calcitonin	Teripara-tide
MOA	Exogenous supplementation; Prevents bone loss	Cytotoxicity to osteoclasts	(-) Binding of RANKL to RANK	Osteoblastic activity through oestrogen receptors	Osteoblastic activity through Calcitonin receptors	Osteoblas-tic activity through PTH receptors
Dose	1200 mg/d (Calcium)	Varies with the drug(s)	60 mg SC/6 months	60 mg/d	200 IU intranasally/d	20 μg/d, SC
Efficacy	++	++++	+	+	+	++
Clinical Implications	First line drugs along with Biphosphonates	First line drugs along with Calcium + Vitamin D	Second/Third line drugs	Second/Third line drugs	Second/Third line drugs	Second/ Third line drugs
Important ADRs	GIT (Abdominal bloating, consti-pation)	Esophagitis, GIT disturbances, Thrombophlebitis, Hypersensitivity	Flue like syndrome, immuno-suppression	(↑) Risk of DVT by 3 folds	-	Leg cramps, headache, dizziness

Biphosphonates and their relative potency is as follows:

Biphosphonates	Relative Potency
FIRST GENERATION	
Etidronate	1
Tiludronate	10
SECOND GENERATION	
Pamidronate	100
Alendronate	100-500
Ibandronate	500-1000
THIRD GENERATION	
Risedronate	1000
Zoledronate	5000

Ans: (c) Biphosphonates

Ref: *Pavone V, Testa G, Giardina SMC, Vescio A, Restivo DA, Sessa G. Pharmacological Therapy of Osteoporosis: A Systematic Current Review of Literature, Front Pharmacol 2017;8(803),Page 1-7*

4. Pegloticase is used for treatment of:

(a) Refractory chronic tophaceous gout
(b) Refractory rheumatoid arthritis
(c) Ankylosing spondylosis
(d) CPPD

Explanation:

- **Pegloticase:** Drug used for treatment of gout.
- The various classes of drugs available for treatment of gout includes:

Mechanism of Action	Drug(s)	Clinical Indication(s)
Relieves pain and inflammation	NSAIDs	Acute gouty arthritis
	Glucocorticoids	
	Colchicine	
Oxidation of uric acid into more soluble and inactive metabolites	Pegloticase	Chronic gout (*Refractory to other drugs*)
	Rasburicase	Malignancy associated hyperuricemia (*Both in children and adults*)

Contd.

Contd.

(-) Reabsorption of uric acid from renal tubules and (↑) its excretion	Probenecid	Chronic gout
	Lesinurad	Chronic gout (*Adjunct therapy to xanthine oxidase inhibitors*)
(-) Synthesis of uric acid by (-) *xanthine oxidase* enzyme	Allopurinol	Hyperuricemia (*Associated with gout and cancer chemotherapy*)
	Febuxostat	Hyperuricemia

Important differences between **Pegloticase** and **Rasburicase** are tabulated as follows:

	Pegloticase	**Rasburicase**
Source	Recombinant pegylated uricase	Recombinant uricase
Clinical Indication	Chronic gout (*Refractory to other drugs*)	Malignancy associated hyperuricemia (*Both in children and adults*)
Plasma $t_{1/2}$	14 days	16-23 hours
ADRs	Development of antibodies against the drug (90%)	Development of antibodies against the drug
	Infusion related reactions	Methemoglobinemia
	Anaphylaxis	Anaphylaxis
	Hemolysis (in G6PD-deficient)	Hemolysis (in G6PD-deficient)
	GIT [Nausea (11%), vomiting, constipation, diarrhea]	GIT (Nausea, vomiting, constipation, diarrhea)
	Chest pain (6%)	Acute renal failure
	Erythema	Fever
	Pruritus	Headache
	Urticaria (11%)	Abdominal pain

Ans: (a) Refractory chronic tophaceous gout

Ref: *Grosser T, Smyth EM, FitzGerald GA. Pharmacotherapy of Inflammation, Fever, Pain and Gout, In: Brunton LL, Hilal-Dandan R, Knollmann BC, Editors, Goodman and Gilman's The Pharmacological Basis of Therapeutics, 13th Edition, New York: McGraw-Hill 2018,Page 685-709*

5. A patient admitted in the ICU was initiated on Warfarin treatment, which of the clotting factor would be affected?

(a) Factor II
(b) Factor VI
(c) Factor XII
(d) Factor V

Explanation:

- **Warfarin:** Most commonly used oral anticoagulant.
- ***Vitamin K Epoxide Reductase* (VKOR)** is responsible for conversion of vitamin K Epoxide (***Oxidized Form***) to vitamin K hydroquinone (***Reduced Form***).
- Vitamin K hydroquinone (Reduced Form) is essential for **γ-carboxylation** of vitamin K dependent factors (**Factor II, VII, IX and X**).
- γ-carboxylation of vitamin K dependent factors is very essential for conversion of **prozymogens to zymogens.**
- These zymogens are very crucial for **binding to Ca^{2+}** and interaction with anionic phospholipids.
- This physiological phenomenon of binding to Ca^{2+} and interaction with anionic phospholipids activates or brings the action as '**coagulation**'.
- **Mechanism of Action of Warfarin:**
  - (-) *Vitamin K Epoxide Reductase* (VKOR).

- **ADME of Warfarin:**
  - Good absorption.
  - Food can interfere the absorption.
  - Peak plasma concentration (2-8 hours).
  - Metabolism (CYP2C9).
  - Excretion (Renal).
- **Genetic Polymorphism Associated with Warfarin:**
  - CYP2C9 polymorphism (Require reduction in dosage of warfarin).
  - VKORC1 gene polymorphism (Require reduction in dosage of warfarin).

Important Facts about Anticoagulants has been summarized in the following table:

	Low Molecular Weight Heparin (LMWH)	**Heparin**	**Fondaparinux**	**Warfarin**
Molecular Target for MOA	Xa, IIa	Xa, IIa	Xa	VKOR (II, VII, IX, X)
Oral Bioavailability (%)	90	30	100	93
Plasma $t_{1/2}$ (h)	4	1 -8	17	37
Renal Excretion	Yes	No	Yes	Yes
Antidote	Protamine Sulfate	Protamine Sulfate	None	Vitamin K
Antidote Effect	Partial	Complete	None	Complete
Incidence of Thrombocytopenia (%)	<1	<5	<0.1	Negligible/None
Monitoring/Lab Control	Not Recommended	aPTT/Clotting Time	Not Recommended	PT/INR

Ans: (a) Factor II

Ref: *Hogg K, Weitz JI. Blood Coagulation and Anticoagulant, Fibrinolytic and Antiplatelet Drugs, In: Brunton LL, Hilal-Dandan R, Knollmann BC, Editors, Goodman and Gilman's The Pharmacological Basis of Therapeutics, 13th Edition, New York: McGraw-Hill 2018,Page 585-603*

6. Which of the following drug acts by inhibiting the transcription of DNA to RNA?

(a) Nitrofurantoin (b) Ciprofloxacin

(c) Rifampicin (d) Novobiocin

Explanation:

Antimicrobial Agents (AMAs) are described in the following table:

	Nitrofurantoin	**Ciprofloxacin**	**Rifampicin**	**Novobiocin**
Class	Urinary antiseptic	Fluoroquinolone	Rifamycin (*Macrocyclic antibiotics*)	Antibiotic (*Streptomyces niveus*)
MOA	Antiseptic	(-) *DNA gyrase* in gram negative bacteria (-) *Topoisomerase IV* in gram positive bacteria	(-) DNA-dependent RNA polymerase leading to (-) RNA synthesis	(-) *DNA gyrase* and (-) *ATPase*

Contd.

Contd.

Indication(s)	UTI	UTI, URTI, Gram negative bacterial infections	TB, leprosy	Clinical utility limited due to availability of safe and efficacious AMAs

Ans: (c) Rifampicin

Ref: *Gumbo T. Chemotherapy of Tuberculosis, Mycobacterium Avium Complex Disease and Leprosy, In: Brunton LL, Hilal-Dandan R, Knollmann BC, Editors, Goodman and Gilman's The Pharmacological Basis of Therapeutics, 13th Edition, New York: McGraw-Hill 2018, Page 1067-86*

7. Which of the following antimicrobials should not be given to a chronic asthmatic patient managed on theophylline therapy?

(a) Erythromycin (b) Cefotaxime

(c) Cotrimoxazole (d) Amoxicillin

Explanation:

- **Theophylline:** Belongs to methylxanthines and forms the adjunctive therapy in the treatment of bronchial asthma.
- **Mechanism of Action of Theophylline:**
  - Non-selective inhibition of '*Phosphodiesterase (PDE) Enzyme.*
  - Antagonism of adenosine receptors.
- Various factors can affect the clearance of theophylline and hence its serum concentration. These factors are tabulated as below**:**

Theophylline: (↑) Clearance and Hence (↓) Serum Concentration	**Theophylline: (↓) Clearance and Hence (↑) Serum Concentration**
Microsomal Enzyme (CYP1A2) Induction (*By Barbiturates, rifampin, ethanol, smoking and marijuana*)	Microsomal Enzyme Inhibition (*By Erythromycin, ciprofloxacin, cimetidine, allopurinol, zafirlukast, zileuton and fluoxamine*)
Pediatric population	Geriatric population
Low carbohydrate diet	High carbohydrate diet
High protein diet	Viral infections
Barbecued meat	Hepatic disorders (*Acute and chronic liver failure*)
	Lung disorders (*Pneumonia*)
	Cardiac disorders (*Congestive cardiac failure*)

Ans: (a) Erythromycin

Ref: *Barnes PJ. Pulmonary Pharmacology, In: Brunton LL, Hilal-Dandan R, Knollmann BC, Editors, Goodman and Gilman's The Pharmacological Basis of Therapeutics, 13th Edition, New York: McGraw-Hill 2018, Page 727-49*

8. Beta lactam group of antimicrobial agents confers resistance by all the following mechanisms *except:*

(a) Alteration of penicillin binding protein (b) Drug efflux

(c) Breakdown of drug structure (d) Alteration of 50S ribosome structure

Explanation:

- **Beta lactam group of antimicrobial agents include:**
  - Penicillins.
  - Cephalosporins.

- Monobactams.
- Carbapenems.

Important facts about beta lactam group of antimicrobial agents are tabulated as follows:

	Penicillins	Cephalosporins	Monobactams	Carbapenems
Presence of 'β-Lactam Ring' in Structure	Present	Present	Present	Present
MOA	(-) Cell wall synthesis	(-) Cell wall synthesis	(-) Cell wall synthesis	(-) Cell wall synthesis
Drug(s)	**Natural Penicillins** • Penicillin-G (Benzyl Penicillin)	**First Generation (Oral)** • Cefadroxil • Cephalexin	Aztreonam	Imipenem Meropenem Faropenem Doripenem Ertapenem
	Acid Resistant Penicillins • Penicillin-V (Phenoxymethyl Penicillin)	**First Generation (Parenteral)** • Cefazolin		
	Penicillinase Resistant Penicillins • Cloxacillin • Dicloxacillin • Methicillin	**Second Generation (Oral)** • Cefuroxime axetil • Cefaclor • Cefprozil		
	Amino-Penicillins • Ampicillin • Becampicillin • Amoxicillin	**Second Generation (Parenteral)** • Cefuroxime • Cefoxitin		
	Ureido-Penicillins • Piperacillin • Mezlocillin	**Third Generation (Oral)** • Cefpodoxime • Cefixime • Ceftibuten • Ceftamet • Cefdinir		
	Carboxy-Penicillins • Carbenicillin • Ticarcillin	**Third Generation (Parenteral)** • Ceftizoxime • Ceftazidime • Ceftriaxone • Cefotaxime • Cefoperazone		
		Fourth Generation (Parenteral) • Cefpirome • Cefepime		
		Fifth Generation (Parenteral) • Ceftobiprole • Ceftaroline		
Cross Hypersensitivity	Present	Present	Absent	Present

Contd.

Contd.

Spectrum of Activity	Gram Positive (Mainly)	Both Gram Positive and Negative	Gram Negative	Both Gram Positive and Negative
Mechanism of Resistance	1. Mutations in Penicillin Binding Proteins (PBPs) 2. Drug efflux 3. Destruction of β-lactam ring by *β-lactamases* 4. (↓) Entry of drug at the site of action			

Ans: (d) Alteration of 50S ribosome structure

Ref: *MacDougall C. Penicillins, Cephalosporins and Other β-Lactam Antibiotics, In: Brunton LL, Hilal-Dandan R, Knollmann BC, Editors, Goodman and Gilman's The Pharmacological Basis of Therapeutics, 13th Edition, New York: McGraw-Hill 2018, Page 1023-38*

9. Which of the following anti-hypertensive drug is avoided in patients with high serum uric acid levels?

(a) Prazosin (b) Enalapril

(c) Atenolol (d) Hydrochlorothiazide

Explanation:

The common ADRs associated with drugs has been listed in the following table:

	Hydrochlorothiazide	Enalapril	Atenolol	Prazosin
Class	Thiazide diuretic	ACE inhibitor	β-Blocker	α-Blocker
ADRs	Hyperglycemia	Hyperkalemia	Bradycardia	Postural hypotension
	Dyslipidaemia	Hypotension	Dyslipidemia	Reflex tachycardia
	Hyperuricemia	Cough (10-16%)	Exacerbation of underlying COPD	Miosis
	Hypercalcemia	Dysgeusia	Exacerbation of underlying variant angina	Nasal stuffiness
	Extracellular volume depletion	GIT disturbances	Exacerbation of underlying DM	Inhibition of ejaculation
	Hypotension	Hypersensitivity (1-4%)	Rebound hypertension	
	Hypokalemia	CNS (Headache, dizziness)	GIT disturbances	
	Hyponatremia	Teratogenicity	Erectile dysfunction	
	Hypochloremia	Proteinuria	CNS (Nightmares, mental depression)	
	Metabolic alkalosis	Hematological (Granulocytopenia)		
	Hypomagnesemia			
	Hypersensitivity			
	Erectile dysfunction			
	CNS (Vertigo, headache)			
	GIT disturbances			
	Dermatological (Photosensitivity, rashes)			

Drugs causing hyperuricemia is listed in the following table:

Drug Induced Hyperuricemia
Loop diuretics (*Furosemide, Ethacrynic acid*)
Thiazide diuretics
Cytotoxics
Aspirin

Ans: (d) Hydrochlorothiazide

Ref: *Jackson EK. Drugs Affecting Renal Excretory Function, In: Brunton LL, Hilal-Dandan R, Knollmann BC, Editors, Goodman and Gilman's The Pharmacological Basis of Therapeutics, 13th Edition, New York: McGraw-Hill 2018, Page 445-70*

10. A patient of biliary colic presented to hospital. Intern gave an injection and the pain worsened. Which is the most likely injection given?

(a) Morphine
(b) Diclofenac
(c) Nefopam
(d) Etoricoxib

Explanation:

- **Opioids:**
  - Centrally acting potent analgesics.
  - Acts through opioid receptors (μ, κ, δ).
  - Can cause biliary spasm.
  - Opioid (Morphine) causes constriction of the sphincter of Oddi and can (↑) biliary pressure in the common bile duct (CBD) by 10 folds within 15 minutes of its parenteral administration.
  - (↑) Biliary pressure due to opioids can further leads to (↑) in serum lipase and amylase levels.
  - This biliary spasm due to opioids is completely antagonized by the opioid antagonists; however, the atropine like drugs can only relieve it partially.
- Other drugs (**like diclofenac, nefopam and etorcoxib**) are NSAIDs.
- NSAIDs do not have any action on the biliary pressure.

Ans: (a) Morphine

Ref: *Yaksh T, Wallace M. Opioids, Analgesia and Pain Management, In: Brunton LL, Hilal-Dandan R, Knollmann BC, Editors, Goodman and Gilman's The Pharmacological Basis of Therapeutics. 13th Edition, New York: McGraw-Hill 2018, Page 355-86*

11. A patient diagnosed with Rheumatoid arthritis was on medications. After 2 years, he developed blurring of vision and was found to have corneal opacity. Which drug is most likely to cause this?

(a) Sulfasalazine
(b) Chloroquine
(c) Methotrexate
(d) Leflunomide

Explanation:

Various **Classes of Drugs in Addition to NSAIDs** for the treatment of rheumatoid arthritis are listed as follows:

Disease-Modifying Antirheumatic Drugs (DMARDs)			
Small Molecules		**Biologicals**	
Drug(s)	**Class/MOA**	**Drug(s)**	**Class/MOA**

Contd.

Contd.

Leflunomide	Pyrimidine synthase inhibitor	**Adalimumab**	TNF-α antagonist
Methotrexate	Antifolate	**Etanercept**	
Azathioprine	Purine synthase inhibitor	**Infliximab**	
Cyclophosphamide	Alkylating agent	**Golimumab**	
Hydroxychloroquine	Antimalarial	**Certolizumab**	
Sulfasalazine	Salicylate	**Anakinra**	IL-1 receptor antagonist
Penicillamine	Chelating agent	**Tocilizumab**	IL-6 receptor antagonist
Cyclosporine	Calcineurin inhibitor	**Abatacept**	T-cell costimulation inhibitor
Auranofin	Gold compound	**Tofacitinib**	Janus kinase inhibitor
Minocycline	5-Lipoxygenase inhibitor, tetracycline antibiotic	**Rituximab**	Ab toward CD20 (cytotoxic toward B cells)

ADRs associated with use of hydroxychloroquine (DMARDs) are listed as follows:

ADRs of Hydroxychloroquine	
Single Fatal Dose	**30 mg/Kg body weight**
Acute Toxicity (*Due to Parenteral Administration*)	Vasodilation
	Myocardial suppression
	Hypotension
	Cardiac arrhythmias
	Cardiac arrest
	Confusion
	Convulsions
	Coma
Acute Toxicity (*Due to Oral Administration*)	GIT disturbances
	Ophthalmic (Visual disturbances)
	Dermatological (Pruritus, Urticaria)
Prolonged Treatment with Suppressive Doses/ Chronic Toxicity	CNS (Headache, Confusion, Convulsions, Neuropsychiatric disturbances, Suicidal thoughts)
	Ophthalmic (Blurring of vision, Diplopia, Corneal opacities)
	Dermatological/Hypersensitivity (Lichenoid skin eruptions, Bleaching of hair, Discoloration of nail beds and mucous membranes)
	CVS (widening of the QRS interval and T-wave abnormalities)
	Hematological (Blood dyscrasias and Hemolysis)
	Retinopathy (Irreversible; For high daily doses >250 mg/d)
	Ototoxicity (Irreversible; For high daily doses >250 mg/d)
	Toxic myopathy
	Peripheral neuropathy
	Cardiopathy

Ans: (b) Chloroquine

Ref: *Vinetz JM. Chemotherapy of Malaria, In: Brunton L, Chabner B, Knollman B, Editors, Goodman and Gilman's The Pharmacological Basis of Therapeutics, 13th Edition, New York: McGraw-Hill 2018, Page 969-86*

12. A boy is planning to travel by bus. Which of the following drug can be used to prevent motion sickness in this person?

(a) Promethazine
(b) Cetirizine
(c) Loratadine
(d) Fexofenadine

Explanation:

- **Drugs Found to be Efficacious for Motion Sickness Include:**
  - Promethazine.
  - Diphenhydramine.
  - Dimenhydrinate.
  - Meclozine.
- **MOA of Drugs Found to be Efficacious for Motion Sickness:**
  - Antagonism of H_1 receptors.
- All the above drugs have **only prophylactic role,** i.e., in prevention of motion sickness.
- Hence these drugs should be taken ***at least one hour prior*** to the planned journey.
- **Promethazine:** Along with its efficacy in motion sickness, it is also effective in ***morning sickness in pregnancy, radiation induced sickness***.

Ans: (a) Promethazine

Ref: *Tripathi KD, Essentials of Medical Pharmacology, 8th Edition, New Delhi, Jaypee Brothers Medical Publishers 2019, Page 183*

13. Theophylline causes diuresis because of:

(a) PDE4 inhibition
(b) Beta-2 agonism
(c) PDE3 inhibition
(d) Adenosine A_1 receptor antagonism

Explanation:

The mechanisms of various ADRs associated with the use of theophylline are tabulated as follows:

Adverse Drug Reaction (ADR)	Mechanism
GIT (*Nausea, vomiting, abdominal discomfort*)	Inhibition of PDE4
CNS (*Headache*)	Inhibition of PDE4
CNS (*Seizures*)	Blockade of A_1 receptors
Renal (*Diuresis*)	Blockade of A_1 receptors
CVS (*Arrhythmias*)	Inhibition of PDE3 and blockade of A_1 receptors

Ans: (d) Adenosine A_1 receptor antagonism

Ref: *Barnes PJ. Pulmonary Pharmacology, In: Brunton LL, Hilal-Dandan R, Knollmann BC, Editors, Goodman and Gilman's The Pharmacological Basis of Therapeutics, 13th Edition, New York: McGraw-Hill 2018, Page 727-49*

14. Which of the following is not a prokinetic?

(a) $5HT_4$ agonist
(b) D_2 Blocker
(c) Macrolides
(d) Diphenoxylate

Explanation:

- **Prokinetics:** Dugs which enhances the gastrointestinal transit and fastens the gastric emptying by intestinal coordinated propulsive motility. However, this definition does not include the cholinomimetics and anti-ChEs (Which increases the intestinal propulsive motility in uncoordinated fashion).

- **Prokinetics Include:**
  - D_2 Receptor Blockers (Metoclopramide, Domperidone).
  - 5-HT_4 Agonists (Cisapride, Mosapride, Itopride, Cinitapride).
- **MOA of Metoclopramide Include:**
  - D_2 Receptor antagonism (Most predominant MOA).
  - 5-HT_4 Agonism.
  - 5-HT_3 Antagonism (At higher concentration).
- **MOA of Cisapride Include:**
  - 5-HT_4 Agonism (Major).
  - 5-HT_3 Antagonism (Minor).
- **MOA of Mosapride Include:**
  - 5-HT_4 Agonism (Major).
  - 5-HT_3 Antagonism (Minor).
- **MOA of Itopride Include:**
  - D_2 Receptor antagonism (Most predominant MOA).
  - Anti-ChE Action.
  - 5-HT_4 Agonism (Minor).
- **MOA of Cinitapride Include:**
  - 5-HT_2 Receptor antagonism (Most predominant MOA).
  - D_2 Receptor antagonism (Most predominant MOA).
  - 5-HT_4 Agonism (Minor).
- **Macrolides:**
  - Antimicrobial agent cats by inhibition of bacterial protein synthesis.
  - They also stimulates the '*Motilin receptors*' in the GIT and enhances the gastrointestinal transit and fastens the gastric emptying by intestinal coordinated propulsive motility.
- **Diphenoxylate:**
  - Synthetic opioid drug (Structure closely related to pethidine).

Ans: (d) Diphenoxylate

Ref: *Tripathi KD. Essentials of Medical Pharmacology, 8th Edition, New Delhi: Jaypee Brothers Medical Publishers 2019, Page 711*

15. Most potent drug in the DRC is:

(a) Only A
(b) Only B
(c) Only C
(d) Only A and B

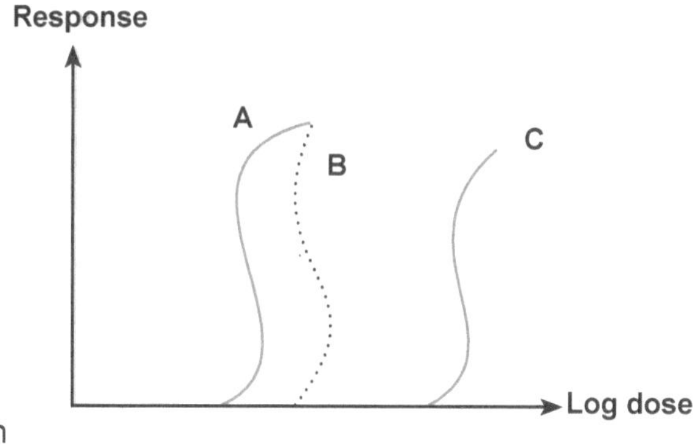

Explanation:

- **Drug Potency:**
  - **Amount of drug** needed to produce a certain response.

- The **position of the 'Dose Response Curve (DRC)'** on the **'X'** axis determines the potency of the drug.
- If the position of the 'Dose Response Curve (DRC)' on the **'X'** axis falls more towards the **'Left side'** then the drug is '**more potent'.**
- In the given graph, 'Dose Response Curve (DRC)' of '**Drug A'** on the **'X'** axis is falling more towards the **'Left side'** hence the drug A is '**more potent'** among all the three drugs.
- In the given graph, the potency of drug(s) A>B>C.

- **Drug Efficacy:**
  - **Maximal response** of the drug that can be elicited at any given dose.
  - The **height of the 'Dose Response Curve (DRC)'** on the **'Y'** axis determines the efficacy of the drug.
  - If the height of the 'Dose Response Curve (DRC)' on the **'Y'** axis falls **'Highest'** then the drug is '**more efficacious'.**
  - In the given graph, 'Dose Response Curve (DRC)' of '**Drug A, B and C'** on the **'Y'** axis is falling have the **'Same Height'** hence the drug A, B and C are '**Equally Efficacious'.**
  - In the given graph, the efficacy of drug(s) A=B=C.
- **Clinical Implications:**
  - **Efficacy of the drug** is an important decisive factor than potency of the drug in the clinical practice.

Ans: (a) Only A

Ref: *Tripathi KD, Essentials of Medical Pharmacology, 8th Edition, New Delhi, Jaypee Brothers Medical Publishers 2019, Page 64*

16. True about non-competitive inhibition is:

(a) Km remains same, Vmax decreases
(b) Km increases, Vmax remains same
(c) Km decreases, Vmax increases
(d) Km increases, Vmax increases

Explanation:

- Enzyme inhibition can be competitive (equilibrium type) or noncompetitive.

The differences between competitive (equilibrium type) or noncompetitive are as follows:

	Competitive (*Equilibrium Type*) Enzyme Inhibition	Noncompetitive Enzyme Inhibition
Drug	Structurally similar to the endogenous ligand(s)	Structurally not similar to the endogenous ligand(s)
Site of Binding	Same site of endogenous ligand(s)	Different site of endogenous ligand(s)
kM	(↑)	Normal/Unchanged
Vmax	Normal/Unchanged	(↓)
Examples	**Carbidopa** *(as competitive inhibitor)* for Levodopa *(Endogenous ligand) at 'Dopa decoboxylase' enzyme*	**Disulfiram** *(as noncompetitive inhibitor)* at *'Aldehyde dehydrogenase'* enzyme
	Physostigmine *(as competitive inhibitor)* for Acetylcholine *(Endogenous ligand) at 'Cholinesterase'* enzyme	**Digoxin** *(as noncompetitive inhibitor)* at *'Na^+ K^+ ATPase'* enzyme
	Captopril (*as competitive inhibitor*) for Angiotensin-1 (*Endogenous ligand*) at *'Angiotensin Converting Enzyme (ACE)'* enzyme	**Omeprazole** *(as noncompetitive inhibitor)* at *'H^+ K^+ ATPase'* enzyme
	Allopurinol *(as competitive inhibitor)* for Hypoxanthine *(Endogenous ligand)* at *'Hypoxanthine oxidase'* enzyme	**Acetazolamide** *(as noncompetitive inhibitor)* at *'Carbonic anhydrase'* enzyme

Contd.

Contd.

	Moclobemide *(as competitive inhibitor)* for Catecholamines *(Endogenous ligand)* at *'Monoamine –Oxidase A (MAO –A)'* enzyme	**Propylthiouracil** *(as noncompetitive inhibitor)* at *'Peroxidase'* enzyme
	Finasteride *(as competitive inhibitor)* for Testosterone *(Endogenous ligand)* at *'5α -Reductase"* enzyme	**Sildenafil** *(as noncompetitive inhibitor)* at *'Phosphodiesterase -5 (PDE5)'* enzyme
	Letrozole *(as competitive inhibitor)* for Testosterone *(Endogenous ligand)* at *'Aromatase'* enzyme	**Aspirin** *(as noncompetitive inhibitor)* at *'Cyclooxygenase'* enzyme

Ans: (a) Km remains same, Vmax decreases

Ref: *Tripathi KD, Essentials of Medical Pharmacology, 8th Edition, New Delhi, Jaypee Brothers Medical Publishers 2019, Page 47*

17. A patient with diabetes and COPD developed post-operative urinary retention. Which of the following drugs can be used for short-term treatment to relieve the symptoms of this person?

(a) Terazosin (b) Tamsulosin

(c) Bethanechol (d) Methacholine

Explanation:

The Contrasting Features of Drug(s):

	Terazosin	Tamsulosin	Bethanechol	Methacholine
Class	α_1 Selective Blocker	α_1 Selective Blocker	Synthetic choline ester	Synthetic choline ester
Uses	Hypertension	Hypertension	Postoperative urinary retention	For diagnosis of bronchial airway hyperreactivity
	Benign hypertrophy of prostate (BHP)	Benign hypertrophy of prostate (BHP)	Diabetic autonomic neuropathic bladder	
			Chronic hypotonic bladder	
			Myogenic bladder	
			Neurogenic bladder	
			Gastric atony (*Former Use*)	
			Postoperative abdominal distention (*Former Use*)	
			Adynamic ileus (*Former Use*)	
			Gastroparesis (*Former Use*)	
			Gastroesophageal reflux Disease (*Former Use*)	

Ans: (c) Bethanechol

Ref: *Brown JH, Brandl K, Wess J. Muscarinic Receptor Agonists and Antagonists, In: Brunton LL, Hilal-Dandan R, Knollmann BC, Editors, Goodman and Gilman's The Pharmacological Basis of Therapeutics, 13th Edition, New York: McGraw-Hill 2018, Page 149-61*

18. A patient on lithium therapy developed hypertension. He was started on thiazides for hypertension. After few days, he developed coarse tremors and other symptoms suggestive of lithium toxicity. Explain the likely mechanism of this interaction.

(a) Thiazides inhibit the metabolism of lithium

(b) Thiazides act as an add on drug to lithium

(c) Thiazides increases the tubular reabsorption of lithium

(d) Thiazides cause loss of water thereby increases lithium levels

Explanation:

- **Lithium:** It is a anti-maniac drug.
- Lithium has **very narrow therapeutic range** and hence Therapeutic Drug Monitoring (**TDM)** is clinically essential to prevent its serous toxicity or therapeutic failure due to its subtherapeutic concentrations.
- Lithium levels are also altered by many co-administered drugs due to **drug-drug interactions:**

Co-administered Drug(s)	Effect on Lithium Levels	Underlying Mechanism
Diuretics *(Thiazides)*	(↑↑↑↑↑)	(↓) Lithium clearance from renal tubules
Diuretics *(K^+ Sparing)*	(↑↑)	(↓) Lithium clearance from renal tubules
Diuretics *(Loop/Furosemide)*	(↑)	(↓) Lithium clearance from renal tubules
Diuretics *(Osmotic/Acetazolamide)*	(↓)	(↑) Lithium clearance from renal tubules
NSAIDs	(↑↑)	(↑) Renal tubular reabsorption of lithium
ACE Inhibitors *(Lisinopril)*	(↑↑)	(↑) Lithium retention

Clinical Implications of Serum Concentration of Lithium:

Serum Concentration of Lithium (mEq/L)	Clinical Implications
0.6-1	Used for bipolar prophylaxis
0.4-0.8	Used for antidepressant augmentation
>1.5	Lithium toxicity
>2	Requires admission of the patient
>3	Indication for hemodialysis
>3.2	Permanent neurological damage
>4.2	Death

Ans: (c) Thiazides increases the tubular reabsorption of lithium

Ref: *Meyer JM, Pharmacotherapy of Psychosis and Mania, In: Brunton LL, Hilal-Dandan R, Knollmann BC, Editors, Goodman and Gilman's The Pharmacological Basis of Therapeutics, 13th Edition, New York: McGraw-Hill 2018, Page 279-302*

19. A woman sleeping in the night develops pain and funny feelings like insect crawling on the legs, which is relieved by shaking her legs. Which of the following drug is used as first line?

(a) Pramipexole

(b) Gabapentin

(c) Vitamin B_{12}

(d) Iron tablets

Explanation:

- The symptoms mentioned in the question are consistent with restless leg syndrome. **Restless leg syndrome** is associated with abnormal sensation in legs, which improves with leg movement.
- **Iron tablets** should be given as **first line drug** in case of iron deficiency and if serum ferritin level is ≤75 mcg/l.

- In case there is no response to iron tablets or there is no iron deficiency, then the first line drug becomes **dopamine agonists** (**pramipexole**, ropinirole and rotigotine) or GABA releasing drugs (pregabalin and gabapentin). Overall dopamine agonists are more effective and are considered drugs of choice. But with increasing dose of dopamine agonists, the effect decreases; a phenomenon known as augmentation.
- In case patient does not respond to above-mentioned drugs, then levodopa or an opioid (oxycodone, methadone, tramadol) is used, i.e., in resistant cases.

Ans: (d) Iron tablets

Ref: *CMDT 2019, Page 1030*

20. A person was given a muscle relaxant that competitively blocks nicotinic receptors. Which of the following drug is used for reversal of muscle relaxation after surgery?

(a) Neostigmine (b) Carbachol
(c) Succinylcholine (d) Physostigmine

Explanation:

- **Reversal of anesthesia/Postoperative decurarization:**
  - ***Neostigmine is preferred.***
  - **Neostigmine:** Reversible anticholinesterase.
  - **Anticholinesterase:** (-) The enzyme AchE.
  - **AchE:** Involved in the degradation of Ach.
  - Hence **Anticholinesterases (Neostigmine),** (↑) the availability of Ach at the post-synaptic cleft and post-synaptic membrane to enhance the cholinergic neurotransmission at the skeletal muscular end-plate to bring the **recovery/normal tone** of the skeletal muscle.
- However, the use of Neostigmine in 'Reversal of anesthesia/Postoperative decurarization' is associated with its **unwanted muscarinic symptoms:**
  - To prevent these unwanted muscarinic symptoms, anti-muscarinic drug (**Atropine/Glycopyrrolate**) is combined with Neostigmine.
  - **Dose:** Neostigmine 0.5–2 mg (30–50 μg/kg) I.V. + Atropine or Glycopyrrolate 10 μg/kg (*To block muscarinic actions*).

Ans: (a) Neostigmine

Ref: *Tripathi KD, Essentials of Medical Pharmacology, 8th Edition, New Delhi, Jaypee Brothers Medical Publishers 2019, Page 122*

21. Anti-glaucoma drug that acts by increasing uveoscleral outflow via ciliary muscles is:

(a) Timolol (b) Pilocarpine
(c) Latanoprost (d) Dorzolamide

Explanation:

- Many classes of drug are available for treatment of glaucoma and include:
  - **Beta Blockers** (*Timolol, Levobunolol, Carteolol, Betaxolol*).
  - **Prostaglandin Analogues** (*Latanoprost, Bimatoprost, Travoprost*).
  - **Adrenergic Agonists** (*Dipivefrine, Brimonidine, Apraclonidine*).
  - **Miotics** (*Pilocarpine, Echothiophate, Physostigmine*).
  - **Carbonic Anhydrase Inhibitors** (*Acetazolamide, Brinzolamide, Dorzolamide*).

- The mechanism of action of above classes of drug(s) used for treatment of glaucoma are tabulated as follows:

Drug Class	Uveoscleral Outflow	Trabecular Outflow	Aqueous Secretion
Beta Blockers	–	–	(↓)
Prostaglandin Analogues	(↑)	(↑)	–
Adrenergic Agonists (Adrenaline, Dipivefrine)	(↑)	(↑)	(↓)
Adrenergic Agonists (Brimonidine, Apraclonidine)	(↑)	–	(↓)
Miotics	–	(↑)	–
Carbonic Anhydrase Inhibitors	–	–	(↓)

Ans: (c) Latanoprost

Ref: *Tripathi KD, Essentials of Medical Pharmacology, 8th Edition, New Delhi, Jaypee Brothers Medical Publishers 2019, Page 168*

22. Which of the following is a late inward sodium channel blocker?

(a) Ivabradine
(b) Ranolazine
(c) Trimetazidine
(d) Fasudil

Explanation:

The Contrasting Features of Drug(s) are depicted in the following table:

	Ranolazine	Trimetazidine	Ivabradine	Fasudil
Class	Antianginal	Antianginal	Antianginal	Rho-kinase inhibitor
MOA	(-) Late Na^+ current (Late I_{Na})	(-) Mitochondrial long chain 3-ketoacyl-CoAthiolase (LC3-KAT)/ pFOX (fatty acid oxidation pathway) inhibition	Blockade of cardiac pacemaker (sino-atrial) cell 'f' channels	Rho-kinase inhibitor
	(-) Mitochondrial long chain 3-ketoacyl-CoAthiolase (LC3-KAT)			
$t_{1/2}$ (h)	7	6	2	-
Dose	0.5-1 g BD	20 mg TID	5-7.5 mg BD	20-80 mg TID
Oral Bioavailability (%)	30-50	-	40	-
ADRs	CNS (Dizziness, Headache)	CNS (Dizziness, Parkinsonism)	CNS (Dizziness, Headache)	CVS (Hypotension)
	CVS (Postural hypotension)	-	CVS (Bradycardia, Prolongation of P-R interval, extra-systoles)	
	GIT (Constipation, dyspepsia)	GIT (Epigastric pain)	GIT (Nausea and vomiting)	
	Others (weakness)	Others (Fatigue, Muscle cramps)	Ophthalmic (Visual disturbances)	

Ans: (b) Ranolazine

Ref: *Tripathi KD, Essentials of Medical Pharmacology, 8th Edition, New Delhi, Jaypee Brothers Medical Publishers 2019, Page 600*

23. At a high altitude of 3000 meters, a person complains of breathlessness. All of the following can be used for management in this case *except:*

(a) Intravenous digoxin
(b) Oxygen supplementation
(c) Immediate descent
(d) Acetazolamide

Explanation:

- **Treatment of Acute Mountain Sickness (AMS):**
  - Immediate stop of ascent.
  - Immediate descent 300–1000 m (Best and first line option).
  - Acetazolamide.
  - Dexamethasone.
  - Supplemental oxygen.
  - Symptomatic (NSAIDs, Anti-emetics).

Ans: (a) Intravenous digoxin

Ref: *Aksel G, Çorbacıoğlu SK, Özen C. High-Altitude Illness: Management Approach, Turk J Emerg Med 2019;19:121-26*

24. Which of the following drugs is used as nail lacquer for onychomycosis?

(a) Fluconazole
(b) Ciclopirox
(c) Itraconazole
(d) Terbinafine

Explanation:

Drugs used for treatment of onychomycosis

Oral	Topical
• Terbinafine – Preferred for dermatophytes Itraconazole – Preferred for candida • Fluconazole – It's an alternative • Griseofulvin – It's not preferred due to resistance	• Ciclopirox lacquer • Efinaconazole solution • Tavaborole solution

Ans: (b) Ciclopirox

Ref: *Goodman and Gilman's The Pharmacological Basis of Therapeutics, 13th Edition, New York, McGraw-Hill 2018, Page1281*

25. Which of the following drugs act by inhibiting DNA replication?

(a) 6-Mercaptopurine
(b) Actinomycin-D
(c) Mitomycin C
(d) Asparaginase

Explanation:

The Contrasting Features of Drug(s):

	6-Mercaptopurine	Actinomycin-D	Mitomycin C	L-Asparaginase
Class	Anti-cancer drug	Anti-cancer drug	Anti-cancer drug	Anti-cancer drug
	Antimetabolite	Cancer Antibiotic	Cancer Antibiotic	
MOA	(-) Purine nucleotide synthesis and metabolism	(-) DNA-dependent RNA polymerase	Alkylating agent	Cell death due to depletion of asparagine
		(-) Transcription (DNA to RNA)	(-) DNA synthesis	
		Breaks in DNA strands		

Ans: (b) Actinomycin-D

Ref: *Wellstein A, Giaccone G, Atkins MB, Sausville EA. Cytotoxic Drugs, In: Brunton LL, Hilal-Dandan R, Knollmann BC, Editors, Goodman and Gilman's The Pharmacological Basis of Therapeutics, 13th Edition, New York, McGraw-Hill 2018, Page 1167-1201*

26. Which of the following factor is targeted by warfarin by inhibiting activity of gamma carboxylase?

(a) Factor VIII
(b) 1 Factor V
(c) Factor II
(d) Factor XI

Explanation:

- **Warfarin** inhibits synthesis of coagulation factors **II, VII, IX and X.**
- It also inhibits synthesis of anticoagulant **protein C and S.**
- **Factor VII** is **shortest** acting and first to disappear, whereas factor II is longest acting and last to disappear after starting warfarin.

Ans: (c) Factor II

Ref: *Hogg K, Weitz JI. Blood Coagulation and Anticoagulant, Fibrinolytic and Antiplatelet Drugs, In: Brunton LL, Hilal-Dandan R, Knollmann BC, Editors, Goodman and Gilman's The Pharmacological Basis of Therapeutics, 13th Edition, New York, McGraw-Hill 2018, Page 585-603*

27. Which of the following fluoroquinolone is contraindicated in liver disease?

(a) Levofloxacin
(b) Pefloxacin
(c) Ofloxacin
(d) Lomefloxacin

Explanation:

- **Fluoroquinolones:** Class of antimicrobial agents acts by the inhibition of bacterial '*DNA gyrase*' enzyme.
- The **'fluoro'** compound is added to them to enhance their antimicrobial spectrum against gram positive microorganisms.
- They have been classified as 'first and second' generations.

	First Generation	**Second Generation**
Year of Introduction	1980s	1990s
Antimicrobial Spectrum of Activity	Gram negative (*Mainly*)	Gram positive (*Mainly*)
Mechanism of Action	(-) '*DNA gyrase*' in gram negative bacteria	(-) '*Topoisomerase IV*' in gram positive bacteria
Examples	Norfloxacin	Levofloxacin
	Ciprofloxacin	Moxifloxacin
	Ofloxacin	Prulifloxacin
	Pefloxacin	Lomefloxacin
		Sparfloxacin
		Gemifloxacin
UNIQUE PROPERTIES		
Food interferes the absorption	Ciprofloxacin	
With 100% oral bioavailability	Levofloxacin	

Contd.

Contd.

Dose reduction required in liver disorders	Ciprofloxacin
	Pefloxacin
	Moxifloxacin
Dose reduction required in kidney disorders	Ciprofloxacin
	Ofloxacin
	Levofloxacin
	Gemfloxacin

Ans: (b) Pefloxacin

Ref: *Tripathi KD, Essentials of Medical Pharmacology, 8th Edition, New Delhi, Jaypee Brothers Medical Publishers 2019, Page 763*

28. Which of the following antiarrhythmic drug is contraindicated in a patient with interstitial lung disease?

(a) Amiodarone (b) Sotalol

(c) Quinidine (d) Lignocaine

Explanation:

Drugs associated with interstitial lung disease and interstitial renal disease are tabulated as follows:

Interstitial Lung Disease or Pulmonary Infiltrates	Cancer Chemotherapeutics	Mitomycin C
		Chlorambucil
		Busulfan
		Cyclophosphamide
		Procarbazine
		Bleomycin
		Melphalan
		Carmustine (BCNU)
	Immunosuppressants	Methotrexate
		Azathioprine
	Microbial Chemotherapeutics	Sulfonamides
		Nitrofurantoin
		Acyclovir
	Others	Amiodarone
		Methysergide
Interstitial Renal Disease or Interstitial Nephritis	Microbial Chemotherapeutics	Methicillin
		Sulfonamides
	Diuretics	Thiazides
		Furosemide
	Others	Phenindione
		Allopurinol

- **Amiodarone:** It is a long acting, highly lipophilic, broad spectrum antiarrhythmic drug.
- ADRs associated with the use of amiodarone are:

Acute/Short Term Use	Chronic Term Therapy
Depressed myocardial activity	**Pulmonary fibrosis** (*Risk is more in individuals with underlying lung disorders and dosage more than 400 mg/d*)
(↓) BP	Hepatotoxicity

Contd.

Contd.

GIT disturbances	**Ophthalmic toxicity** (*Corneal microdeposits*)
	Neuromuscular toxicity (*Proximal muscle weakness, peripheral neuropathy*)
	Thyrotoxicity (*Hypo/Hyperthyroidism*)
	Phototoxicity
	Cardiotoxicity (*QT prolongation, bradycardia*)

Ans: (a) Amiodarone

Ref: *Knollmann BC, Roden DM. Antiarrhythmic Drugs, In: Brunton LL, Hilal-Dandan R, Knollmann BC, Editors, Goodman and Gilman's The Pharmacological Basis of Therapeutics, 13th Edition, New York, McGraw-Hill 2018, Page 547-72*

PATHOLOGY

1. A 35-year-old woman with a long history of dyspnea, chronic cough, sputum production and wheezing dies of respiratory failure following a bout of lobar pneumonia. She was not a smoker or alcoholic. The lung at autopsy is shown in the image. Which of the following underlying conditions was most likely associated with the pathologic changes shown here?

(a) Mutation in dynein arms
(b) Cystic fibrosis
(c) Alpha 1 antitrypsin deficiency
(d) Antibodies against type 4 collagen

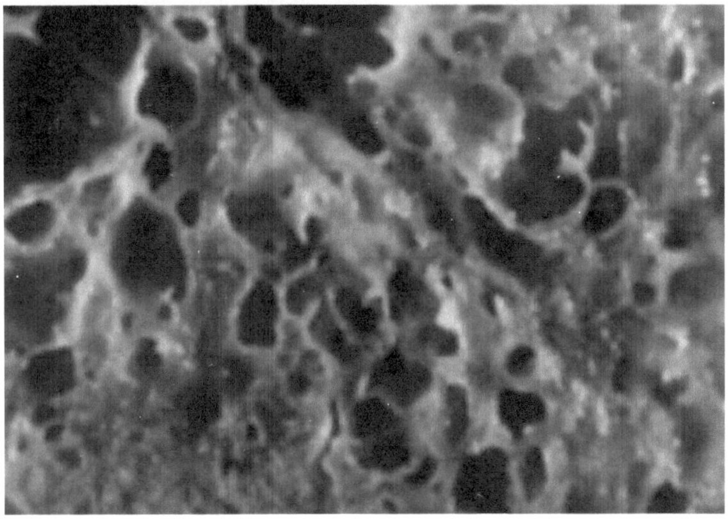

Explanation:

EMPHYSEMA

- **Definition:** Permanent enlargement of air spaces distal to the terminal bronchioles, accompanied by destruction of their walls without significant fibrosis.
- **Four types:** (1) centriacinar, (2) panacinar, (3) distal acinar, (4) irregular.
- **Centriacinar (centrilobular) emphysema**
  - **Site: Central or proximal parts** of acini.
  - Distal alveoli are spared.
  - Apical segments will be affected.
  - Common in cigarette smokers.
- **Panacinar (panlobular) emphysema**
  - Acini are **uniformly** enlarged.
  - Lower zones are involved.
  - Associated with **α1-anti-trypsin deficiency.**
- **Distal acinar (paraseptal) emphysema**
  - **Distal part** of acini are involved.
  - Prominent adjacent to pleura, areas of fibrosis, scarring, atelectasis.
  - Severe in upper half of lungs.
  - **Characteristic feature: Bullae.**
  - **Complication:** spontaneous pneumothorax.

- **Irregular emphysema**
  - Associated with scarring.
  - Most common form.

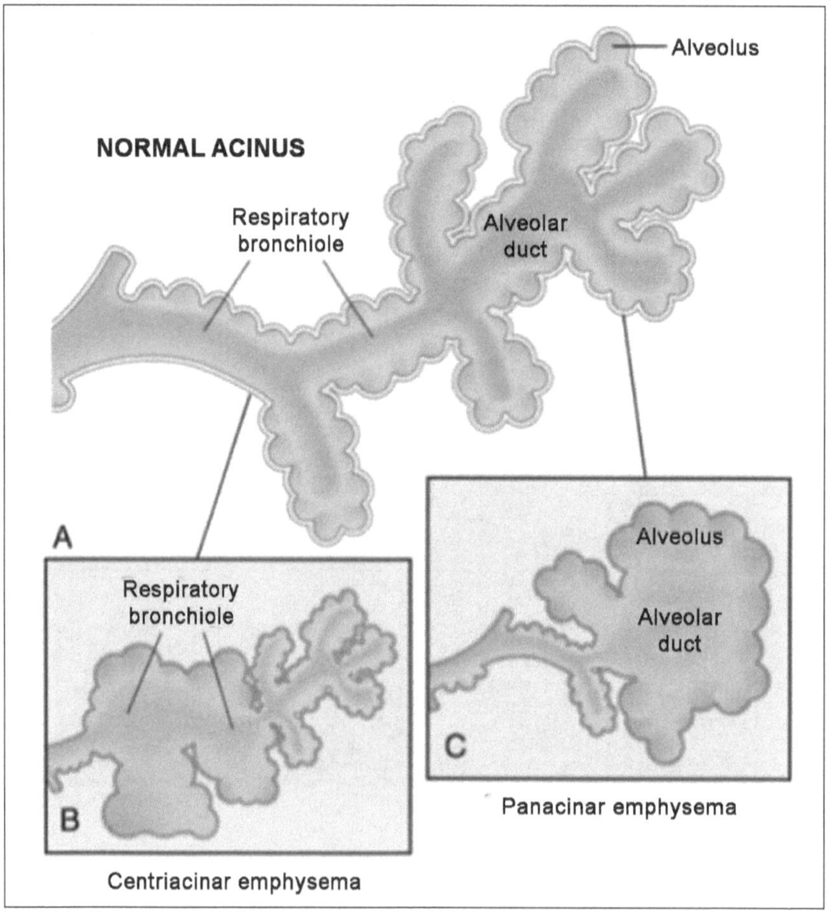

Pattern of emphysema

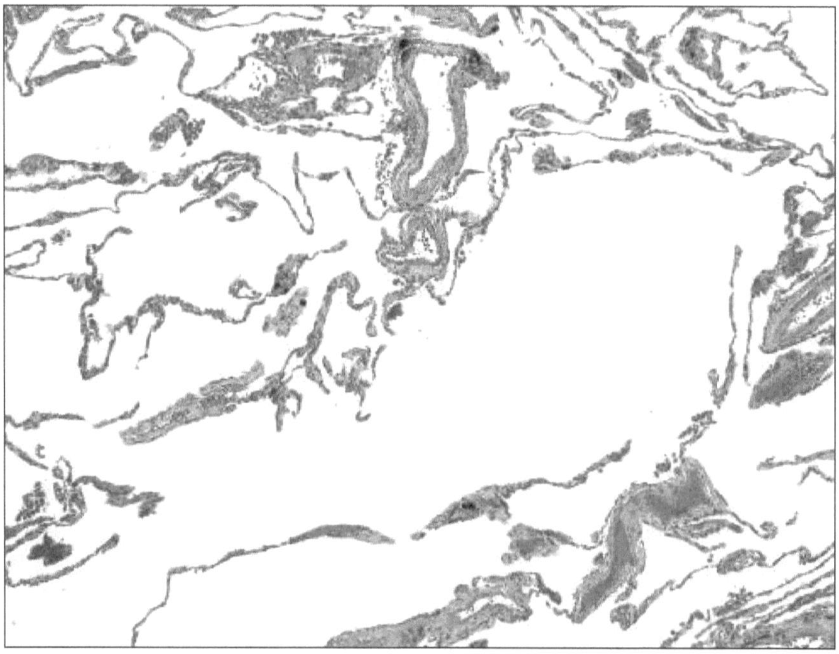

Enlargement of air spaces, with destruction of alveolar septa

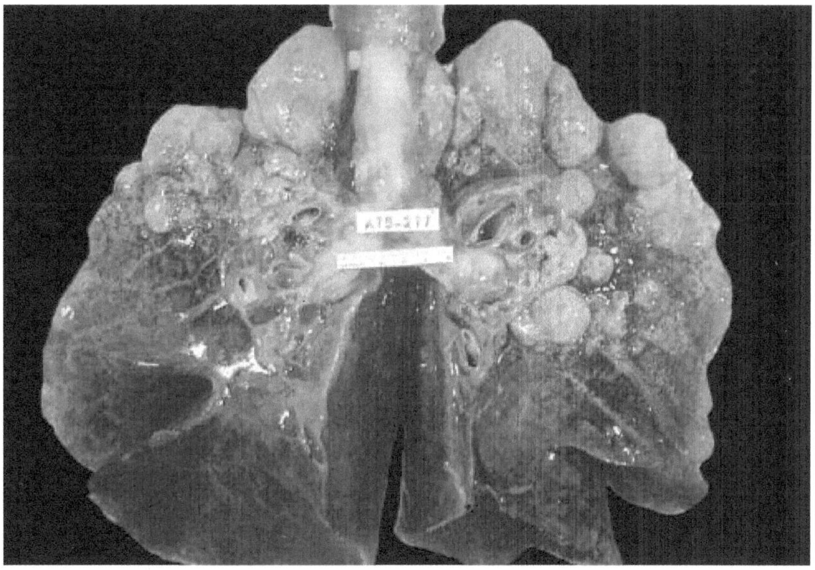

Bullous emphysema

Clinical Features

- Dyspnea.
- Barrel–chest.
- "Pink puffers".

Complications

- Secondary pulmonary hypertension.
- Cor pulmonale.

Conditions Related to Emphysema

- Compensatory emphysema.
- Bullous emphysema.
- Mediastinal (interstitial) emphysema.

Ans: (c) Alpha 1 antitrypsin deficiency

Ref: *Robbins and Cotrans Pathologic Basis of Disease, 10th Edition, Chapter 13: Lung 7, Page 498*

2. A 20-year-old person presented with history of diarrhea, vomiting and poor appetite. Duodenal biopsy of the patient showed crypt hyperplasia, villi atrophy, CD8+ cells in lamina propria. Your most probable diagnosis is:

(a) Environmental enteropathy
(b) Celiac disease
(c) Whipple's disease
(d) Chronic pancreatitis

Explanation:

- The clinical presentation and lab findings suggest **Celiac disease.**

Celiac Disease

- AKA celiac sprue or gluten sensitive enteropathy.
- Immune-mediated enteropathy triggered by ingestion of gluten-containing cereals, such as **wheat, rye, or barley**, in genetically predisposed individuals.

- **Primary treatment: Gluten-free diet.**
- **Association: HLA-DQ2 or HLA-DQ8.**
- **Pathogenesis:** Antibodies against tissue transglutaminase, deamidated gliadin, and anti-endomysial antibodies.
- **Biopsy site:** Second portion of duodenum/proximal jejunum.
- **Histopathology:**
  - Increased numbers of T lymphocytes.
  - Intraepithelial lymphocytosis.
  - Crypt hyperplasia.
  - Villous atrophy.

  Other histologic features of celiac disease: Increased mast cells, plasma cells and eosinophils in upper lamina propria.
- Associated with **dermatitis herpetiformis.**
- **Sensitive tests:** IgA antibodies to tissue transglutaminase/IgA or IgG antibodies to deamidated gliadin.
- **Anti-endomysial antibodies: Specific.**
- **Complications:**
  - Enteropathy-associated T cell lymphoma.
  - Small-intestinal adenocarcinoma.

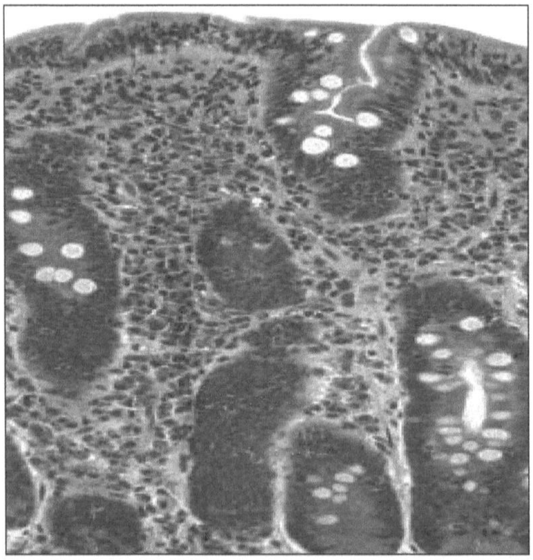

Total villous atrophy with dense plasma cell infiltrate in lamina propria

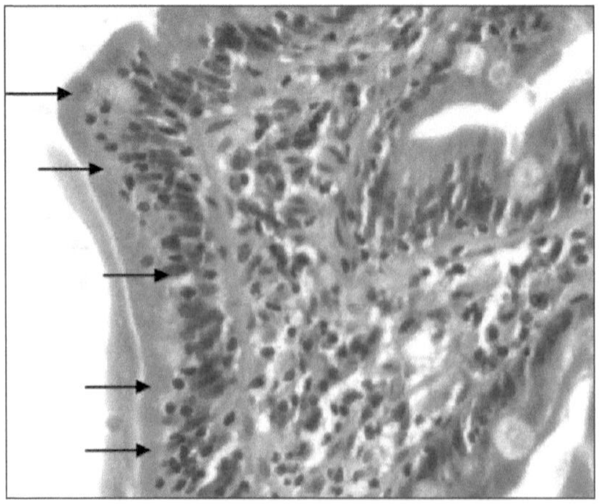

Intraepithelial lymphocytes (arrows)

Whipple's Disease also known as Intestinal Lipodystrophy

- **Etiology:** Bacterium Tropheryma whipplei.
- Manifests as malabsorption, steatorrhea, protein-losing enteropathy.
- **Histopathology:**
  - Foamy macrophages in lamina propia.
  - PAS-positive, diastase resistant macrophages in the lamina propria containing non-acid-fast Gram-positive bacilli.
- **Treatment:** Penicillin, ampicillin, tetracycline, co-trimoxazole.

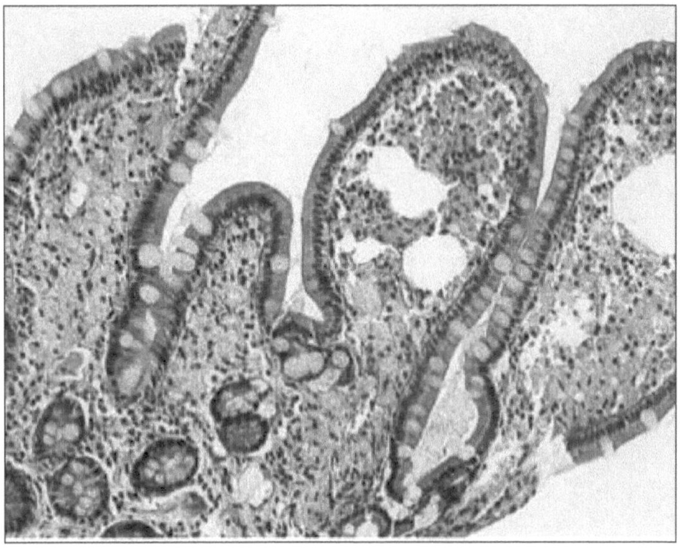

Foamy macrophages in lamina propia

Ans: (b) Celiac disease

Ref: *Robbins and Cotrans Pathologic Basis of Disease, 9th Edition, Chapter 15: Oral Cavities and Gastrointestinal Tract, Page 612*

3. Which of the following is true about Polyarteritis nodosa (PAN)?

(a) Microscopy shows fibrinoid necrosis in large arteries
(b) ANCA is positive
(c) 30% people have HBsAg positive
(d) Patient has hypogammaglobulinemia

Explanation:

Polyarteritis Nodosa (PAN)

- Systemic vasculitis of small/medium-sized muscular arteries.
- No association with ANCA.
- 30%: HBsAg - HBsAb complexes.
- **Microscopy:**
  - Segmental transmural necrotizing inflammation.
  - Transmural inflammation.
  - Fibrinoid necrosis.
  - Fibrous thickening.
  - All stages of activity coexist.

- **C/F:**
  - *Age:* Young.
  - *Hypertension:* Renal artery involvement.
  - Abdominal pain, bloody stools.
  - Peripheral neuritis.
  - Renal involvement–prominent.

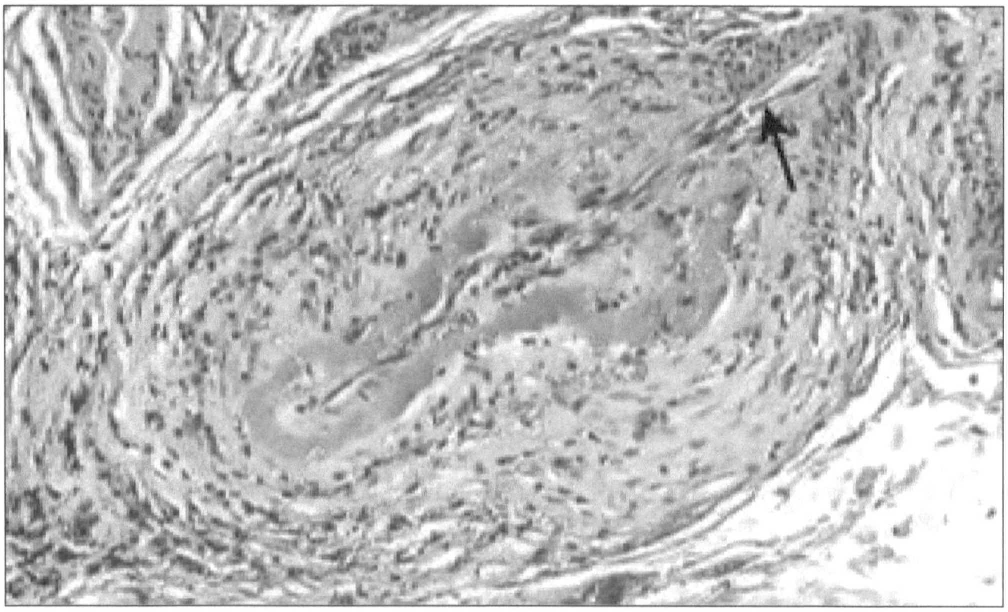

Segmental transmural fibrinoid necrotising vasculitis. Spared vessel fragment shown by arrow

Ans: (c) 30% people have HBsAg positive

Ref: *Robbins and Cotrans Pathologic Basis of Disease, 9th Edition, Chapter 11: The Blood Vessels, Page 509*

4. Which of the following is the correct statement related to Huntington's chorea?

(a) It is a tri-nucleotide expansion mutation related disorder

(b) There is loss of function type of mutation

(c) There are abnormal repeats of CUG

(d) Abnormality is seen due to mutation in Chromosome 6

Explanation:

Huntington Disease (HD)

- Autosomal dominant.
- Movement disorder with degeneration of striatum (caudate and putamen).
- **C/F:** Involuntary jerky movements, dementia, behavioural changes, risk for suicide.
- **Clinical triad:** Motor, cognitive and psychiatric symptoms.
- **Pathogenesis: CAG trinucleotide repeat expansions** in a gene located on 4p16.3 that encodes protein huntington.
- **Normal:** 11 to 34 copies.
- Paternal transmission.
- **Anticipation:** Earlier onset in next generations.
- **Gross:** Atrophy of the caudate nucleus and putamen, loss of neurons, intranuclear inclusions containing ubiquitin.

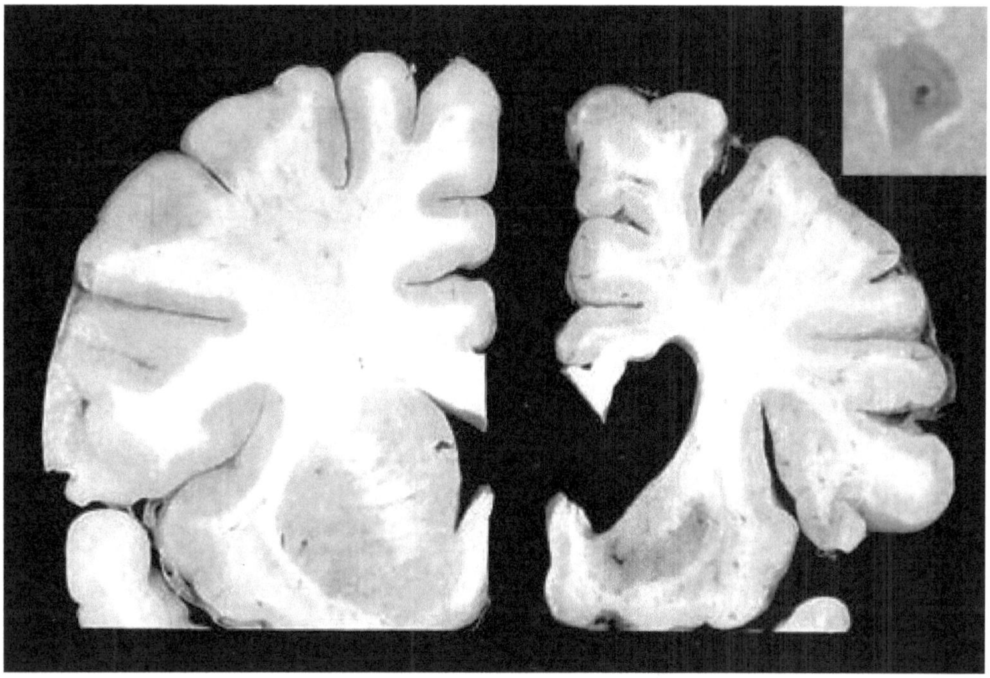

Atrophy of striatum and ventricular dilation. Inset: An intranuclear inclusion in a cortical neuron reactive for ubiquitin

Ans: (a) It is a tri-nucleotide expansion mutation related disorder

Ref: *Robbins and Cotrans Pathologic Basis of Disease, 10th Edition, Chapter 23: Central Nervous System, Page 879*

5. A 25-year-old man presents for a routine physical examination. The patient is tall (6 ft, 5 in) and on examination he was found to have an early diastolic murmur. His family pedigree is as given below. Which of the following is the mode of inheritance by which the disease is likely to be transmitted?

(a) AD
(b) AR
(c) XLR
(d) XLD

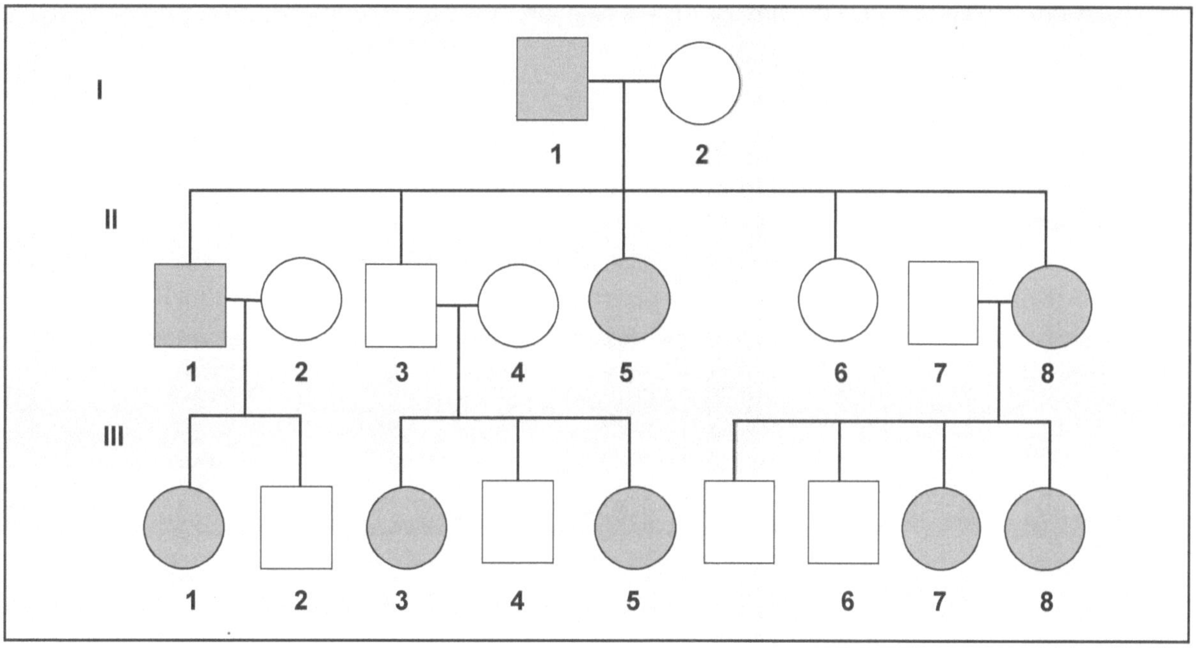

Explanation:

- Manifested in heterozygous state. Hence at least one parent in an index case usually is affected.
- Both males and females can be affected.
- Both sexes can transmit.
- **Features:**
  - Reduced penetrance.
  - Variable expressivity.
  - Dominant negative–in case of osteogenesis imperfecta.
- **Examples:**
  - *Nervous system:* Huntington disease, Neurofibromatosis, Myotonic dystrophy, Tuberous sclerosis.
  - *Urinary system:* Polycystic kidney disease.
  - *GIT:* Familial polyposis coli.
  - *Hematopoietic:* Hereditary spherocytosis, von Willebrand disease.
  - *Skeletal:* Marfan syndrome, Ehlers-Danlos syndrome (some variants), Osteogenesis imperfect, Achondroplasia.
  - *Metabolic:* Familial hypercholesterolemia, Acute intermittent porphyria.

Autosomal Recessive Disorders

- Trait does not usually affect parents of the affected individual, but siblings may show disease.
- Recurrence risk is 25% for each birth.
- Complete penetrance.
- Onset is early in life.
- Include almost all inborn errors of metabolism.
- **Examples:**
  - *Metabolic:* Cystic fibrosis, Phenylketonuria, Galactosemia, Homocystinuria, Lysosomal storage diseases, α1-Antitrypsin deficiency, Wilson disease, Hemochromatosis, Glycogen storage diseases.
  - *Hematopoietic:* Sickle cell anemia, Thalassemias.
  - *Endocrine:* Congenital adrenal hyperplasia.
  - *Skeletal:* Ehlers-Danlos syndrome (some variants), Alkaptonuria.
  - *Nervous system:* Neurogenic muscular atrophies, Friedreich's ataxia, Spinal muscular atrophy.

Ans: (a) AD

Ref: *Robbins and Cotrans Pathologic Basis of Disease, 10th Edition, Chapter 7: Genetic and Pediatric Diseases, Page 879*

6. A 10-year-old boy, presents with complaints of fatigue and abdominal pain after playing football. On detailed history taking, he also complaints of painful swelling of digits in the past. On USG of abdomen he was found to have a small spleen. Which of the following is the most likely diagnosis?

(a) Acute pancreatitis (b) Sickle cell anemia
(c) Iron deficiency anemia (d) Hereditary spherocytosis

Explanation:

- The clinical presentation of fatigue (due to Anemia) with painful swelling of digits (dactylitis) and small spleen is suggestive of sickle cell anemia.

Sickle Cell Disease

- Common hemoglobinopathies–HbS, HbC and HbE.
- **Pathogenesis:** Point mutations at the 6th codon of β globin gene→substitution of lysine for glutamic acid at position 6 of globin chain→Polymerization of HbS molecules→sickling.
- These patients are resistant to P. falciparum.
- HbS common in Central and Southern India.
- Tests for HbS:
  - **Sickling test:** 2% sodium metabisulfite or sodium dithionite.
  - Hemoglobin electrophoresis.
- **Types:**
  - *Sickle cell anemia:* Homozygous.
  - *Sickle cell β thalassaemia:* Double heterozygous.
  - *Sickle cell trait:* Heterozygous carrier.
- **Factors which influence sickling:**
  - Intracellular concentration of HbS.
  - *Other hemoglobins:* HbF protective.
  - Association with thalassemias.
  - *Other abnormal hemoglobins:* HbC or HbD retards sickling.
  - *Decreased oxygen tension:* Induces sickling.
  - Cold increases sickling.
  - Acidosis increases sickling.
- **Clinical Features:**
  - Autosplenectomy.
  - **Infections:** *Streptococcus pneumoniae* (sepsis, meningitis), *Salmonella* (osteomyelitis).
  - **Vasa-occlusive crises:** 'Hand foot syndrome' or dactylitis.
  - **Hematologic crises:** Aplastic crisis, Megaloblastic crisis, Hemolytic crisis, Splenic sequestration crisis.
  - Stroke.
  - **Acute chest syndrome.**
  - Bilirubin gallstones.
  - Chronic leg ulcers.
  - Proliferative retinopathy.

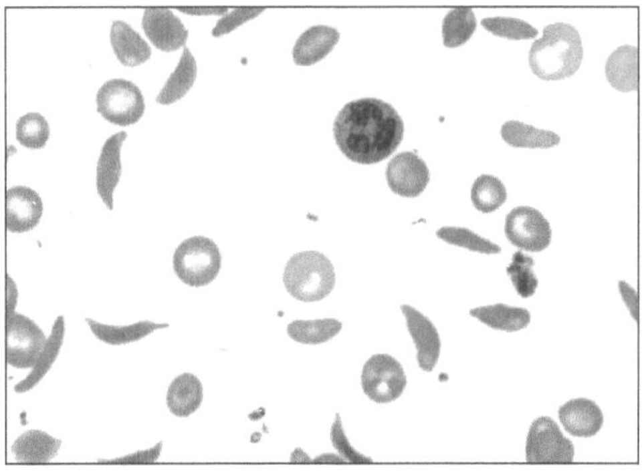

Sickle cells on peripheral smear

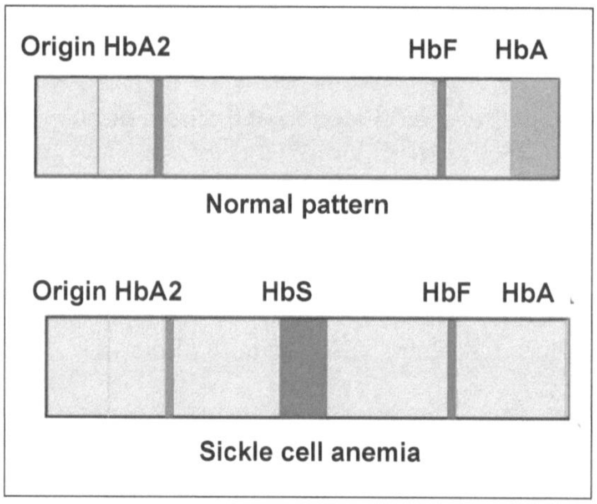

Hb electrophoresis

Ans: (b) Sickle cell anemia

Ref: *Essentials of Haematology*, *Shirish M Kawthalkar, 1st Edition, Chapter 4: Anaemias Due to Impaired Red Cell Production, Page 75*

7. A 30-year-old woman came with complaints of easy fatigability, exertional dyspnea and weight loss. She also complaints of frequent fall. Physical examination revealed there were bilateral decreases in vibration sense. Her hemoglobin levels were 8.2gm%. She was treated with folate. Her anemia improved but neurological symptoms worsened. Which of the following is the most probable reason for her condition?

(a) Folate not absorbed

(b) Unmasked pyridoxine deficiency

(c) Deficiency of folate reductase in CNS

(d) Folate therapy caused use of B_{12} stores aggravating symptoms

Explanation:

- Folic acid or vitamin B_{12} deficiency–common cause for megaloblastic anemia.

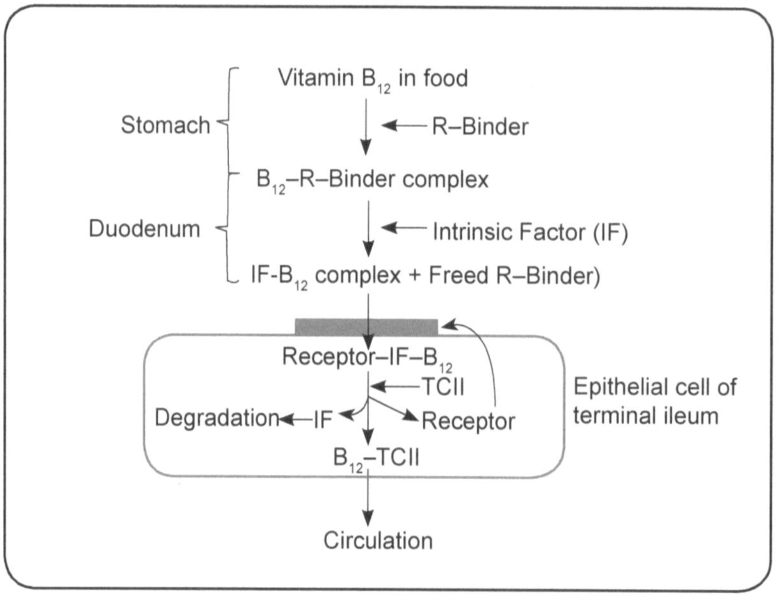

Absorption of vitamin B_{12}

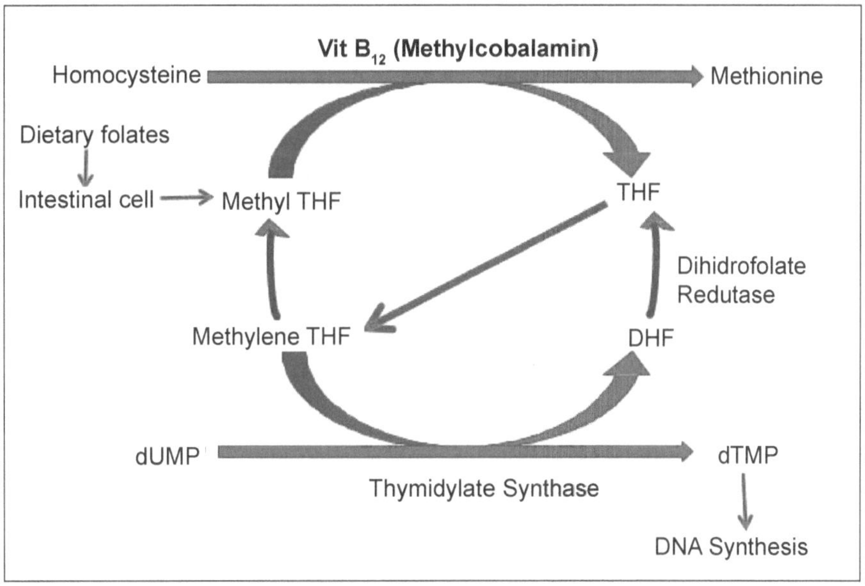

Role of vitamin B_{12} and folate in synthesis of DNA

- **Clinical Features:**
  - Peripheral neuropathy.
  - Subacute combined degeneration of spinal cord.
  - Cerebral changes-dementia, psychosis.
- **Peripheral Blood:**
  - Oval macrocytosis–earliest sign.
  - Hypersegmented neutrophils.
  - Basophilic stippling.
  - Howell-Jolly bodies.
  - Cabot's rings.
- **Bone Marrow:**
  - Megaloblasts.
  - Giant metamyelocytes.
- **Laboratory Features**
  - Serum vitamin B_{12} assay.
  - Methylmalonic acid (MMA) and homocysteine in serum.
  - Schilling test.

Pernicious Anemia:

- Common cause
- Autoimmune disease→chronic atrophic gastritis.
- Autoantibodies (IgG) to parietal.

Ans: (d) Folate therapy caused use of B_{12} stores aggravating symptoms

Ref: *Essentials of Haematology*, Shirish M Kawthalkar, 1st Edition, Chapter 4: Anaemias Due to Impaired Red Cell Production, Page 85

8. A 24-year-old male presented with history of fatigue and tiredness. On investigation he was found to have Hb values of– 9 gm%, mean corpuscular volume (MCV) of 101 FL. Peripheral smear examination showed macrocytic red blood cells (RBC) and hypersegmented neutrophils. Which of the following is the most likely etiology?

(a) Lead poisoning
(b) Iron deficiency anemia
(c) Chronic alcoholism
(d) Hemolytic anemia

Explanation:

- Defective synthesis of DNA in proliferating cells.
- **Peripheral Blood:**

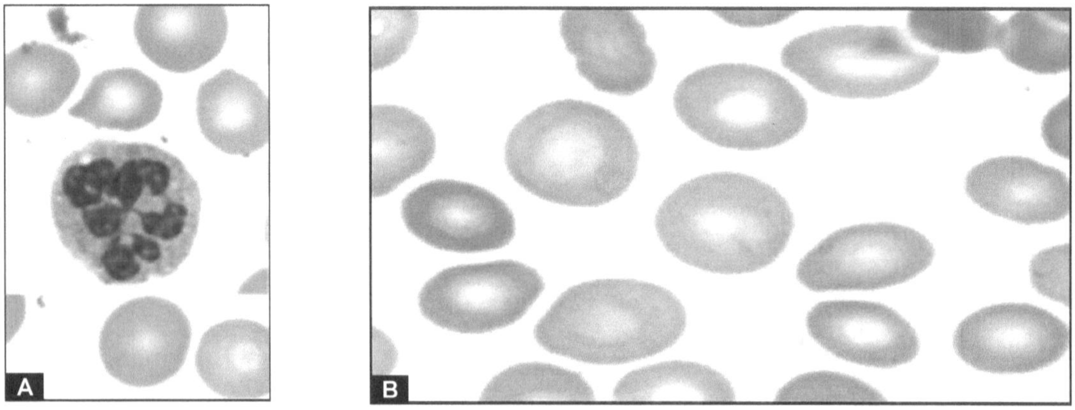

A. Hypersegmented neutrophils, B. Macrocytes

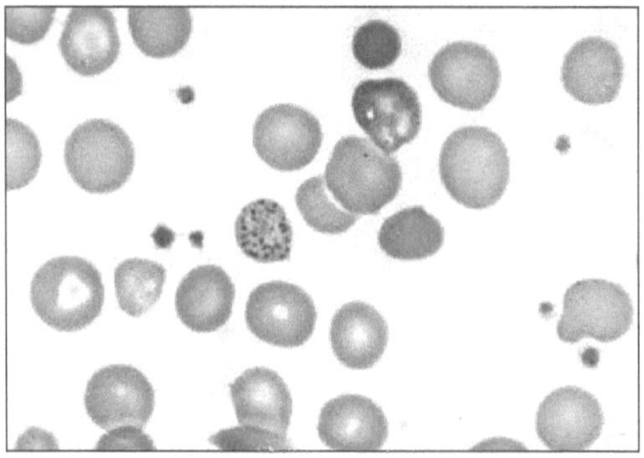

Basophilic stippling

- **Bone Marrow:**

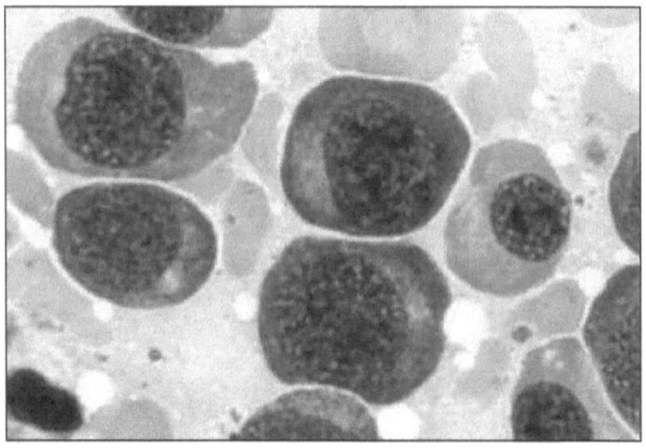

Megaloblast with sieve like chromatin

- **Causes of Macrocytosis:**
  - Alcoholism.
  - Hepatic disease.

- Hypothyroidism.
- Chemotherapeutic drugs.

Evaluation of Macrocytic Anemia

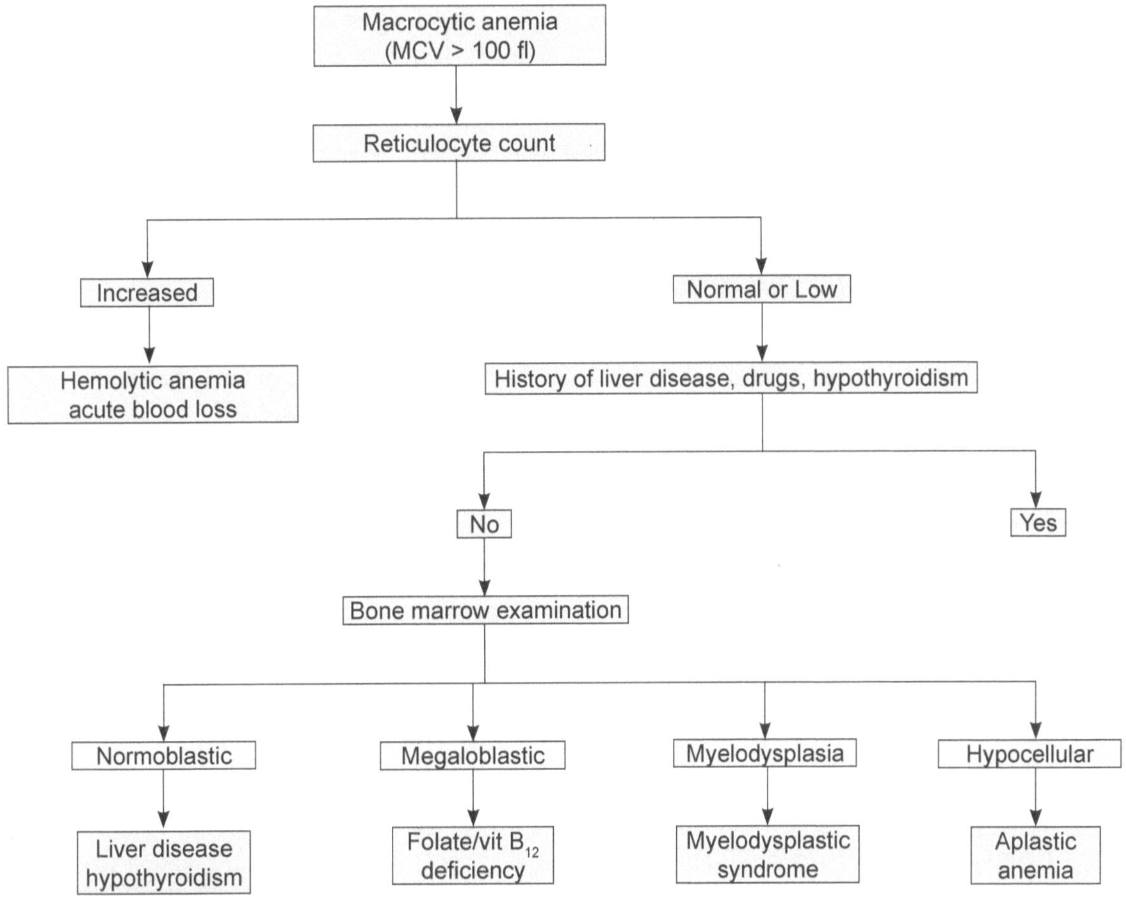

Ans: (c) Chronic alcoholism

Ref: *Essentials of Haematology*, *Shirish M Kawthalkar, 1st Edition, Chapter 4: Anaemias Due to Impaired Red Cell Production, Page 85*

9. A 35-year-old heterosexual patient diagnosed with HIV history of chronic watery diarrhea. Colonoscopic biopsy is shown as below. Which of the following is your most probable diagnosis?

(a) Giardia
(b) Cryptosporidium
(c) Microspora
(d) CMV

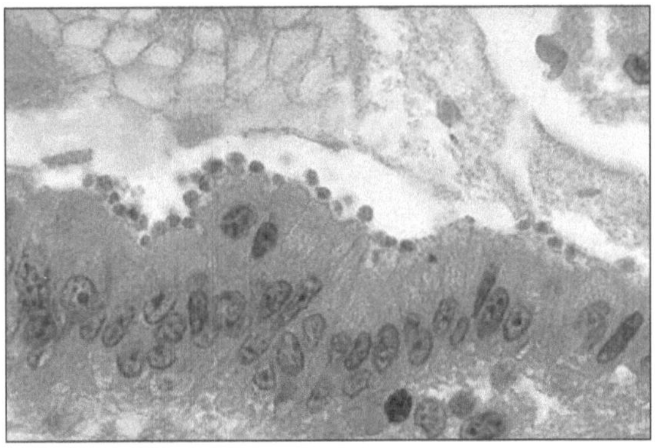

Explanation:

Cryptosporidium Diarrhea

- *Cryptosporidium* is a protozoa.
- Main cause of chronic diarrhea in AIDS.
- Cause of persistent diarrhea in developing countries.
- Worldwide distribution except Antarctica.
- *Source:* Contaminated water.
- Oocysts are resistant to chlorine.
- Common cause of waterborne disease in recreational water.
- *Common site of infection:* Terminal ileum and proximal colon.
- 10 oocysts are sufficient to cause symptomatic infection.
- Sporozoites released are motile and attach to enterocyte brush border and enterocyte cytoskeleton changes.
- Sodium malabsorption, chloride secretion, increased tight junction permeability→nonbloody, watery diarrhea.
- **Histology:**
  - *Blue beads:* 2 - 5 μm basophilic round bodies protruding from the apex of enterocytes.
  - Villous atrophy, crypt hyperplasia, cryptitis, mixed inflammatory cells in lamina propria.
  - *Special stain:* Giemsa stain, Modified AFB.
- **Diagnosis:**
  - Detection of cysts in stool by immunofluorescence or modified acid fast stain.
  - Biopsy.
- **Differential Diagnosis:**
  - **Cyclospora:** Oocysts are 8 μm.
  - **Isospora:** Oocysts are 20 - 30 μm.
  - **Microsporidium:** Intracellular fungus, non-acid fast.

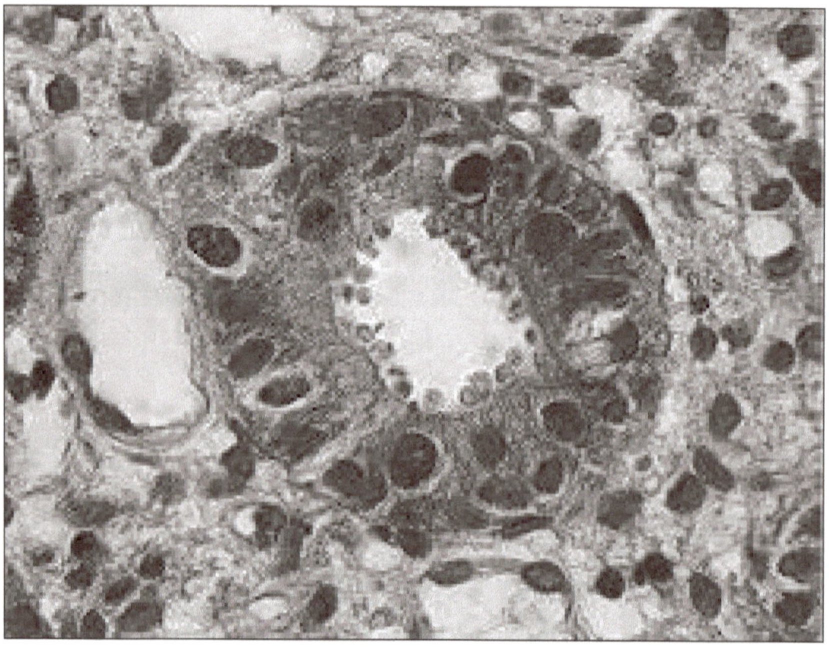

Blue beads

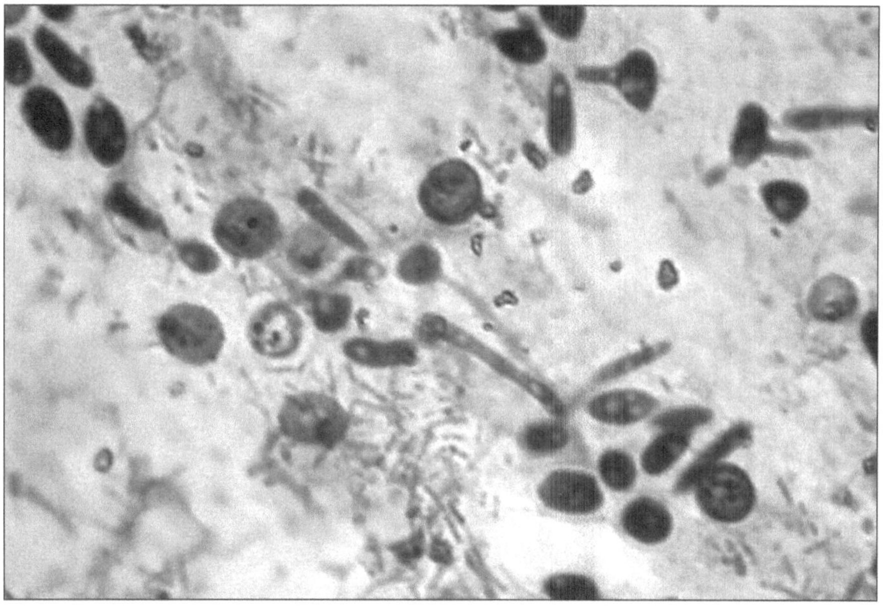

Acid fast positive

Ans: (b) Cryptosporidium

Ref: *Robbins and Cotrans Pathologic Basis of Disease, 9th Edition, Chapter 17: The Gastrointestinal Tract, Page 795*

10. A 5-year-old kid presented with history of blood in stools. On examination there was a polypoidal mass in rectum, biopsy of which is shown here. Your most probable diagnosis is:

(a) Villous adenoma
(b) Juvenile polyp
(c) Vascular malformation
(d) Serrated adenoma

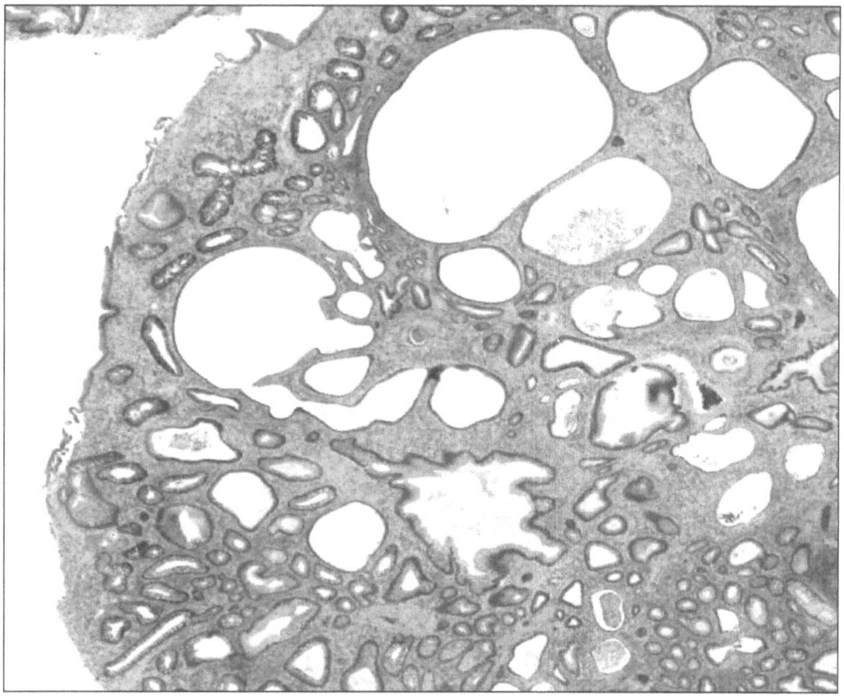

Explanation:

Juvenile Polyps

- Common type of hamartomatous polyp.
- **Sporadic:** Solitary.
- **Juvenile polyposis syndrome:** 3 to 100 polyps, autosomal dominant, TGF-β mutation.
- **Common site:** Rectum.
- **Common presentation:** Rectal bleeding.
- Increased risk of adenocarcinoma.
- **Gross:**
  - Pedunculated, smooth-surfaced,< 3 cm
  - **C/S:** Cystic spaces.
- **Microscopy:**
  - Dilated glands filled with mucin, inflammatory debris.

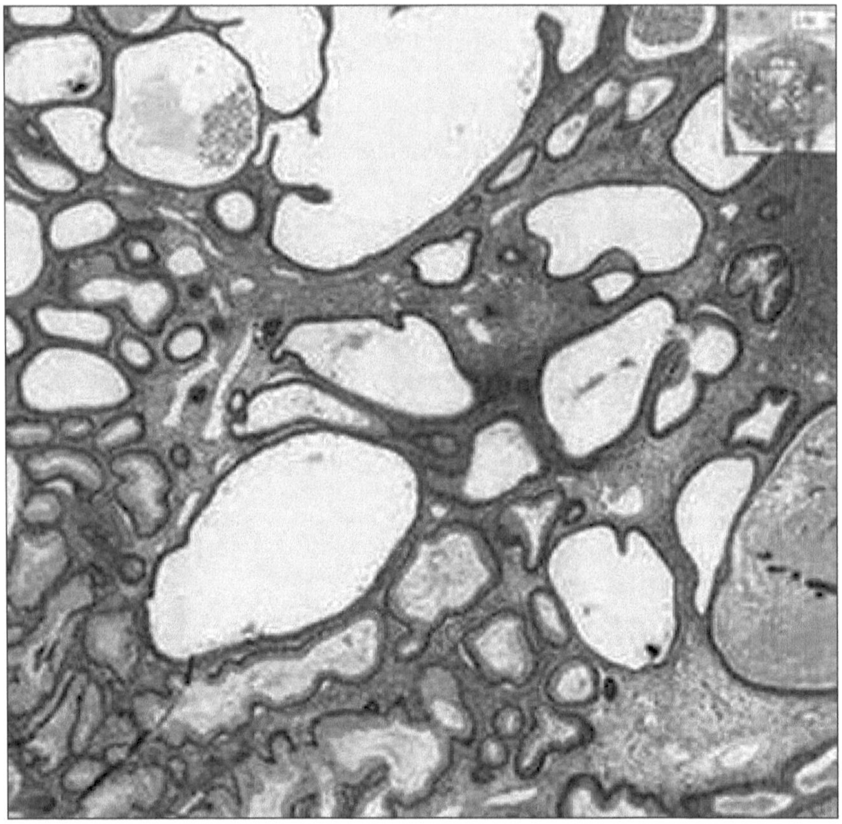

Juvenile polyp: dilated glands

Solitary Rectal Ulcer Syndrome

- **Triad:** Rectal bleeding, mucus discharge, inflammatory lesion of anterior rectal wall.

Peutz-Jeghers Syndrome

- Autosomal dominant.
- Multiple hamartomatous polyps.
- Mucocutaneous hyperpigmentation.

- Increased risk for **malignancies:** Colon, pancreas, breast, lung, ovaries, uterus, testes.
- Mutation in *LKB1/STK11* gene.
- **Histology:**
  - Arborizing network of connective tissue, smooth muscle, lamina propria.
  - Glands lined by normal-appearing intestinal epithelium.

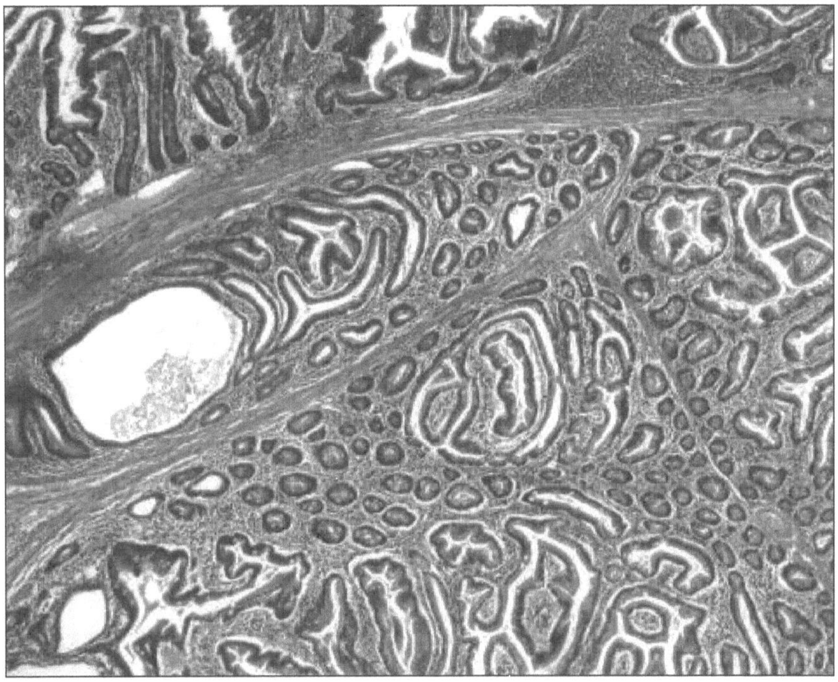

Complex glandular architecture and bundles of smooth muscle

Ans: (b) Juvenile polyp

Ref: *Robbins and Cotrans Pathologic Basis of Disease, 10th Edition, Chapter 15: Oral Cavities and Gastrointestinal Tract, Page 626*

11. A 40-year-old person presented with 10 × 8 cm swelling in retroperitoneum, lesion biopsy is as shown below. Molecular analysis demonstrated t(12, 16). Which of the following is your most probable diagnosis?

(a) Myxoid liposarcoma (b) Lipoma

(c) Synovial sarcoma (d) Pleomorphic sarcoma

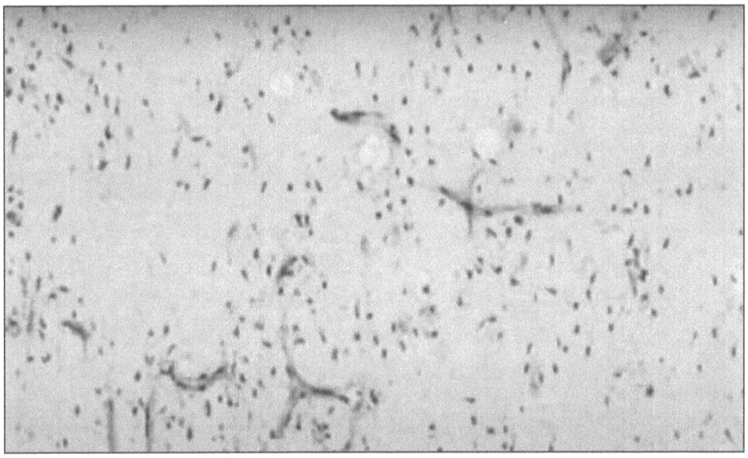

Explanation:

LIPOSARCOMA

- Frequent soft tissue sarcoma in adults.
- **Sites:** Lower extremities, retroperitoneal, perirenal and mesenteric region, shoulder.
- **Pathognomonic feature: Lipoblast.**
- **Types:**
  - Myxoid.
  - Round cell.
  - Well differentiated.
  - Pleomorphic.
- **Myxoid liposarcoma:**
  - Common type.
  - Predilection for lower extremities.
  - *Microscopy:* Lipoblasts, **anastomosing capillary network**, mucoid matrix rich, few/no mitosis.
  - *Genetics:* (12;16)→FUS–DDIT3 fusion.

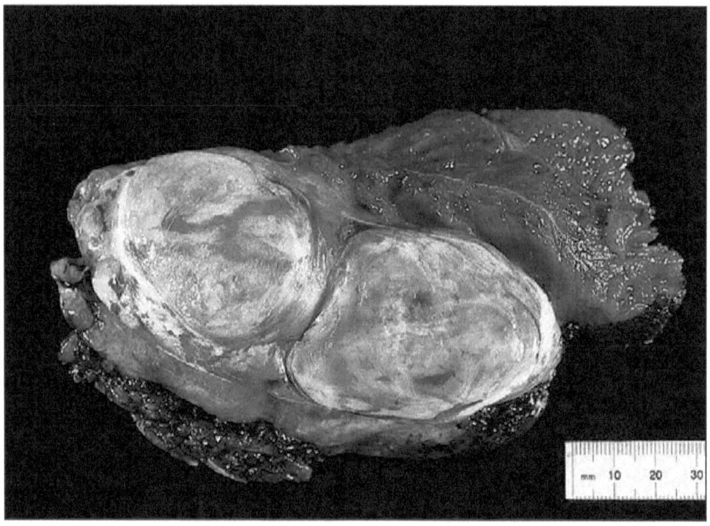

Gross: Myxoid liposarcoma

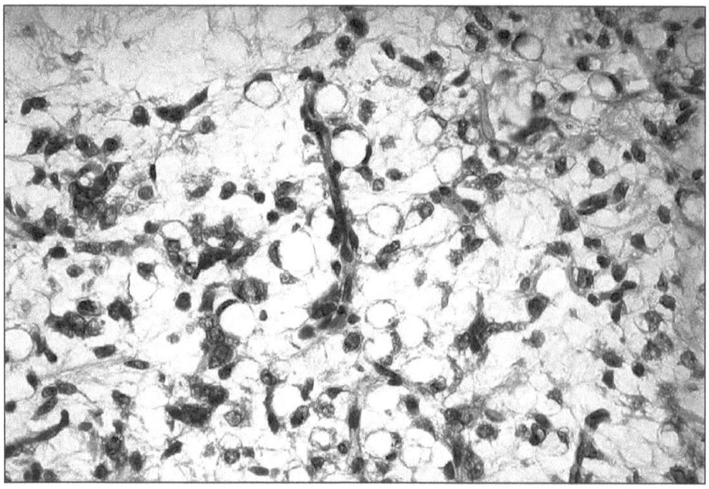

Microscopy: Myxoid liposarcoma

- **Round cell type:**
  - Small tumor cells, scattered lipoblasts, frequent mitoses, less prominent vessels.
  - **S-100:** Diagnostic.
- **Well differentiated liposarcoma:**
  - Includes atypical lipomatous tumor.
- **Spindle cell liposarcoma:**
  - Rare.
  - Variant of atypical lipomatous tumor.
- **Pleomorphic liposarcoma:**
  - Poorly differentiated.
  - *Microscopy:* Cellular, tumor giant cells, lipoblasts, necrosis, many mitoses.
  - S100 positive.
- **Dedifferentiated liposarcoma:**
  - Nonlipogenic component within an atypical lipomatous tumor.
  - *Common site:* Retroperitoneum.
  - PPAR–Gamma positive.
- **IHC for liposarcomas:**
  - S-100.
  - Caveolin.
  - Leptin.

Ans: (a) Myxoid liposarcoma

Ref: *Rosai and Ackerman's Surgical Pathology, 10th Edition, Chapter 25: Soft Tissue, Page 2145*

12. Which of the following infection is common within 1- 4 months post-transplant?

(a) CMV (b) Herpes

(c) Varicella (d) EBV

Explanation:

CYTOMEGALOVIRUS

- **Family:** Herpesvirus.
- Associated with immunosuppression, such as HIV/AIDS, organ transplantation.
- **Cytopathic changes:**
  - Cytomegaly.
  - Nucleomegaly.
  - *Large intranuclear inclusions:* Owl's eye appearance (Cowdry type A inclusion).
  - *Inclusions:* Basophilic/amphophilic, stain positive for PAS and GMS.
  - AKA cytomegalic inclusion disease.
- **Transmission:**
  - *Congenital:* Transplacental.
  - *Perinatal:* Cervical or vaginal secretions.

- Through saliva.
- Iatrogenic.

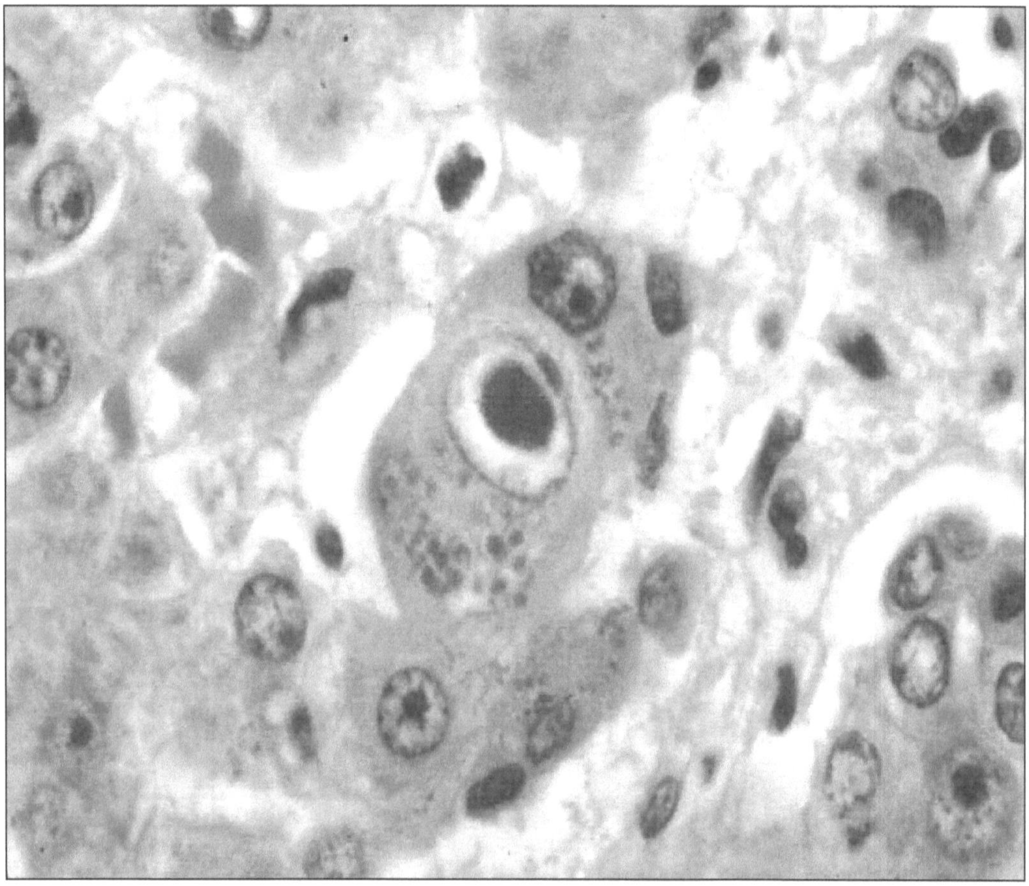

Nuclear inclusion and multiple cytoplasmic inclusions

Cytomegalovirus Mononucleosis

Infectious mononucleosis–like illness marked by fever, atypical lymphocytosis, lymphadenopathy and hepatomegaly accompanied by abnormal liver function test.

Diagnostic Tests

- Tissue sections for inclusions.
- Viral culture.
- Anti-viral antibody titer.
- PCR assay–for CMV DNA.

Ans: (a) CMV

Ref: *Robbins and Cotrans Pathologic Basis of Disease, 10th Edition, Chapter 13: The Lung, Page 533*

13. A 51-year-old person came with complaints of hematuria to the clinic. On examination he was normotensive and had pedal edema. Investigations revealed the patient had no glycosuria and had a creatinine value of 9 mg%. Renal biopsy is as shown below. Which of the following investigations one should do to identify the etiology of the disease?

(a) ANA
(b) Anti-GBM antibodies
(c) HIV RNA
(d) Urine immunoelectrophoresis

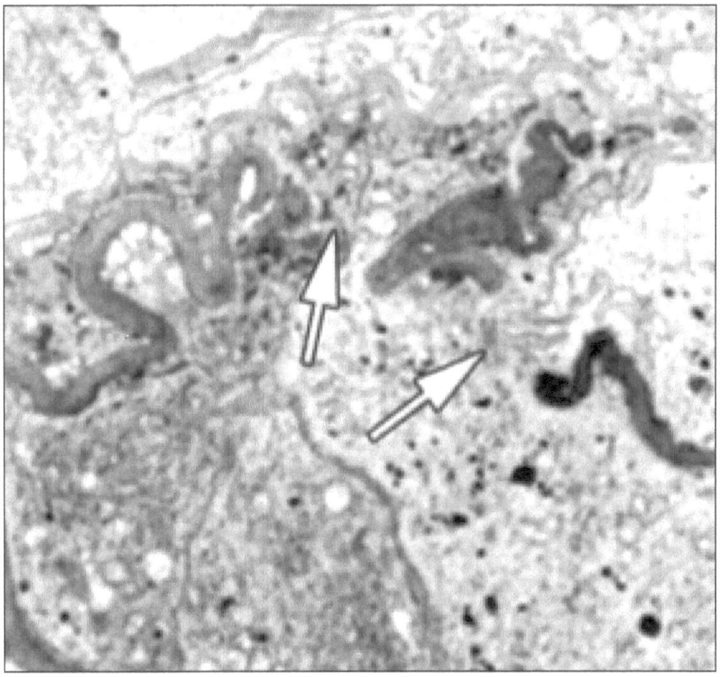

Explanation:

ANTI-GBM ANTIBODIES

- AKA *Goodpasture disease.*
- Deposition of autoantibodies directed against protein components of glomerular basement membrane.
- **Target antigen:** α3 chain of type IV collagen of GBM.
- **Sites:** Lung and kidney.
- In kidney results in RPGN and pulmonary hemorrhage in lungs.
- **Treatment:** Plasmapheresis, immunosuppression.
- **Gross:** Flea bitten kidney.
- **Histology:**
  - Crescents.
- **Immunofluorescence:** Linear pattern GBM fluorescence for Ig and complement.
- **EM: Ruptures in GBM.**

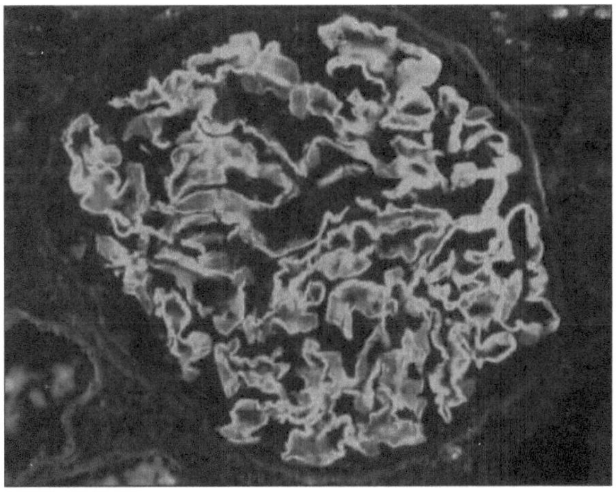

Linear pattern: Direct immunofluorescence

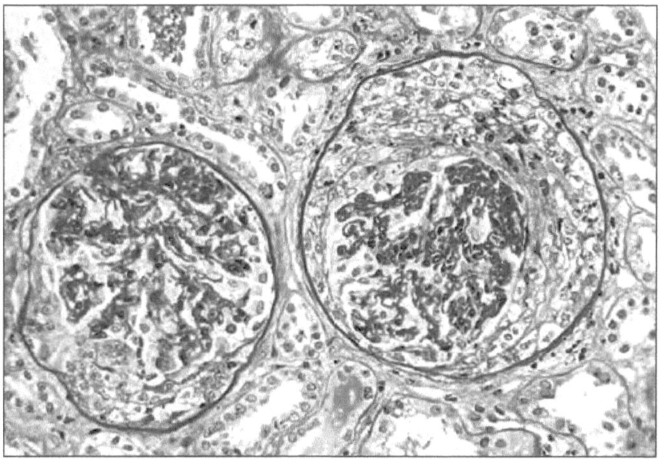

Crescents: PAS stain

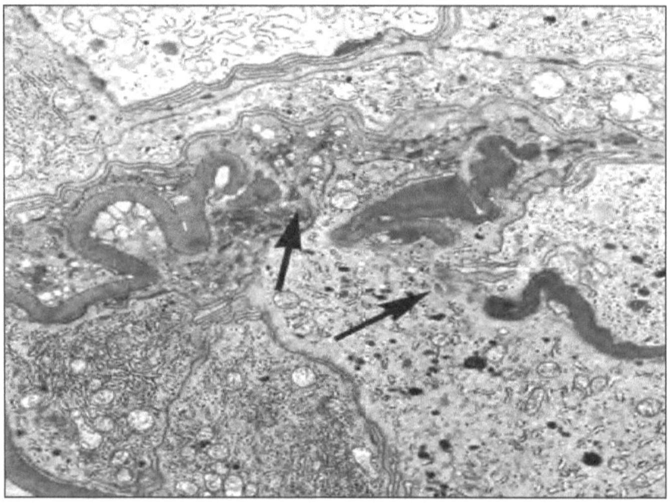

Wrinkling of glomerular basement membrane with focal disruptions ***(arrows)***

Ans: (b) Anti-GBM antibodies

Ref: *Robbins and Cotrans Pathologic Basis of Disease, 10th Edition, Chapter 14: Kidney and Its Collecting System, Page 554*

14. Why is CPD better than ACD for storage of blood?

(a) Because it's less acidic
(b) Improves oxygen transport
(c) Hypertonicity of blood
(d) More citrate ions

Explanation:

ACD

- **ACD:** Acid citrate dextrose.
- **Uses:**
  - To preserve blood for tissue typing.
  - Plasmapheresis.
- **Shelf life:** 21 days.

CPD

- **Components:**
  - *Citrate:* Anticoagulation by binding of calcium in plasma.
  - *Phosphate:* Acts as a buffer to minimize the effects of decreasing pH.
  - *Dextrose:* Maintenance of red cell membrane and metabolism.
- **Shelf life:** 21 days.

CPDA-1

- **49 ml of CPDA:** 1 for 350 ml of blood.
- **Mechanisms:**
  - Prevents clotting of blood.
  - Provides nutrients to maintain metabolism and viability of red cells.
- **Temperature of storage:** 2-6°C.

- **Maximum shelf life:** 35 days.
- **Function of each component:**
  - *Citrate:* Anticoagulation by binding of calcium in plasma.
  - *Phosphate:* Acts as a buffer to minimize the effects of decreasing pH.
  - *Dextrose:* Maintenance of red cell membrane and metabolism.
  - *Adenine:* Generation of ATP (energy source).

SAGM

- Commonly used additive solution.
- **SAGM:** Saline, adenine, glucose, mannitol.
- Shelf life increases from 35 days to 42 days.

Ans: (b) Improves oxygen transport

Ref: *Essentials of Haematology*, *Shirish M Kawthalkar, 1st Edition, Chapter 19: Collection of Donor Blood, Processing and Storage, Page 447*

15. A patient presented with gastritis symptoms and his peripheral smear image is shown. What is the probable diagnosis?

(a) Autoimmune gastritis (b) Celiac disease

(c) Tropical sprue (d) Ulcerative colitis

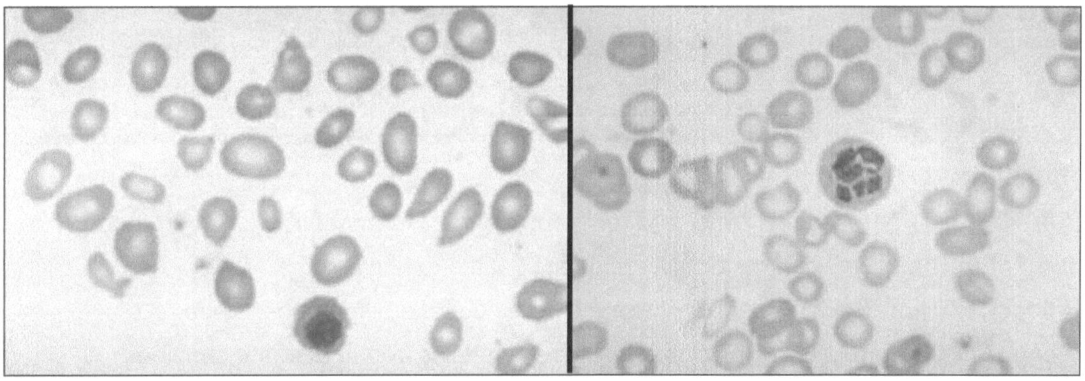

Explanation:

PERNICIOUS ANEMIA

- Common cause of reduced absorption of vitamin B_{12}.
- Described by Thomas Addison.
- Autoimmune disease characterised by:
  - Chronic atrophic gastritis.
  - Failure of secretion of intrinsic factor (IF).
  - Vitamin B_{12} deficiency.
- Autoantibodies against IFand parietal cells.
- **C/F:**
  - Megaloblastic anemia.
  - Neurological complications.

- *Associated autoimmune disorders:* Graves' disease, Hashimoto's thyroiditis, diabetes mellitus, Addison's disease, myasthenia gravis.

- **Lab Investigations:**
  - *PS:* Macrocytic anemia, hypersegmented neutrophils.
  - Raised MCV.
  - *Bone marrow:* Megaloblasts, erythroid hyperplasia.
  - Reduced S. vitamin B_{12} levels.
  - Abnormal Schilling test.
  - Pentagastrin-fast achlorhydria.
  - Anti-IF and anti-parietal cell antibodies.
- Risk of gastric cancer.
- **Interpretation of Schilling test:**
  - **Stage I Normal:** Dietary deficiency.
  - **Stage I Abnormal, Stage II Normal:** Pernicious anemia, gastrectomy.
  - **Stage I Abnormal, Stage II Abnormal:** Ileal disease.

Ans: (a) Autoimmune gastritis

Ref: *Essentials of Haematology*, *Shirish M Kawthalkar, 1st Edition, Chapter 3: Anaemias Due to Impaired Red Cell Production, Page 96*

16. Graft used from an identical twin is called:

(a) Homograft (Allograft) (b) Autograft
(c) Isograft (d) Heterograft (Xenograft)

Explanation:

- **Autografts:** Grafts in which donor and recipient is same individual, E.g., skin graft.
- **Isografts:** Grafts between donor and recipient of same genotype.
- **Allografts (Homograft):** Donor is of same species but of a different genotype.
- **Xenografts (Heterograft):** Donor is of a different species from that of the recipient.
- **HLA matching:** Important to prevent graft rejection.
- **Common grafts:** Skin grafting, kidney and bone marrow transplantation.
- **Graft-versus-host (GVH) reaction:**
  - Occur when immunocompetent cells are transplanted to immunodeficient recipient.
  - **Mechanisms:** Cell mediated/ humoral.
  - **Types:** Hyperacute, acute, chronic.

Ans: (c) Isograft

Ref: *Textbook of Pathology, Harshmohan, 6th Edition, Page 65, Chapter: Immunopathology Including Amyloidosis*

17. Effacement of foot processes is pathognomonic of which disease?

(a) Membranous glomerulonephritis
(b) Minimal change disease
(c) IgA nephropathy
(d) Diabetic nephropathy

Explanation:

MINIMAL CHANGE DISEASE

- **Characteristic feature: Diffuse effacement of foot processes of podocytes.**
- Detected only by **Electron microscopy.**
- **Light microscopy:** Glomeruli appear normal.
- MCC of **nephrotic syndrome** in children.
- **Age:** 2 to 6 years.
- Also known as **lipoid nephrosis.**
- **Immunofluorescence:** No Ig or complement deposits.
- Responds well to corticosteroids.
- **Adults:** Can be associated with **Hodgkin's lymphoma.**

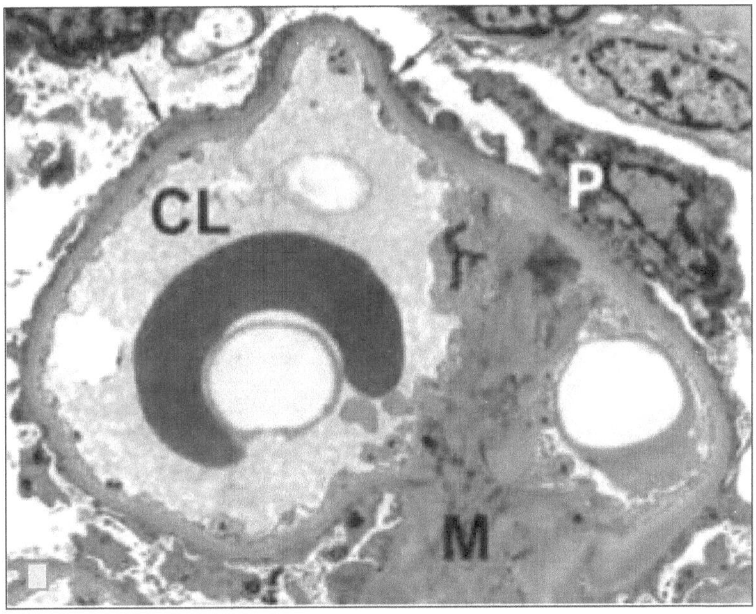

EM: Effacement of foot processes (arrows) and absence of deposits.
CL: Capillary lumen; M: Mesangium; P: Podocyte

EXTRA EDGE

- **Membranous glomerulonephritis:** "Spike and dome" appearance with subepithelial deposits seen in electron microscope.
- **IgA nephropathy:** Prominent IgA deposits in the mesangial regions, often with C3, properdin, IgG or IgM.
- **Diabetic nephropathy:** Capillary basement membrane thickening; diffuse mesangial sclerosis and nodular glomerulosclerosis.

Ans: (b) Minimal change disease

Ref: *Robbins and Cotrans Pathologic Basis of Disease, 9th Edition, Page 917*

18. A 46-year-old man who is a chronic smoker presented with complaints of cough. The physician examines the patient and takes a bronchoscopy biopsy. The picture in the biopsy represents the following. Which of the following cellular changes has happened in this patient?

(a) Hyperplasia (b) Dysplasia

(c) Metaplasia (d) Atrophy

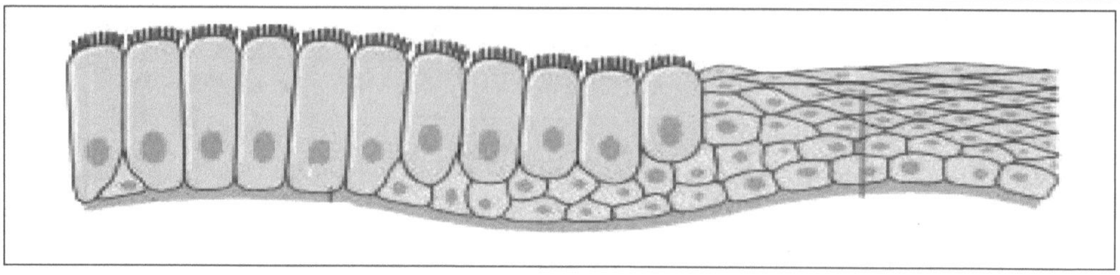

Explanation:

- The given picture shows characteristic **Metaplasia** of columnar epithelium (left) to squamous epithelium (right).

METAPLASIA

- **Definition:** Metaplasia is a reversible change in which one differentiated cell type (epithelial or mesenchymal) is replaced by another cell type.
- **Squamous metaplasia–**E.g., In respiratory tract due to smoking or chronic bronchitis, due to stones in biliary tract, salivary duct or pancreatic duct.
- If risk factor persists malignant transformation occurs in metaplastic epithelium.
- **Columnar metaplasia**–E.g.**,** Barrett esophagus.
- **Connective tissue metaplasia**–E.g.**,** Myositis ossificans.
- **Pathogenesis:** Reprogramming of stem cells.

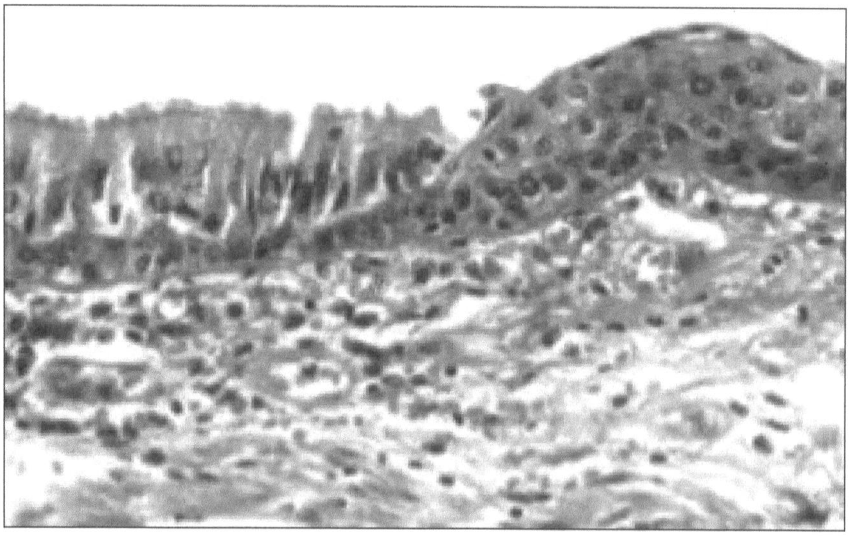

Metaplasia of columnar epithelium (left) to squamous epithelium (right) in a bronchus

Ans: (c) Metaplasia

Ref: *Robbins and Cotrans Pathologic Basis of Disease, 9th Edition, Cellular Responses to Stress and Toxic Insults: Adaptation, Injury and Death, Page 37*

19. A 31-year-old patient came with complaints of thyroid swelling. Her thyroid stimulating hormone (TSH) levels were found to be elevated. Post- operative HPE reports showed lymphocytic infiltration and Hurthle cells. Which of the following is the most likely diagnosis?

(a) Graves' disease
(b) Follicular carcinoma thyroid
(c) Hashimoto thyroiditis
(d) Medullary carcinoma thyroid

Explanation:

- The clinical picture is consistent **with Hashimoto thyroiditis.**

HASHIMOTO THYROIDITIS

- **Autoimmune disease** resulting in thyroid gland destruction and thyroid failure.
- Common cause of hypothyroidism in iodine sufficient areas.
- Known as **struma lymphomatosa.**
- Common in women.
- Major cause of nonendemic goiter in children.
- **Pathogenesis:** Autoantibodies against thyroglobulin and thyroid peroxidase.
- **Genetics:** CTLA4 and PTPN22.
- **Histology:** Mononuclear infiltrate, atrophic thyroid follicles, Hurthle cell.
- **Hashitoxicosis:** Transient thyrotoxicosis due to disruption of thyroid follicles.
- **Complication:** Extranodal marginal zone B-cell lymphoma and papillary carcinoma thyroid.

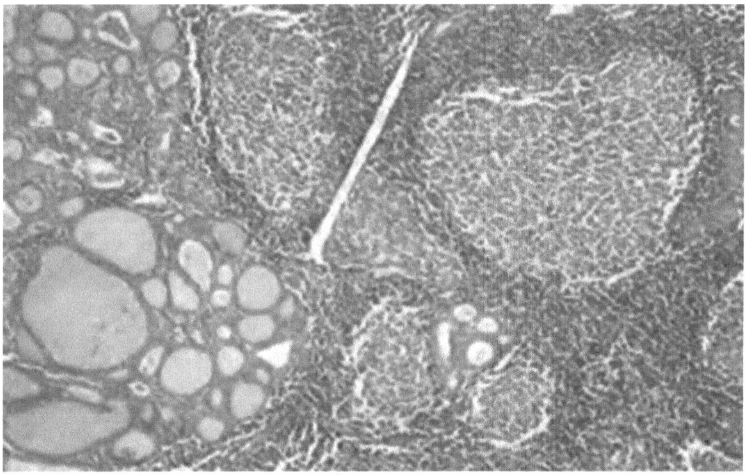

Thyroid parenchyma with dense lymphocytic infiltrate with germinal centres

- **Fibrous variant:** Extensive fibrosis which doesn't extend beyond capsule (unlike Riedel's thyroiditis).
- **Schmidt syndrome:** Hashimoto thyroiditis + lymphocytic adrenalitis.

Ans: (c) Hashimoto thyroiditis

Ref: *Robbins and Cotrans Pathologic Basis of Disease, 9th Edition, Chapter 24: The Endocrine System, Page 1086*

20. A 20-year-old patient presented with swelling in the wrist joint for 2 years duration. HPE showed spindle-shaped cells and Verocay bodies. Which of the following is the diagnosis?

(a) Neurofibroma (b) Schwannoma

(c) Lipoma (d) Dermoid cyst

Explanation:

SCHWANNOMA

- **Syn: Neurilemoma.**
- Benign neural tumor.
- Truly encapsulated.
- Solitary/multiple when associated with Recklinghausen disease type 2.
- **Site:** Flexor surfaces of limbs, neck, mediastinum, retroperitoneum, posterior spinal roots, cerebellopontine angle.
- **Genetics:** NF2 gene located on 22q12, coding for **merlin.**
- **Microscopy:**
  - Antoni A (cellular) and B (hypocellular).
  - Verocay bodies.
- **Types:**
  - **Ancient schwannomas:** Bizarre nuclei.
  - **Plexiform schwannomas.**
  - **Epithelioid schwannoma.**
  - **Melanotic schwannoma.**
  - **Cellular schwannoma:** Verocay bodies absent.
  - **Psammomatous melanotic schwannoma:** Component of the Carney complex.
- **IHC:** S-100 protein, calretinin (in contrast to neurofibromas), calcineurin.

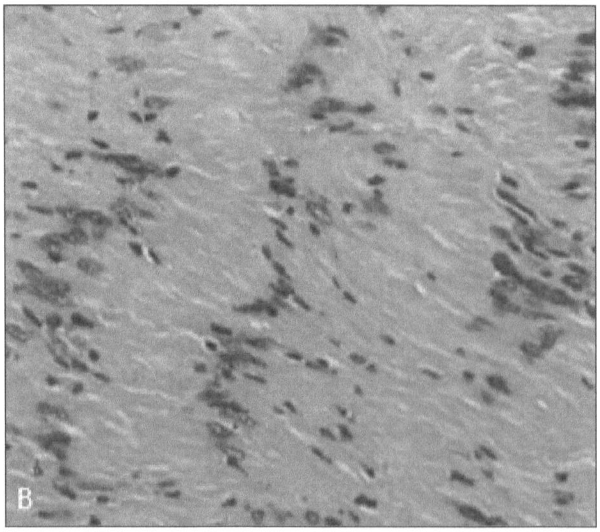

Antoni A area with palisading rows of tumor cell and Verocay bodies

Ans: (b) Schwannoma

Ref: *Rosai and Ackerman's Surgical Pathology, 10th Edition, Chapter 25: Soft Tissue, Page 2130*

21. A 25-year-old male presented with a 2 cm thyroid nodule. A thyroidectomy surgery was done. The histology picture is shown here. What could be the diagnosis?

(a) Papillary carcinoma thyroid
(b) Follicular adenoma
(c) Graves' disease
(d) Adenomatous goitre

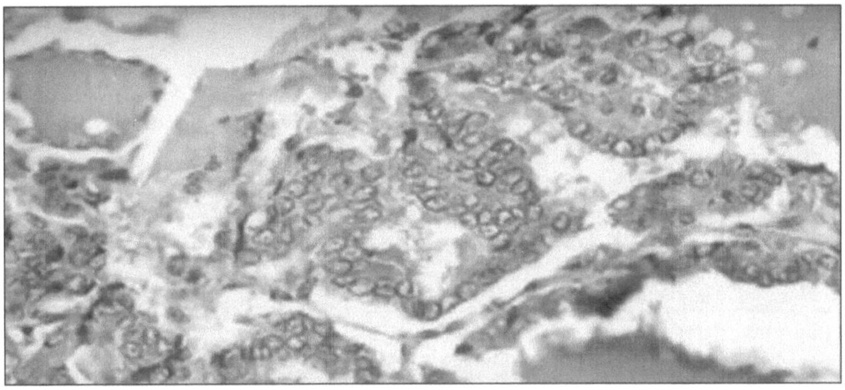

Explanation:

PAPILLARY CARCINOMA THYROID

- Common type of thyroid malignancy.
- Females > males.
- 90% of thyroid malignancies in children.
- **5–10%:** History of irradiation exposure.
- History of hashimoto thyroiditis.
- **Size:** Microscopic to huge.
- Solid/cystic.
- **Microscopy:** Complex, branching true papillae.
- **Nuclear features:**
  - Ground glass (optically clear) nuclei –**Orphan annie nuclei/Coffee Bean appearence.**
  - Nuclear pseudoinclusions.
  - Nuclear grooves.
- Psammoma bodies.
- **IHC:** CK7+/CK20–, thyroglobulin + and TTF-1 +.
- **Genetics:** MAPK pathway activation, RET/PTC, BRAF rearrangements.
- **Variants:**
  - *Papillary microcarcinoma:* 1 cm or less in diameter.
  - Encapsulated variant.
  - Follicular variant.
  - Diffuse sclerosing variant.
  - Oncocytic (oxyphilic) variant.
  - Tall cell and columnar cell carcinoma.
  - Cribriform–Morular variant.
  - Papillary carcinoma with exuberant nodular fasciitis-like stroma.

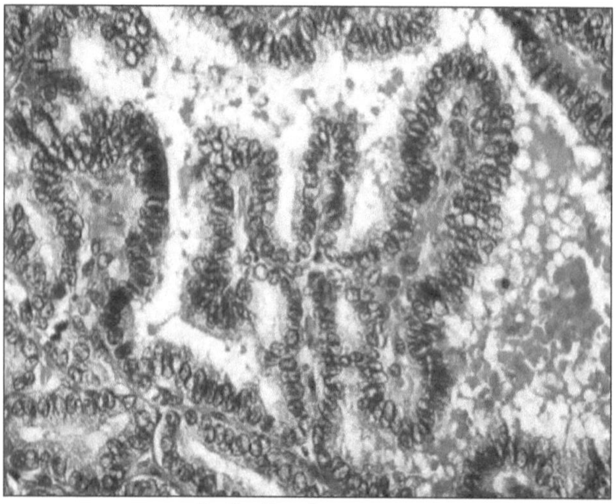

Optically clear nuclei

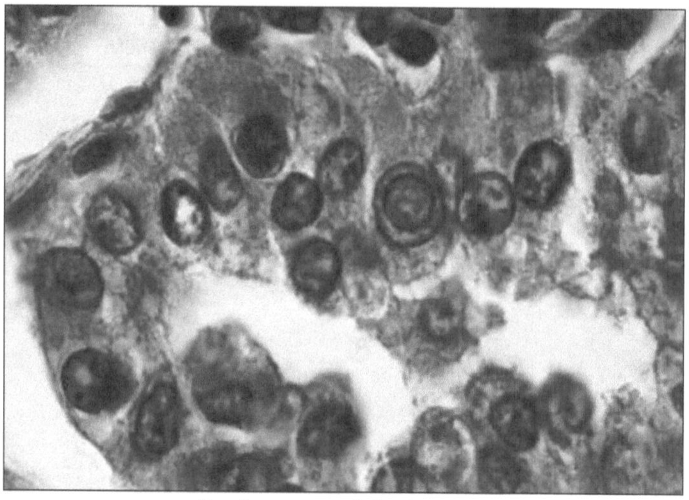

Nuclear pseudoinclusions

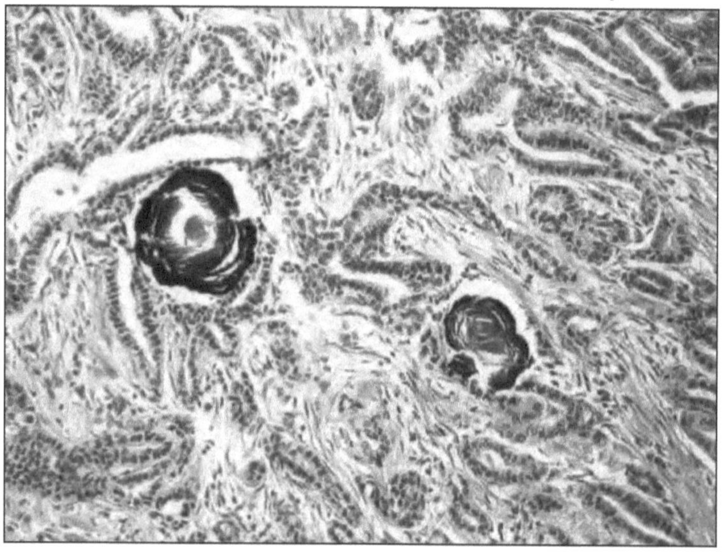

Psammoma bodies

Ans: (a) Papillary carcinoma thyroid

Ref: *Rosai and Ackerman's Surgical Pathology, 10th Edition, Chapter 9: Thyroid Gland, Page 504*

22. Which of the following disease will have bulky friable cardiac vegetations?

(a) Libman-Sachs endocarditis
(b) Infective endocarditis
(c) Rheumatic carditis
(d) Nonbacterial thrombotic endocarditis (NBTE)

Explanation:

INFECTIVE ENDOCARDITIS

- Microbial infection of heart valves/mural endocardium with formation of vegetations composed of thrombotic debris and organisms with destruction of cardiac tissues.
- **Types: Acute and Subacute.**
  - **Acute infective endocarditis:** Infection of normal heart valve by a highly virulent organism (e.g., **Staphylococcus aureus**).
  - **Subacute IE:** Caused by lower virulent organisms (e.g., **viridans streptococci**).
- **S. Aureus:** Seen in **intravenous drug abusers.**

- **HACEK group:** Hemophilus, Actinobacillus, Cardiobacterium, Eikenella and Kingella.
- **Prosthetic valve endocarditis:** Coagulase negative Staphylococci, e.g., **S. Epidermidis.**
- Friable, bulky, destructive vegetations–**hallmark.**
- **Dukes criteria.**
- **Complications:** Palms or soles **(Janeway lesions),** subcutaneous nodules in the pulp of the digits **(Osler nodes),** retinal hemorrhages in the eyes (**Roth spots).**

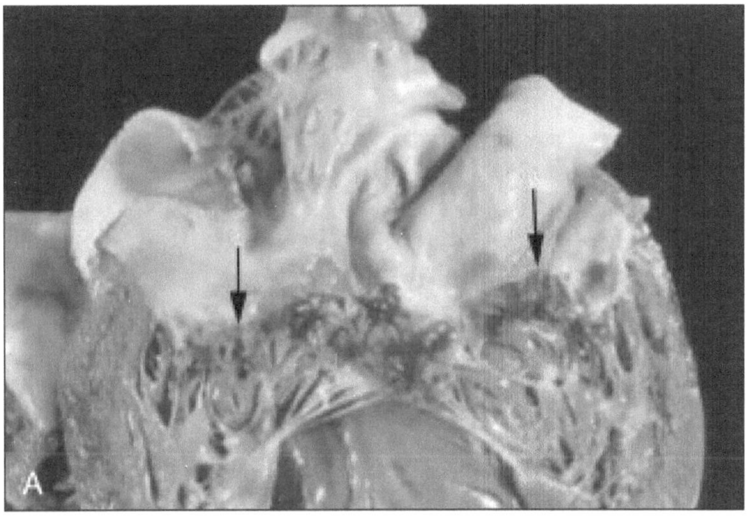

Bulky friable vegetations (arrows)

- **Libman-Sacks endocarditis:**
  - Nonbacterial thrombotic endocarditis in **SLE.**
  - AKA **marantic endocarditis.**
  - Small (1 to 4 mm in diameter), single or multiple, sterile, pink verrucous/warty vegetations.

Ans: (b) Infective endocarditis

Ref: *Robbins and Cotrans Pathologic Basis of Disease, 9th Edition, Chapter 12: The Heart, Page 559*

23. A 40-year-old woman presented with a 4 cm mass in the upper outer quadrant of breast. Biopsy from the mass showed densely-packed cells with bland nuclei and mucin infiltrating the stroma. Which of the following is your diagnosis?

(a) Colloid carcinoma
(b) Tubular carcinoma
(c) Papillary carcinoma
(d) Medullary carcinoma

Explanation:

COLLOID CARCINOMA OF BREAST

- AKA mucoid, colloid, or gelatinous carcinoma.
- **Age:** Postmenopausal women.
- **Gross:** Well circumscribed, crepitant, currant jelly-like mass.
- **Microscopy:**
  - Small clusters of tumor cells 'floating in a sea of mucin'.
  - Clusters-solid/acinar/micropapillary structures.
  - Mucin-extracellular, acid/neutral type.
- **IHC:** MUC2 +ve, WT1 +ve, ER and PR +ve, c-erbB-2 negative.
- **25-50%:** Endocrine differentiation.

- **Pure mucinous carcinoma:** Low incidence (2–4%) of nodal metastases.
- **Diagnostic criteria:** >50% extracellular mucin.

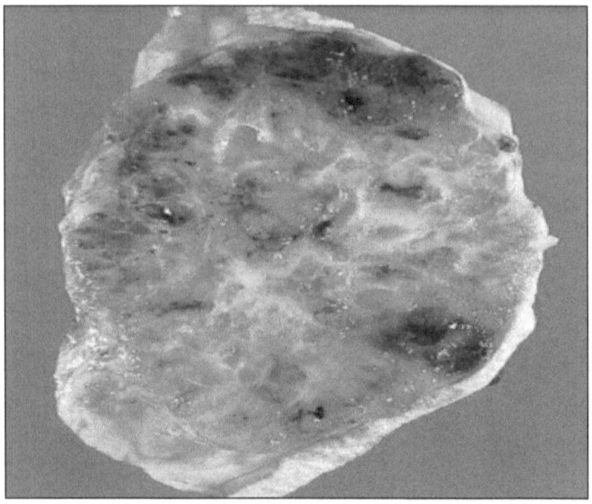

Gelatinous gross appearance – mucinous carcinoma

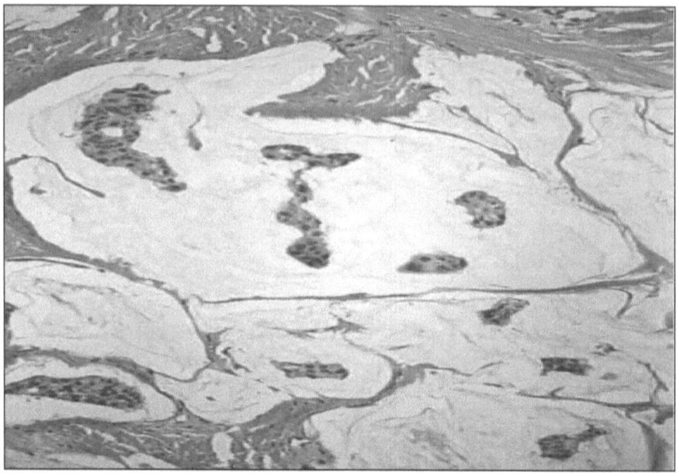

Clusters of well differentiated tumour cells floating in sea of mucin

MEDULLARY CARCINOMA OF BREAST

- **Age:** <50 years.
- Common in Japanese women.
- **Genetics: BRCA1 mutations.**
- **Basal-like carcinoma.**
- **Gross:** Well circumscribed, large, solid, homogenous, **brain like consistency.**
- **Microscopy:**
  - *Borders:* 'Pushing' type.
  - Synctium growth pattern.
  - Minimal or no glandular differentiation.
  - Absence of mucin.
  - *Tumour cells:* Large, pleomorphic, large nuclei, prominent nucleoli, numerous mitoses.
  - Prominent lymphoplasmacytic infiltrate.
- **IHC: 'Triple negative'.**
- **Express HLA-DR antigen.**
- **Axillary lymph node metastases: Common.**
- **Prognosis:** Good.

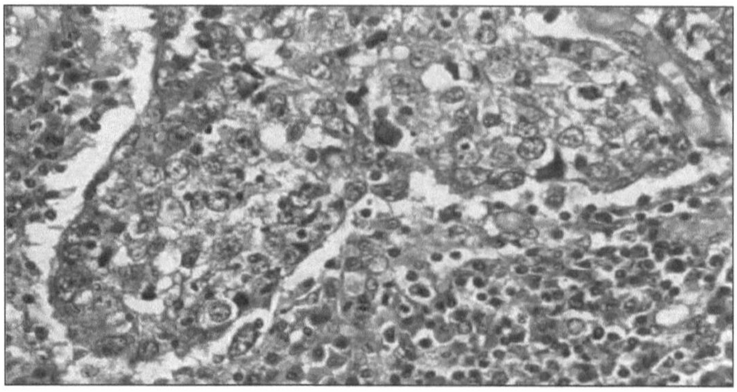

The large tumour cells in syncytium infiltrated by lymphocytes and plasma cells

Ans: (a) Colloid carcinoma

Ref: *Rosai and Ackerman's Surgical Pathology, 10th Edition, Chapter 20: Breast, Page 1699*

24. All Trans Retinoic Acid (ATRA) is used in the treatment of tumour associated with:

(a) BCR-ABL (b) PML-RARA
(c) cMYC (d) CEBPA

Explanation:

- **AML**–Most common form of acute leukemia in adults.
- Predominant form of leukemia before **1 year.**
- **DIC:** Most common in AML **M3.**
- **AML with recurrent genetic abnormalities:**
  - Occurs in young.
  - Favourable response to therapy and longer survival.
  - Reverse transcriptase-polymerase chain reaction (RT-PCR)–Sensitive.
  - *AML with t(8;21)(q22;q22) (AML1/ETO):* Blasts are large, Auer rods are frequent.
  - AML with inv(16).
  - *AML with t(15;17) (PML/RARα):* Abnormal promyelocytes, faggots–bundles of Auer rods, MPO–strong +ve, treatment with all-trans retinoic acid.
  - *AML with 11q23 (MLL):* Monocytic or myelomonocytic leukemia.

AML with t(15;17) ***(PML/RARα):***

- Correlate with **Acute promyelocytic leukemia** (**APML**, **APL**).
- Sensitive to **all-trans retinoic acid** (**ATRA**; tretinoin).
- ATRA induces the terminal differentiation of the leukemic promyelocytes.
- **ATRA therapy:** Unique side effect of differentiation syndrome.
- **Arsenic trioxide:** Used for relapsed/refractory disease.

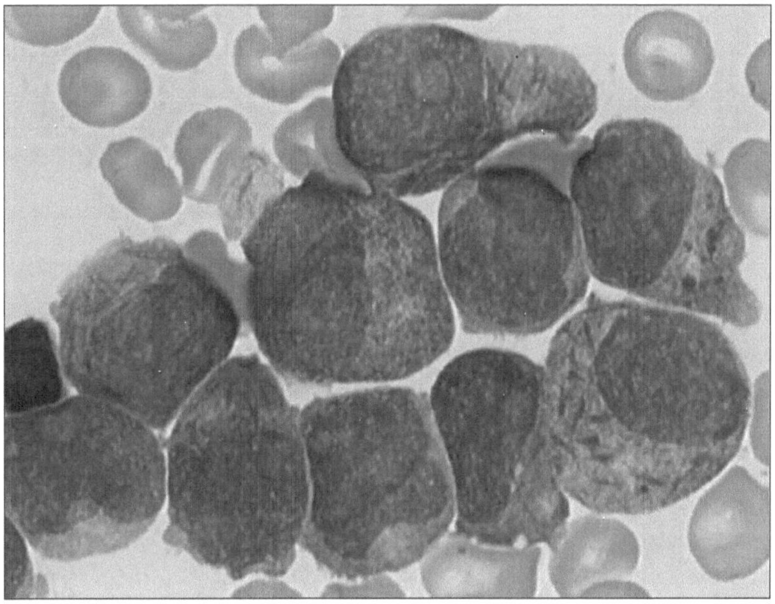

AML with t(15;17) (*PML/RARα*): Abnormal promyelocytes with Auer rods

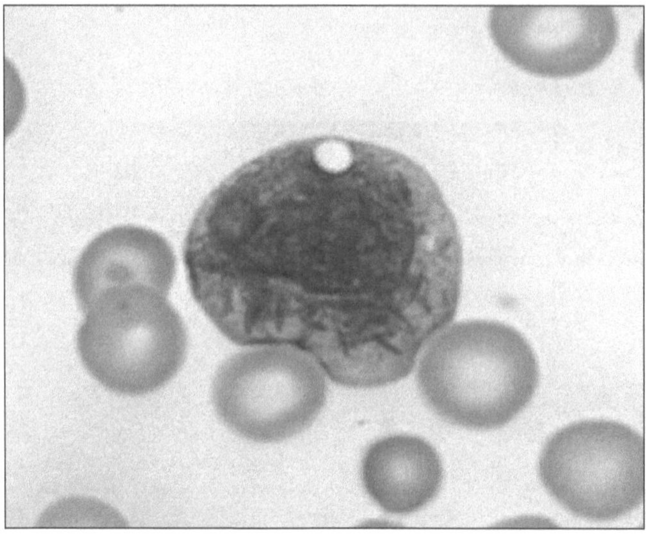

AML with faggots

Ans: (b) PML-RARA

Ref: *Essentials of Haematology*, *Shirish M Kawthalkar, 1st Edition, Chapter 5: Acute Leukemia, Page 223*

25. Which of the following factors play a major role in initiation of thrombus formation?

(a) Vasoconstriction (b) Coagulation cascade activation
(c) Platelets activation (d) Endothelial injury

Explanation:

- **Thrombus:** The intravascular mass formed from the constituents of blood.
- **Virchow triad:** (1) Endothelial injury, (2) Stasis or turbulent blood flow, and (3) Hypercoagulability of the blood.
- **Endothelial injury:** Leading to platelet activation almost inevitably underlies thrombus formation.
- Endothelial activation or dysfunction.

Hypercoaguability:

Hypercoagulable States
Primary (Genetic) **Common**
• Factor V mutation (Arg to Glu substitution in amino acid residue 506 leading to resistance to activated protein C; factor V Leiden) • Prothrombin mutation (G20210A non-coding sequence variant leading to increased prothrombin levels) • Increased levels of factors VIII, IX, XI, or fibrinogen (Genetics unknown)
Rare
• Antithrombin deficiency • Protein C deficiency • Protein S deficiency
Very Rare
• Fibrinolysis defects • Homozygous homocystinuria (deficiency of cystathione β-synthetase)
Secondary (Acquired) **High Risk for Thrombosis**

Contd.

Contd.

• Prolonged bed rest or immobilization • Myocardial infarction • Atrial fibriliation • Tissue injury (surgery, fracture, burn) • Cancer • Prosthetic cardiac valves • Disseminated intravascular coagulation • Heparin-induced thrombocytopenia • Antiphospholipid antibody syndrome
Lower Risk for Thrombosis
• Cardiomyopathy • Nephrotic syndrome • Hyperestrogenic states (pregnancy and postparturn) • Oral contraceptive use • Sickle cell anemia • Smoking

- **Types:** Arterial or cardiac and venous.
- **Lines of Zahn:** Pale platelet and fibrin deposits alternating with darker red cell-rich layers.
- **Mural thrombi:** Thrombi occurring in heart chambers/in aortic lumen.
- **Postmortem clots:** "Chicken fat" upper portion, red currant jelly appearance of dependent part.
- **Vegetations:** Thrombi on heart valves.
- **Fate of the Thrombus:**
  - Propagation.
  - Embolization.
  - Dissolution.
  - Organization and recanalization.

Ans: (d) Endothelial injury

Ref: *Robbins and Cotrans Pathologic Basis of Disease, 9th Edition, Chapter 4: Hemodynamic Disorders, Thromboembolic Disease and Shock, Page 122*

26. A 5-year-old male child presented to the clinic with history of recurrent infections. On examination the child had rashes as shown below. Routine blood investigations revealed the patient had low platelets. Which of the following is the probable diagnosis in the kid?

(a) Job's syndrome
(b) Wiskott-Aldrich syndrome
(c) Henoch-Schönlein purpura
(d) Hyper IgM syndrome

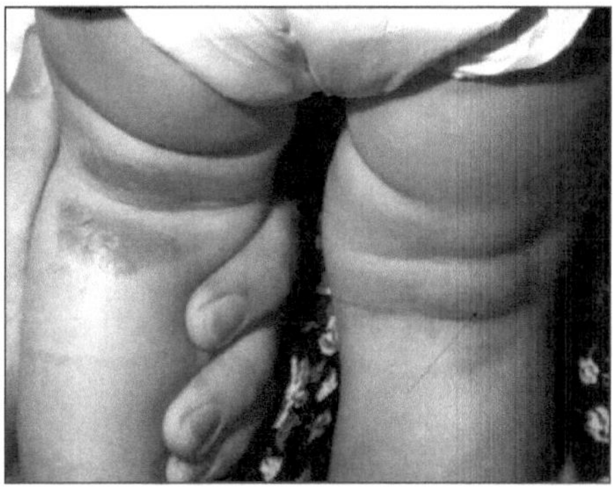

Explanation:

WISKOTT-ALDRICH SYNDROME

- **X-linked disease.**
- **Triad:** Thrombocytopenia, Eczema, Recurrent infection.
- **Defect:** In cellular immunity.
- **IgM:** Low, IgG – Normal, IgA and IgE – Elevated.
- **Mutation:** Gene coding Wiskott-Aldrich syndrome protein (WASP), located at **Xp11.23.**
- **Treatment:** HSC transplantation.

JOB'S SYNDROME

- **Hyper:** IgE syndrome.
- **Triad:** Atopic dermatitis, recurrent skin and pulmonary infections.
- **Two types:**
  - **Type I**–Autosomal dominant.
  - **Type II**–Autosomal recessive.
- **Mutation:** STAT3 gene.
- **Treatment:** Interferon gamma.

Henoch-Schönlein purpura

- **AKA IgA vasculitis.**
- **Triad:** Palpable purpura, arthritis, abdominal pain.
- **Hematuria: 40%.**
- Platelet count normal or elevated.

Ans: (b) Wiskott-Aldrich syndrome

Ref: *Robbins and Cotrans Pathologic Basis of Disease, 9th Edition, Chapter 6: Diseases of the Immune System, Page 242*

27. A 33-year-old man presents with a 5-week history of calf pain, swelling and low grade fever. Serum levels of creatine kinase are elevated. A muscle biopsy reveals numerous eosinophils and hemogram shows peripheral blood eosinophilia. Which of the following interleukins is primarily responsible for the increase in eosinophils in this patient?

(a) IL5 (b) IL4

(c) IL1 (d) IL6

Explanation:

- Major maturation and differentiation factor for eosinophils in humans.
- Pivotal role in innate and acquired immune responses and eosinophilia.
- Its specific receptor is **IL-5R.**
- **IL-5Rα:** Expressed on mature **eosinophils** and **basophils.**
- **Eosinophils' granules contain:** Major basic protein, eosinophil peroxidase, eosinophil-derived neurotoxin.
- **Functions of IL-5:**
  - Induces maturation of eosinophils.
  - Prolongs eosinophil survival.

   - Eosinophil chemotactic activity.
   - Increases eosinophil adhesion to endothelial cells.
- Peripheral eosinophilia is characterized as:
   - *Mild:* 500 to 1500/mcl (0.5 to 1.5 × 10^9/l).
   - *Moderate:* 1500 to 5000/mcl (1.5 to 5 × 10^9/l).
   - *Severe:* > 5000/mcl (> 5 × 10^9/l).
- **Causes of eosinophilia:**
   - *Allergic disorders:* Asthma, Hay fever, drug allergies, allergic skin diseases (Pemphigus, Dermatitis herpetiformis).
   - Parasitic infections.
   - Addison's disease.
   - *Malignancy:* Chronic myelogenous leukemia, Eosinophilic leukemia, Hodgkin's lymphoma.
   - Systemic autoimmune diseases–SLE.
   - Kimura disease.
   - Eosinophilic granulomatosis with polyangiitis.
   - Eosinophilic myositis.
   - Eosinophilic myocarditis.
   - Fungal infection.

Ans: (a) IL5

Ref: *Interleukin-5 and IL-5 Receptor in Health and Diseases. Proc Jpn Acad Ser B Phys Biol Sci 2011, Oct 11;87(8), Page 463-85*

28. Which of the following will be seen on cardiac biopsy of a patient who had a post-MI reperfusion injury?

(a) Waviness of fibers
(b) Eosinophilic contraction bands
(c) Neutrophils in cardiac muscle
(d) Swelling of cells

Explanation:

- **Reperfusion** is restoration of blood flow to ischemic myocardium threatened by infarction.
- It improves myocardial function.
- **Methods available:** Thrombolysis, angioplasty, stent placement, CABG.
- Benefits of reperfusion depends on:
   - Rapidity of re-establishing coronary blood flow.
   - Extent of restoration of blood flow.
- **Morphology:**
   - Hemorrhagic.
   - *Eosinophilic contraction bands:* Closely packed sarcomeres.
- **Reperfusion injury:** Can result in arrhythmias due to oxidative stress, calcium overload and inflammatory cells.

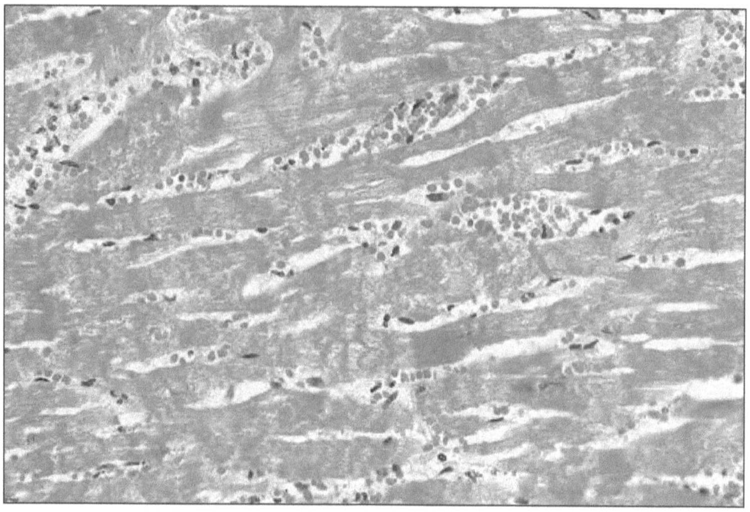

Myocardial necrosis with contraction bands

Ans: (b) Eosinophilic contraction bands

Ref: *Robbins and Cotrans Pathologic Basis of Disease, 9th Edition, Chapter 12, The Heart, Page 546*

29. An 11-year-old boy came with history of cough for 15 days. On examination he was found to have cervical lymphadenopathy. Lymph node biopsy showed the below finding. Which of the following is the most appropriate diagnosis?

(a) Leprosy
(b) Sarcoidosis
(c) TB
(d) Syphilis

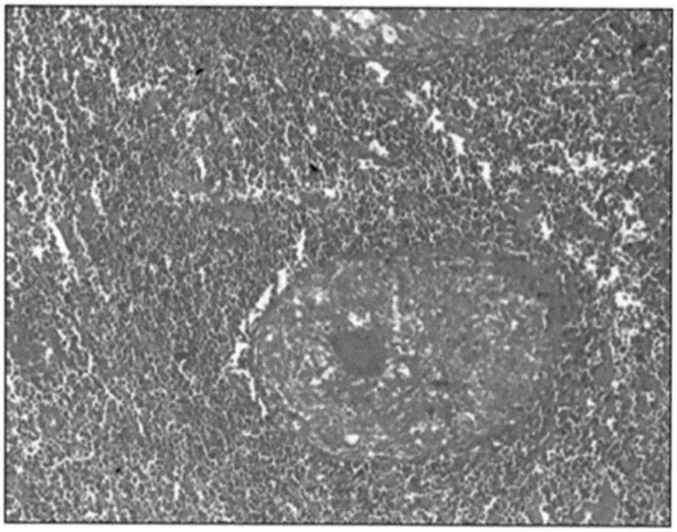

Explanation:

- **Granuloma** is defined as a circumscribed, tiny lesion, about 1 mm in diameter, composed predominantly of collection of modified macrophages called epithelioid cells, and rimmed at the periphery by lymphoid cell.
- **Infection associated granulomas:**
  - TB.
  - Leprosy.
  - Histoplasmosis.
  - Cryptococcosis.

- Cocccidioidomycosis.
- Blastomycosis.
- Cat-sratch disease.

- **Non-infectious granulomas:**
  - Sarcoidosis.
  - Crohn's disease.
  - Foreign body granuloma.
  - Rheumatoid nodules.
- **Caseating granulomas: TB*.**
- **Non-caseating granulomas:**
  - Sarcoidosis.
  - Crohn's disease.
  - Fungal infections.
  - Foreign body granuloma.
  - Silicosis.
  - Berylliosis.
- **Suppurative granulomas:** Cat-scratch disease, actinomycosis.
- **Naked granuloma: Sarcoidosis.**

TUBERCULOSIS

- **Types: Primary Tuberculosis and Secondary Tuberculosis.**
- **Primary Tuberculosis**
  - **Ghon's complex:** Ghon's focus, Lymphatic vessel, Lymph node.
  - **Ghon's focus:** Subpleural focus in the upper part of lower lobe/lower part of upper lobe.
  - **Fate:** Fibrosis,calcification (Ranke complex)/progressive primary tuberculosis/primary miliary tuberculosis/progressive secondary tuberculosis.
  - **Tabes mesenterica:** Enlarged mesenteric lymph nodes.
  - **Simons focus:** Post primary scarred lesion at apex.
  - **Assman focus:** Reactivated Simon focus.
  - **Rich focus:** Seen in cerebral cortex.
- **Secondary Tuberculosis**
  - Infection of an individual who has been previously infected or sensitised.
  - **Lesion:** Apex of lung as oxygen tension is high.
  - **Fate:** Heal/Fibrocaseous tuberculosis/Tuberculous caseous pneumonia/Miliary tuberculosis.
- **Diagnosis:**
  - Acid-fast (Ziehl-Neelsen) staining.
  - Fite-Faraco staining.
  - Gomori methenamine silver.
  - PCR.
  - IgM antibodies to PGL-1 antigen.

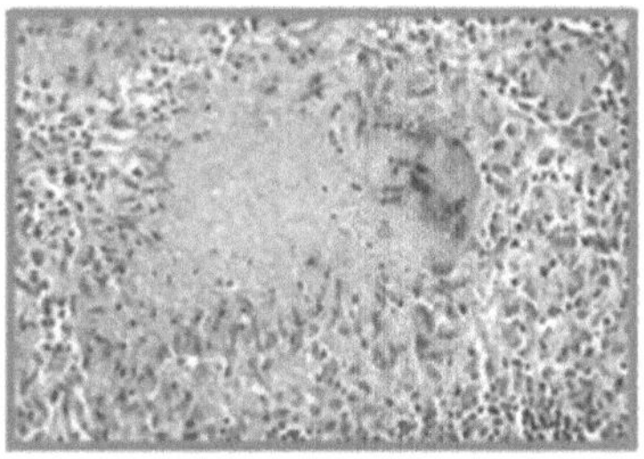

Caseating granulomas TB

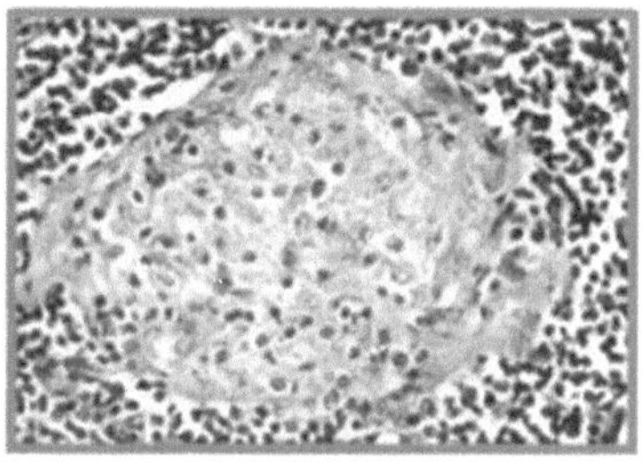

Non caseating granulomas Sarcoidosis

Ans: (c) TB

Ref: *Textbook of Pathology, Harshmohan, 6th Edition, Chapter 6: Inflammation and Healing, Page 148*

30. Which of the following is the etiology of Werner syndrome with premature aging?

(a) Increased length of telomere

(b) Short telomere with damaged DNA and loss of helicase

(c) Increased advanced glycation end products

(d) Decreased lipid peroxidation

Explanation:

- Cellular aging-results from decline in cellular function and viability.
- **Factors:** DNA damage.

WERNER SYNDROME

- Also known as "**adult progeria**".
- Premature aging.
- Autosomal recessive disorder.
- Defect in DNA helicase.
- **Six cardinal symptoms:**
  - Premature graying of hair or hair loss.
  - Bilateral cataracts.
  - Atrophied skin.
  - Soft tissue calcification.
  - Sharp facial features.
  - Abnormal high-pitched voice.
- **Cellular Senescence: State of terminally non-dividing cells after fixed number of divisions**.
- **Cause: Telomere shortening.**
- **Telomeres:** Short repeated sequences of DNA at ends of chromosomes, important for replication of chromosome ends and for protecting ends from degradation.
- Telomere length is maintained by **telomerase.**

Ans: (b) Short telomere with damaged DNA and loss of helicase

Ref: *Robbins and Cotrans Pathologic Basis of Disease, 9th Edition, Chapter 2: Cellular Responses to Stress and Toxic Insults: Adaptation, Injury and Death, Page 66*

MICROBIOLOGY

1. A 30-year-old man reports 4 hours after acquiring a clean wound without laceration. He had received TT vaccination 10 years back. What do you advice regarding tetanus prophylaxis?

(a) Full course tetanus vaccine to be given
(b) Single dose TT
(c) Full course TT with TIG
(d) No need of any vaccine

Explanation:

PREVENTION OF TETANUS

(A) Active Immunization

- Most effective method.
- **Tetanus Toxoid (TT)** given as deep intramuscular route in anterolateral aspect of thigh in children and deltoid in adults.
- Monovalent vaccine – Plain formol toxoid (incubating toxin with formalin).
- Adsorbed form (formol toxoid adsorbed into alum).
- Combined vaccine – DPT (Diphtheria toxoid, Pertussis whole cell killed preparation, Tetanus toxoid).
- Protective anti-tetanus toxoid titre is >=**0.01unit/ml.**

Immunization Schedule

- Primary immunisation according to National Immunization schedule:
  - 1st dose @ 6 weeks of birth.
  - 2nd dose @ 10 weeks of birth.
  - 3rd dose @ 14 weeks of birth.
  - 1st booster dose @16-24 months.
  - 2nd booster dose @ 5-6 years.
  - Additional doses @ 10 years and 16 years.
- Adult immunization in case of defaulter of primary immunization in childhood:
  - 2 doses at one month interval.
  - 2 booster doses @ 1 and 6 years.

National Immunization Schedule (NIS) for Infants, Children and Pregnant Women				
Vaccine	**When to give**	**Dose**	**Route**	**Site**
For Pregnant Women				
TT-1	Early in pregnancy	0.5 ml	Intramuscular	Upper Arm
TT-2	4 weeks after TT-1*	0.5 ml	Intramuscular	Upper Arm
TT-Booster	If received 2 TT doses in a pregnancy within the last 3 years*	0.5 ml	Intramuscular	Upper Arm
For Infants				
BCG	At birth or as early as possible till one year of age	0.1 ml (0.05 ml until 1 month age)	Intradermal	Left Upper Arm

Contd.

Contd.

Hepatitis B–Birth dose	At birth or as early as possible within 24 hours	0.5 ml	Intramuscular	Anterolateral side or mid-thigh
OPV-0	At birth or as early as possible within the first 15 days	2 drops	Oral	Oral
OPV 1, 2 and 3	At 6 weeks, 10 weeks and 14 weeks (OPV can be given till 5 years of age)	2 drops	Oral	Oral
Pentavalent 1, 2 and 3	At 6 weeks, 10 weeks and 14 weeks (can be given till one year of age)	0.5 ml	Intramuscular	Anterolateral side of mid-thigh
Rotavirus#	At 6 weeks, 10 weeks and 14 weeks (can be given till one year of age)	5 drops	Oral	Oral
IPV	Two fractional dose at 6 and 14 weeks of age	0.1 ml	Intradermal two fractional dose	Intradermal: Right Upper Arm
Measles/MR 1st dose$	9 completed months-12 months (can be given till 5 years of age)	0.5 ml	Subcutaneous	Right Upper Arm
JE-1**	9 completed months-12 months	0.5 ml	Subcutaneous	Left Upper Arm
Vitamin A (1st dose)	At 9 completed months with measles-Rubella	1 ml (1 lakh IU)	Oral	Oral
For Children				
DPT booster-1	16-24 months	0.5 ml	Intramuscular	Anterolateral side of mid-thigh
Measles/MR 2nd dose$	16-24 months	0.5 ml	Subcutaneous	Right Upper Arm
OPV booster	16-24 months	2 drops	Oral	Oral
JE-2	16-24 months	0.5 ml	Subcutaneous	Left Upper Arm
Vitamin A* (2nd to 9th dose)**	16-18 months. Then one dose every 6 months up to the age of 5 years	2 ml (2 lakh IU)	Oral	Oral
DPT booster-2	5-6 years	0.5 ml	Intramuscular	Upper Arm
TT	10 years and 16 years	0.5 ml	Intramuscular	Upper Arm

* Give TT-2 or Booster doses before 36 weeks of pregnancy. However, give these even if more than 36 weeks have passed. Give TT to a woman in labour, if she has not previously received TT.

** JE Vaccine is introduced in select endemic districts after the campaign.

*** The 2nd to 9th doses of Vitamin A can be administered to children 1-5 years old during biannual rounds, in collaboration with ICDs.

Phased introduction, at present in Andhra Pradesh, Haryana, Himachal Pradesh and Orissa from 2016 and expanded in Madhya Pradesh, Assam, Rajasthan and Tripura in February 2017 and planned in Tamil Nadu and Uttar Pradesh in 2017.

$ Phased introduction, at present in five states namely Karnataka, Tamil Nadu, Goa, Lakshadweep and Puducherry (As of February 2017).

(B) Passive Immunisation

- Human Tetanus Immunoglobulin (HTIG).
- Equine derived Antitetanus serum (ATS).
- **Dose:** 250IU HTIG or 1500 IU ATS as SINGLE IM dose.
- Duration of protection:
  - HTIG: 30 days.
  - ATS: 7-10 days.

Tetanus Prophylaxis After Injury

Wound category	Simple wound	Other wounds
Category A	Nothing required	Nothing required
Category B	Toxoid 1 dose	Toxoid 1 dose
Category C	Toxoid 1 dose	Toxoid 1 dose + HTIG
Category D	Toxoid complete dose	Toxoid complete dose + HTIG

- **Category A:** Taken complete course of TT/booster within past 5 years.
- **Category B:** Taken complete course of TT/booster within past > 5 years to < 10 years.
- **Category C:** Taken complete course of TT/booster within past >10 years.
- **Category D**: Not taken complete course of TT/booster or immunity status unknown.
- **Simple wound:** < 6 hours, clean, not penetrating, no/negligent tissue damage.
- **Treatment of Choice for Tetanus** – *Passive Immunization (Tetanus antiserum).*
- **Choice for Prophylaxis** – *Active Immunization (Tetanus toxoid).*

Also Note:

- Recent guidelines for pregnant women with regards to tetanus prophylaxis during the antenatal period is administration of dT instead of TT, with same dosage and scheduling guidelines.

Ans: (b) Single dose TT

Ref: *mohfw.gov.in/sites/default/files/24545352106148966 3873.pdf*

2. Which of the following is vector for Zika virus?

(a) Aedes aegypti (b) Anopheles stephens
(c) Culex pipiens (d) Phlebotomus papatasi

Explanation:

Zika Virus

- Zika virus is a member of the Flaviviridae family.
- Single stranded RNA virus.
- First isolated from a Rhesus monkey from the Zika forest of Uganda.
- **Vector: Aedes aegypti, Aedes albopictus.**
- **Routes of transmission:**
  - Mosquito bite.
  - Transplacental transmission.

- Sexual transmission from infected partner.
- Transmission via blood transfusion.

- **Incubation period:** 3-12 days.
- **Clinical Features:**
  - 80% of infected individuals remain asymptomatic.
  - Maculopapular rash with/without fever.
  - Headache.
  - Arthralgia/arthritis.
  - Conjunctivitis (non-purulent/hyperaemia).
  - Joint and muscle pain.

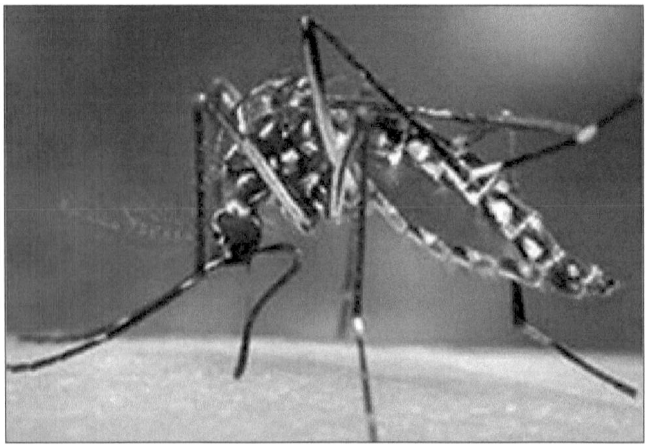

Aedes aegypti

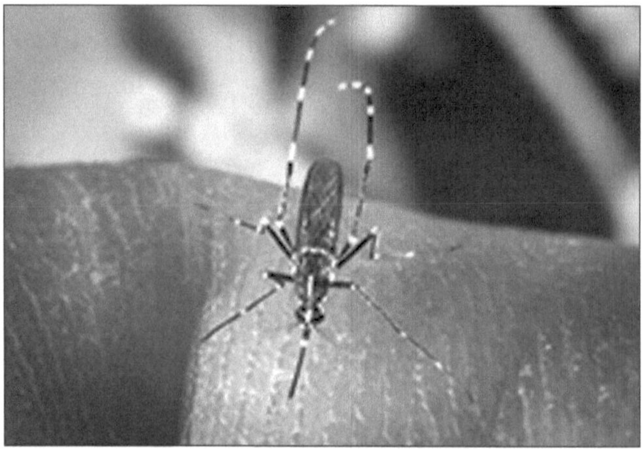

Aedes albopictus

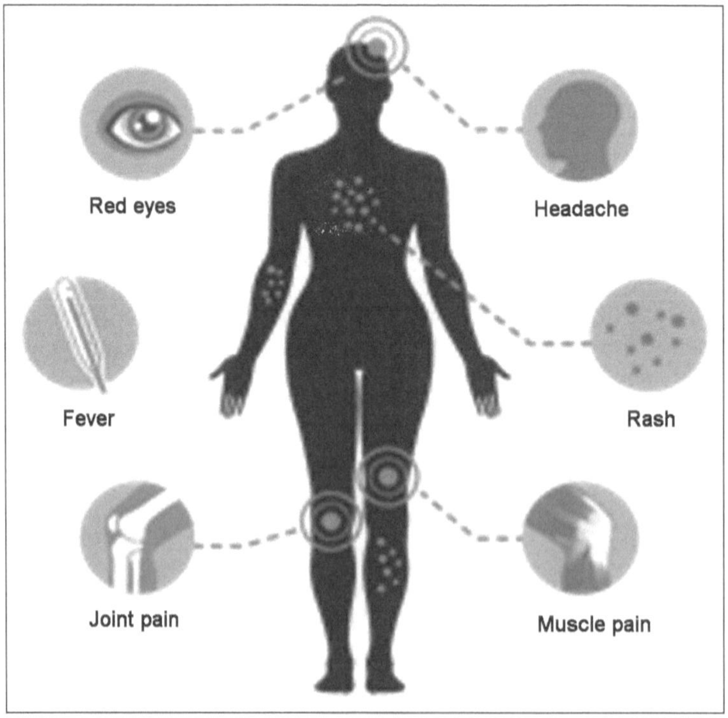

Clinical features

Diagnosis

- Sample – Serum, urine, blood, CSF, amniotic fluid.
- Serology.
- Detection of Zika specific IgM antibodies.
- IgM antibodies against Zika virus detectable from day 5 after onset of symptoms.
- Detection of Zika-specific IgM antibodies requires confirmation by plaque-reduction neutralisation tests because of cross-reactivity with antibodies against other flaviviruses.

Complications

- Microcephaly in foetuses and newborns.
- Guillain-Barré syndrome.

Treatment

- Symptomatic treatment.
- No specific antiviral.
- No specific vaccine.

Prevention

- Mosquito control.

Anopheles Stephensi

- It is an important vector of **Plasmodium falciparum and Plasmodium vivax malaria** in urban India.
- Peak in the biting activity is found to be in the early hours of morning (3-6 am).
- Larvae of An. stephensi breed in various artificial containers in homes and collections of water associated with construction sites and other industrial locations.

Culex Pipiens

- It has been found to be an active vector for:
  - West Nile encephalitis virus (Flaviviridae).
  - Usutu virus (Flaviviridae).
  - Sindbis virus (Togaviridae).

Phlebotomus Papatasi (Sand fly).

- It is a vector for **Sand fly fever virus (Bunyaviridae).**

Ans: (a) Aedes aegypti

Ref: *Paniker's Textbook of Medical Parasitology, 8th Edition, Page 67*

3. A female from a tribal area of Jharkhand reports with fever for the last 3 days. Peripheral blood is collected and stained with Giemsa stain. A diagnosis of Malaria is made. The smear is shown in the figure. What is the likely cause?

(a) P. vivax

(b) P. malariae

(c) P. ovale

(d) P. falciparum

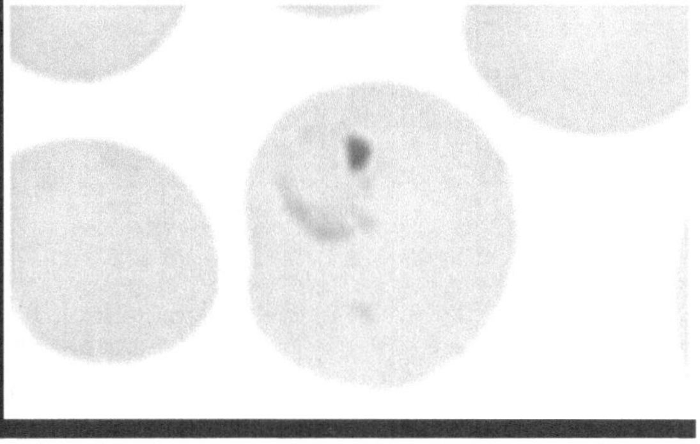

Explanation:

- The picture shows the **ring form or young trophozoite**. Multiple ring forms are found within the RBC in P. falciparum infection.

Plasmodium Species

- Plasmodium species are protozoan parasites causing malaria.
- It belongs to:
  - **Phylum:** Apicomplexa.
  - **Class:** Sporozoa.
  - **Order:** Hemosporidia.
  - **Genus:** Plasmodium.
- 4 species are known to cause human infections:
  - Plasmodium falciparum.
  - Plasmodium vivax.
  - Plasmodium malariae.
  - Plasmodium ovale.
- **Vector:** Female Anopheles mosquito. Major species transmitting malaria in India are: An. culicifacies. An. fluviatilis, An. stephensi, An. minimus, An. philippinensis, An. sundaicus.
- Plasmodium completes its life cycle in 2 hosts:
  - **Definitive host:** Female Anopheles mosquito (sexual phase or Gametogony).
  - **Intermediate host:** Man (asexual phase or Schizogony).
- **Asexual phase** is also called endogenous or intrinsic phase. In humans, schizogony takes place:
  (i) **Within red blood cells (RBC):** Erythrocytic schizogony; and
  (ii) **Within liver:** Exo erythrocytic/pre erythrocytic schizogony. Products of schizogony are called merozoites.
- **Sexual phase** is also called extrinsic or exogenous phase. Products of gametogony are called sporozoites.

Schizogony

- Human gets infected by the bite of infected female anopheles mosquito.
- Sporozoites enter the bloodstream through bite of the mosquito.

Pre-Erythrocytic Stage

- Spindle shaped sporozoites enter the hepatocytes and become rounded, forming schizont or meront.
- Each mature liver schizont contains 2000-50000 uninucleate merozoites.
- After 6-15 days, these schizonts rupture to release the merozoites.

Erythrocytic Stage

- Merozoites invade the RBCs by attaching to the glycophorin receptor on the RBC cell wall. Merozoites enter the RBC through the process called invagination.
- Inside the RBC, the merozoites enlarge, with a vacuole in the centre, pushing the cytoplasm to the periphery and the nucleus to one pole. This is the ring form or young trophozoite. Multiple ring forms called accollé ring forms are found within the RBC in P. falciparum infection, as shown in the picture.
- The parasite breaks down the hemoglobin and releases hemazoin pigment. Pigmented RBCs are characteristic of erythrocytic phase of malaria. The appearance of the pigments varies with respect to the Plasmodium species.

- **P. falciparum:** 1-3 solid black pigments.
- **P. vivax:** Multiple golden-brown pigments.
- **P. malariae:** Multiple dark brown pigments.
- **P. ovale:** Multiple blackish-brown pigments.

- Merozoite enlarges and acquires amoeboid motility and forms trophozoite, whose nucleus undergoes mitosis and forms schizont or meront. This bursts and releases 8-12 merozoites into circulation, which in turn affects other RBCs.
- Certain trophozoites develop into male and female gametocytes. Mature gametocytes are crescent shaped in P. falciparum malaria, while in other species, it is rounded.
- Person with the gametocytes in circulation become the carrier or reservoir of infection.
- These gametocytes are taken in by the mosquito while taking a blood meal.

Gametogony

- Male gametocyte divides to form 8 actively motile, whip-like gametocytes.

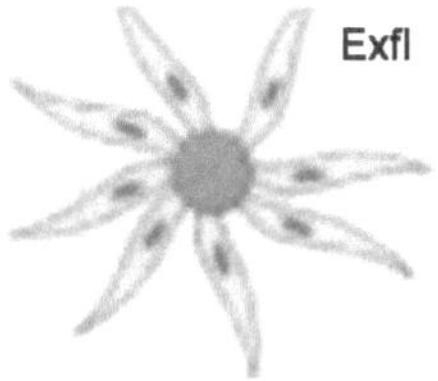

Exfl

- Male and female gametocytes fertilise to form zygote, within 30-120 mins of the blood meal. Motionless, round zygote becomes elongated and motile within 18-24 hours to form the ookinete (travelling vermicule). Numerous sporozoites are formed within the ookinete, making it the oocyst. The mature oocyst ruptures, releasing the sporozoites into the body cavity of the mosquito. These sporozoites move to the salivary gland of the mosquito and are injected into the humans, initiating human infection.

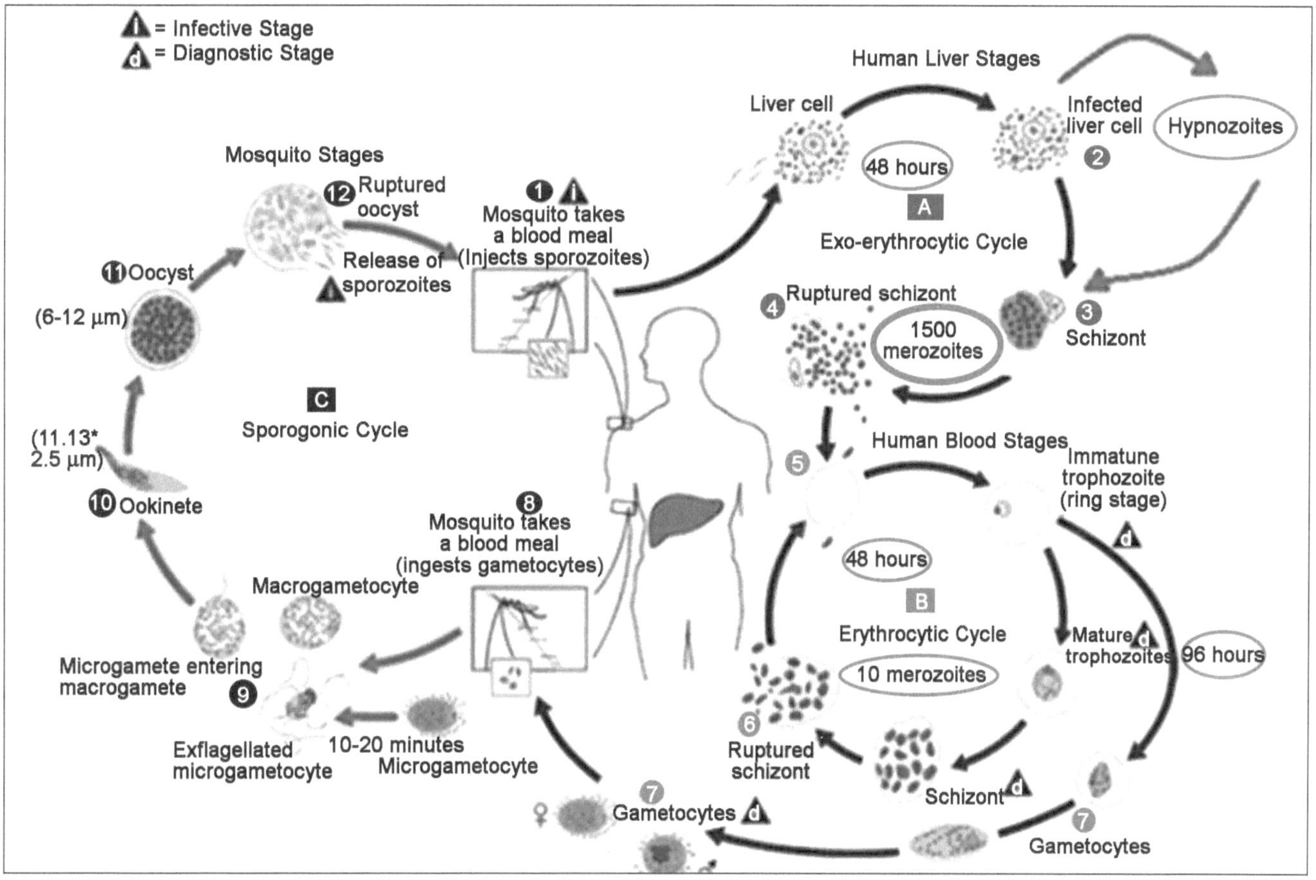

- **Hypnozoites:** In P. vivax and P. ovale, certain sporozoites remain dormant in the latent phase (resting phase). These are called hypnozoites, which when activated releases merozoites and initiate an infection.

Relapse

- In P. falciparum and P. malariae, no hypnozoites are found. However, certain merozoites persists in the circulation and sometimes causes short term relapse or **recrudescence.**

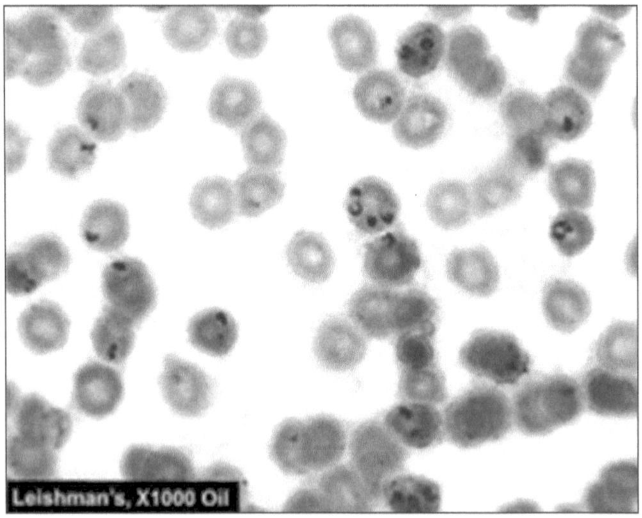

Ring forms of P. falciparum in blood film

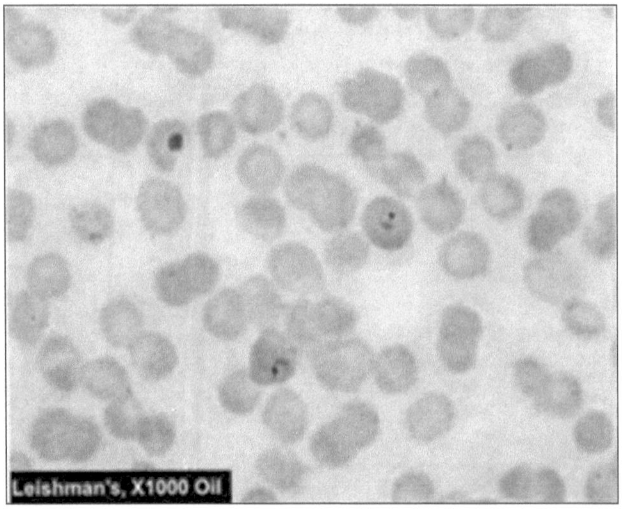

Ring forms of P. vivax in blood film

Characteristics of Ring Forms

- **P. falciparum malaria:** Rings are tiny and seen attached to the margin of the RBC, called accole or form applique. Binucleate rings, due to double chromatin, resembling stereo headphones are seen. Multiple ring forms are seen within a single RBC. **Maurer's dots** are characteristic of falciparum.
- **P. vivax malaria:** Ring forms are well defined, with prominent central vacuole. One side of the ring is thicker and other side thinner, with the nucleus seen on the thin side (Signet ring appearance). Numerous pigments (**Schuffner's dots**) seen within the RBCs.
- **P. malariae malaria:** Ring forms are well defined and thick walled, with prominent central vacuole. The old trophozoites are seen stretched over the RBCs forming band forms. Numerous large pigments are seen within the RBC.
- **P. ovale malaria:** Ring forms are well defined and compact, with prominent central vacuole. **Schuffner's** dots are very prominent and abundant.

Also Note:

- **Plasmodium Knowlesi** is the fifth known malarial parasite to infect human beings.

Ans: (d) P. falciparum

Ref: *Paniker's Textbook of Medical Parasitology, 8th Edition, Page 66 and Mohan H. Textbook of Pathology, 6th Edition, Page 189*

4. Shown in the figure is HBV card test. Which of the following is the principle of the test?

(a) ELISA
(b) Immunofluorescence
(c) Chemiluminescence
(d) None of the above

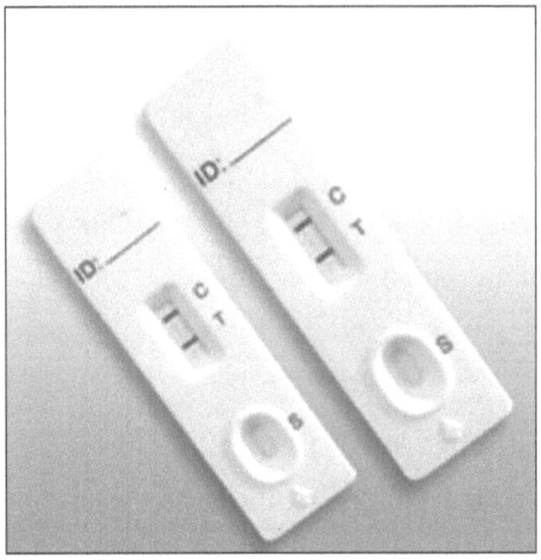

Explanation:

- The given test is a cassette form of immunochromatographic test.

Hepatitis B Virus (HBV)

- Classified as a Hepadnavirus.
- 3 major antigens:
  - HBsAg – Surface antigen. Present on the envelope.
  - HBcAg – Core antigen.
  - HBeAg – Nucleocapsid antigen.

HBsAg

- Also called Australian antigen.
- Appears as spherical and tubular form.
- Major antigen in HBV infection. Detectable 2-6 weeks prior to the appearance of clinical and biochemical evidence of hepatitis.
- HBsAg persists throughout the HBV infection.
- HBV chronic carrier – patients in whom HBsAg persists > 6 months.
- HBV card test is a **immunochromatographic** test.
- It is based on **Lateral flow technique.**
- Immunochromatographic tests are used as point of care tests for detection of antigen or antibody in the sample.
- It is an *in vitro*, rapid, qualitative test to detect Hepatitis B surface antigen (HBsAg) in serum.
- It is available in cassette form and strip form.

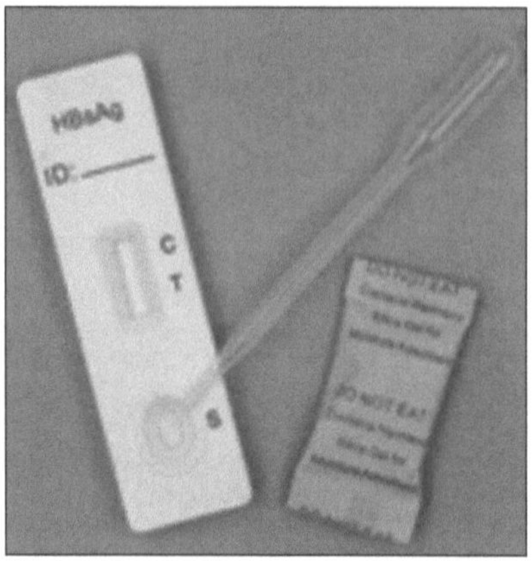

Structure of the Cassette:

- It consists of a nitrocellulose membrane (NCM) and an absorbent pad.
- NCM has 2 lines.
- Test line – coated with monoclonal antibody targeted against the test antigen.
- Control line – coated with anti-human immunoglobulin.
- Sample window is infiltrated with specific antibody against the target antigen (HBSAg), labelled with chromogenic marker (colloidal gold or silver).

Principle of Immunochromatographic Assay:

- The sample (serum) containing the antigen is added to the sample well.
- The sample flows along the NCM by capillary action. Antigen (Ag) reacts with the antibody (Ab) labelled with the chromogenic marker, to form "Ag-specific Ab-colloidal gold complex".
- Moving along the NCM, "Ag-specific Ab-colloidal gold complex" is immobilized by the antigen specific monoclonal antibody in the test line, to form a colored band–**Test Band.**
- Free colloidal gold labelled is bound to the anti-human immunoglobulin in the control line, and forms a colored line – **Control band.**
- Test is considered invalid if the control band is not formed, irrespective of the test band formation or not.

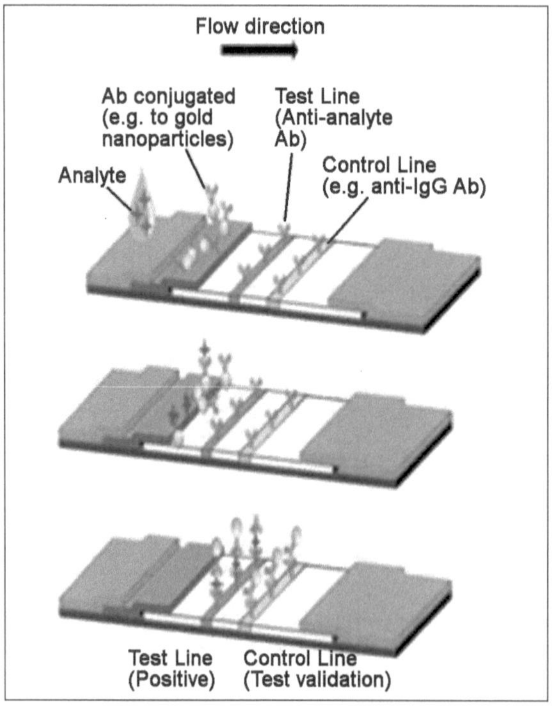

Ans: (d) None of the above

Ref: *Essentials of Medical Microbiology, 1st Edition, Page 136 and Jawetz, Melnick and Adelberg's Medical Microbiology, 26th Edition, Page 509*

5. A 12-year-old boy presents with vomiting within 3 hours of consumption of food at a party. What is the likely organism responsible for the symptoms?

(a) Clostridium botulinum (b) Staphylococcus aureus

(c) Salmonella (d) Clostridium perfringens

Explanation:

Incubation period, Organism	Symptoms	Common food sources
1-6 hours		
Staphylococcus aureus	Nausea, vomiting, diarrhea	Ham, poultry, potato or egg salad, mayonnaise, pastries
Bacillus cereus	Nausea, vomiting, diarrhea	Fried rice
Clostridium botulinum	Nausea, vomiting, diarrhea	Canned food
8-16 hours		
Clostridium perfringens	Abdominal cramps, diarrhea (vomiting rare)	Beef, poultry, legumes, gravies
B. cereus	Abdominal cramps, diarrhea (vomiting rare)	Meats, vegetables, dried beans, cereals
> 16 hours		
Vibrio cholerae	Watery diarrhea	Shellfish, water
Enterotoxigenic *E.coli*	Watery diarrhea	Salads, cheese, meat, water
Enterohemorrhagic *E.coli*	Bloody diarrhea	Ground beef, salami, milk, raw vegetables, apple juice
Salmonella species	Inflammatory diarrhea	Beef, poultry, eggs, dairy products
Campylobacter jejuni	Inflammatory diarrhea	Poultry, raw milk
Shigella species	Dysentery	Potato or egg, salad, lettuce, raw vegetables
Vibrio parahaemolyticus	Dysentery	Mollusks, crustaceans

Staphylococcal Food Poisoning

- Caused by Staphylococcal enterotoxin. It is a superantigen.
- It is a preformed toxin. Hence incubation period is **1-6 hours.**
- Heat and acid stable toxin.
- 12 serotypes: A-E, G-I, R-T and V. Serotype A is most common cause of food poisoning. **Serotype F** does not cause food poisoning but causes **Toxic shock syndrome.**
- Most common source: Food handlers.
- Most common food items: Milk, bakery items, custards, salads, processed meats.

Clostridium Botulinum

(See Figure on the Next Page)

- Anaerobic gram positive bacilli with **subterminal spore**.
- Produces botulinum toxin, a powerful neurotoxin.

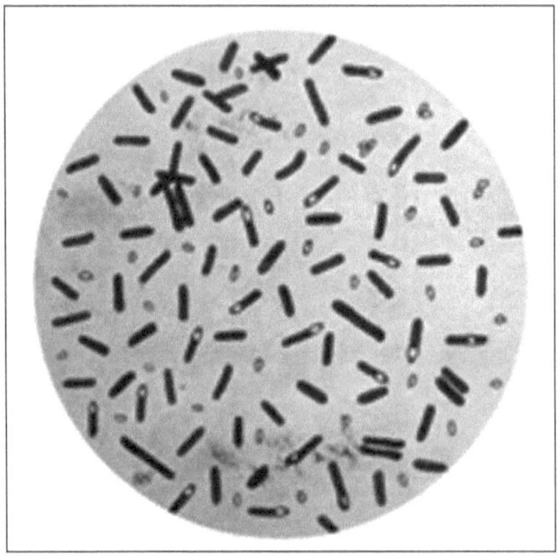

- Causes **botulism** (reversible flaccid paralysis).
- **Botulinum toxin** (BT), is an exotoxin, produced **intracellularly**, released from the bacterial cell only after autolysis.
- BT has 8 serotypes (A,B,C1,C2,D,E,F,G). Most common infection is caused by **serotype A**. All are neurotoxins except **serotype C2**, which is an **enterotoxin**.
- BT is synthesized in inactive form, and requires trypsin to convert into active form.

Mechanism of Action

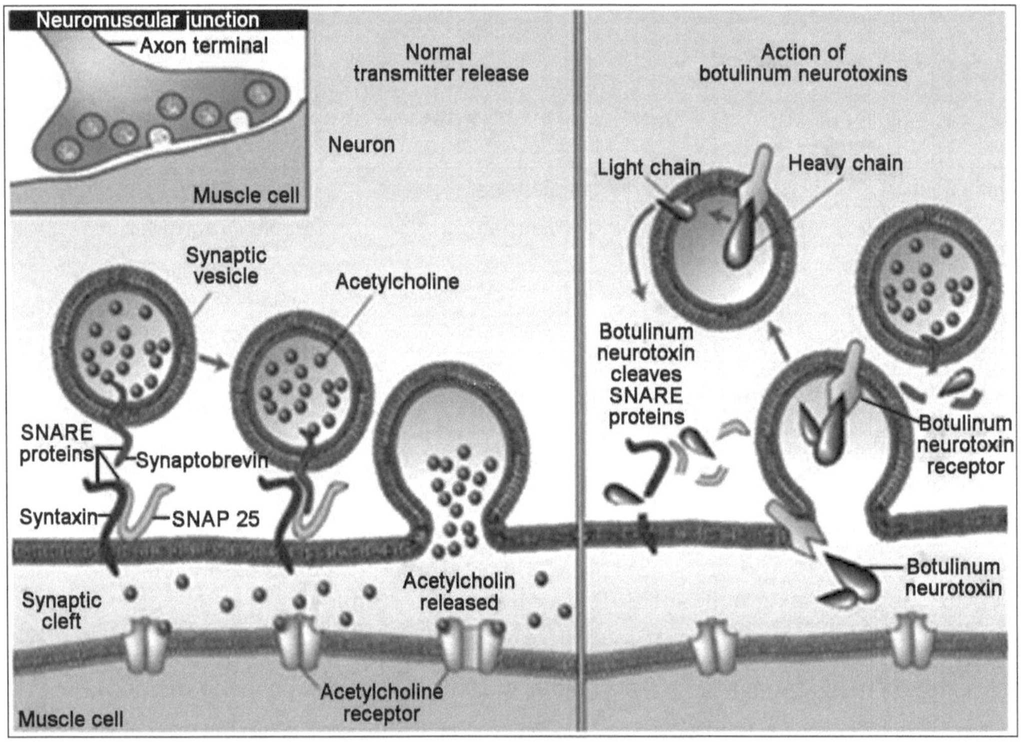

- BT is transported to the peripheral cholinergic nerve terminals.
- BT binds to the **acetylcholine receptors** on the nerve terminals at the neuromuscular junction. This results in blockade of release of acetylcholine, leading to **flaccid paralysis.**

Types of Botulism

- Food borne botulism – due to ingestion of preformed toxin in canned foods and honey.

- Incubation period 12-36 hours.
- Vomiting and diarrhea are rarely seen. It is followed by progressive muscle weakness.

Types

- **Wound botulism**–due to contamination of wounds with spores of Cl. botulinum.
- **Infant botulism**–due to ingestion of spores of Cl. botulinum in contaminated honey in children < 1 year. Results in floppy child syndrome (can also be caused by Benzodiazepine toxicity)

Treatment

- Botulinum antitoxin – neutralize unbound free BT in circulation.
- No treatment in case BT is already bound to nerve terminals.

Clostridium Perfringens

- Previously called **Clostridium welchii**.
- It is a commensal in human large intestine.
- Capsulated, non-motile, anaerobic, gram positive bacillus, with subterminal bulging spores.
- Spores are heat resistant.
- Classified into 5 types based on the toxin production.
- Produces 4 major toxins and 8 minor toxins.
- Produces a heat labile enterotoxin, responsible for food poisoning and necrotizing enterocolitis.
- Food poisoning occurs within **6-24 hours** of ingestion of contaminated food and not characterized by fever or vomiting.
- Food poisoning is caused by **type A enterotoxin.**
- Food source – contaminated meat.
- **MOA:** Enterotoxin forms pores in intestinal mucosal membrane.
- Beta toxin produces by Cl. perfringens type C, causes enteritis necroticans (gas gangrene of bowel).

Salmonella

- Non-typhoidal Salmonella like S. typhimurium and S. enteritidis, causes gastroenteritis, characterized by nausea, vomiting, watery diarrhea, fever and abdominal cramps within **6-48 hours** of ingestion of contaminated food.

Ans : (b) Staphylococcus aureus

Ref: *Textbook of Medical Microbiology by Dr. CP Baveja*

6. The active disinfectant property of bleaching powder is due to:

(a) Chlorine (b) Chloramine

(c) Hypochlor acid (d) Hypochlorous acid

Explanation:

- **Bleaching powder or calcium hypochlorite (CaOCl2)** is produced by passing chlorine through calcium chloride.
- When bleaching powder dissolves, it reacts with water to **hypochlorous acid (HOCl)** and **hypochlorite ions** (OCl-). Hypochlorous acid (HOCl, which is electrically neutral) and hypochlorite ions (OCl-, electrically negative) will form free chlorine when bound together. This results in disinfection. Both substances have very distinctive behaviour.

- The disinfecting properties of chlorine in water are based on the **oxidizing power** of the **free oxygen atoms** and on chlorine substitution reactions.
- The disinfectant action of chlorine is mainly due to hypochlorous acid and to a small extent due to hypochlorite ions. Hypochlorous acid is **70-80 times** more effective than hypochlorite ions.

Ans: (d) Hypochlorous acid

Ref: *Park Textbook of Social and Preventive Medicine, 23rd Edition, Page 714*

7. Which of the following is the cause of donovanosis?

(a) H. ducreyi
(b) Klebsiella granulomatis
(c) Leishmania donovanosis
(d) Treponema pallidum

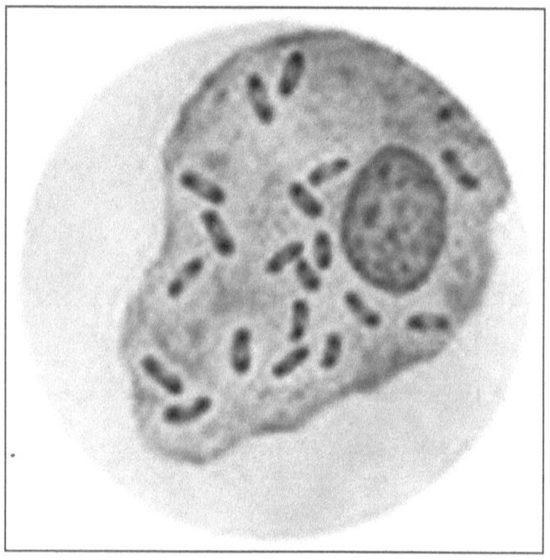

Explanation:

DD for Genital Ulcers

Painless Genital Ulcers	
Syphilis	*Treponema pallidum*
Lymphogranuloma Venereum	*Chlamydia trachomatis (L1, L2, L3)*
Donovanosis	*Klebsiella granulomatis*
Painful Genital Ulcers	
Chancroid	*Hemophilus ducreyi*
Herpes Genitalis	*Herpes simplex virus 2 and 1*
Urethral Discharge	
Gonorrhea	*Neisseria gonorrhoeae*
Non-Gonococcal Urethritis	*Chlamydia trachomatis*
	Ureaplasma urealyticum
	Mycoplasma genitalium
	Mycoplasma hominis

Donovanosis

- Also called **Granuloma Inguinale.**
- Caused by **Klebsiella (Calymmatobacterium) granulomatis.**
- Painless, Hypertrophic ulcer, margins are rolled and elevated.
- **Diagnosis**
  - Presence of "**Donovan body**" confirmatory in Giemsa stain.

- **Donovan bodies**
  - 1-2 mm, rounded coccobacilli, within cystic spaces in large mononuclear cells.
  - Safety-pin appearance.

Hemophilus Ducreyi

- Causes soft chancre or chancroid.
- Lesion is tender with foul purulent and hemorrhagic discharge, with enlarged, tender inguinal lymph nodes.
- Hemophilus ducreyi is a pleomorphic gram negative cocco-bacillus.
- Take up **bipolar staining**.
- **School of fish or railroad track appearance**.

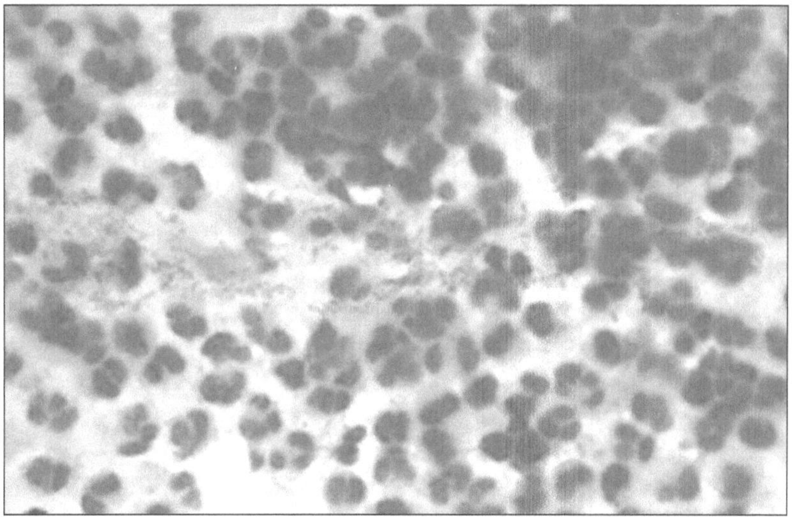

School of fish or railroad track appearance

Treponema Pallidum

- Causes syphilis.
- Transmitted through sexual contact or vertical transmission
- 4 clinical stages: Primary, secondary, latent and tertiary.
- **Primary syphilis** (hard chancre) presents as hard, painless, solitary chancre.
  - Associated with bilateral, hard, painless, non-tender inguinal lymphadenopathy.
- **Secondary syphilis** may be present as condyloma lata.
- **Latent syphilis** is characterized by absence of clinical symptoms but with positive serological tests.
- **Tertiary syphilis** is characterized by gummatous lesions.

Ans: (b) Klebsiella granulomatis

Ref: *Ananthanarayanan and Paniker's Textbook of Microbiology*

8. Urethritis in male is not caused by:

(a) H. ducreyi (b) Gonococcus

(c) Trichomonas (d) Chlamydia

Explanation:

AGENTS CAUSING URINARY TRACT INFECTIONS

- **Gram Negative Organisms**

- Escherichia coli.
- Klebsiella pneumoniae.
- Proteus spp.
- Pseudomonas aeruginosa.
- Acinetobacter sp.
- Enterobacter sp.
- Serratia sp.
- Neisseria gonorrhoeae.

- **Gram Positive Organisms**
  - Enterococcus fecalis.
  - Staphylococcus saprophyticus
    (restricted to infections in young sexually active women).
  - Staphylococcus aureus.
  - Staphylococcus epidermidis (commonly found as a contaminant in urine, pathogen in immunocompromised).

Non bacterial urethritis	Chlamydia spp. Ureaplasma spp.
Fungi	Candida albicans
Parasites	Trichomonas vaginalis Schistosoma hematobium
Viruses	Herpes simplex virus Adenovirus BK virus Cytomegalovirus

Hemophilus Ducreyi

- Hemophilus ducreyi causes a venereal disease, **soft chancre** or **chancroid**.
- It is characterized by multiple, painful, non-indurated irregular ulcers on the genitalia, associated with painful regional lymphadenopathy (usually unilateral).

Gonococci

- Neisseria gonorrhea is a gram-negative diplococcus with adjacent sides concave (kidney shaped).
- Gonorrhea is a sexually transmitted disease characterized by cervicitis, urethritis and conjunctivitis.
- It affects both male and female.
- In males, acute urethritis is most common manifestation, characterized by purulent urethral discharge.
- Complications include epididymitis, prostatitis, balanitis and seminal vesiculitis.
- If left untreated, it may spread to periurethral tissues causing multiple abscesses with discharging sinuses, forming water can perineum.
- In women, it may lead to pelvic inflammatory disease, leading to peritonitis and perihepatitis. This is called **'Fitz Curtis Hugh' syndrome**.

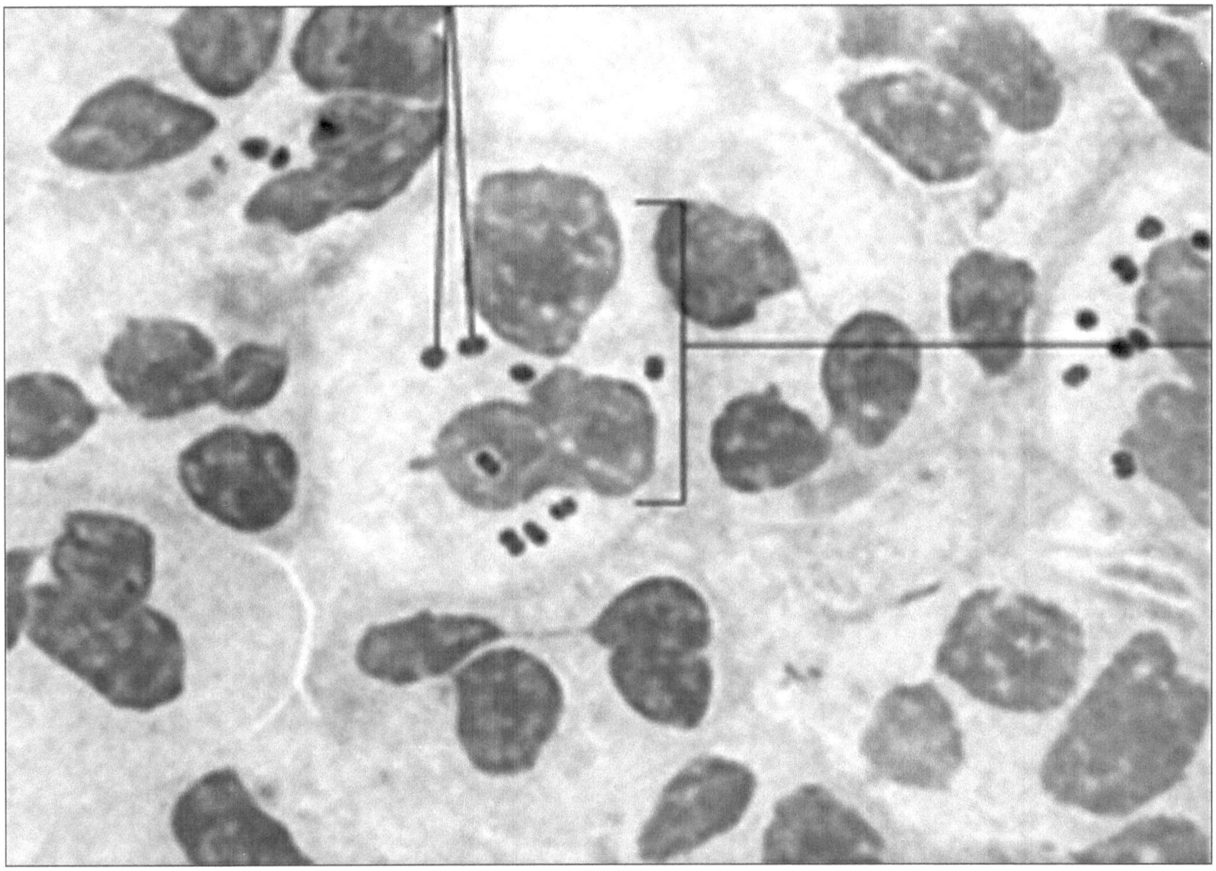

Gonococci

Chlamydia

- Chlamydia trachomatis is an obligate intracellular bacterium.
- Based on major outer membrane proteins, it is divided into 18 serotypes, causing the following:
  - **Trachoma:** Serotype A,B,Ba and C.
  - **Genital infections:** Serotype D-K.
  - **Lymphogranuloma venereum: Serotype: L1,L2,L3.**
- C. trachomatis is the most common cause of Non-Gonococcal Urethritis (NGU).
- It also causes **Reiter's syndrome**, characterized by conjunctivitis, urethritis, reactive arthritis and characteristic mucocutaneous lesions.

Trichomonas Vaginalis

- It is a genital protozoan flagellate transmitted through sexual contact.
- It exists only in **trophozoite form**. Cystic stage is not seen. Trophozoite is pear shaped. It shows rapid jerky or twitching motility.
- High vaginal pH (>4.5) favors trichomoniasis.
- In females, it causes pruritic vaginitis.
- In males, it is usually asymptomatic but may cause urethritis, epididymitis and prostatitis.
- Culture is the gold standard for diagnosis. Cysteine-Peptone-Liver-Maltose (CPLM) is the medium preferred.
- Metronidazole is the treatment of choice. Both partners should be treated simultaneously.

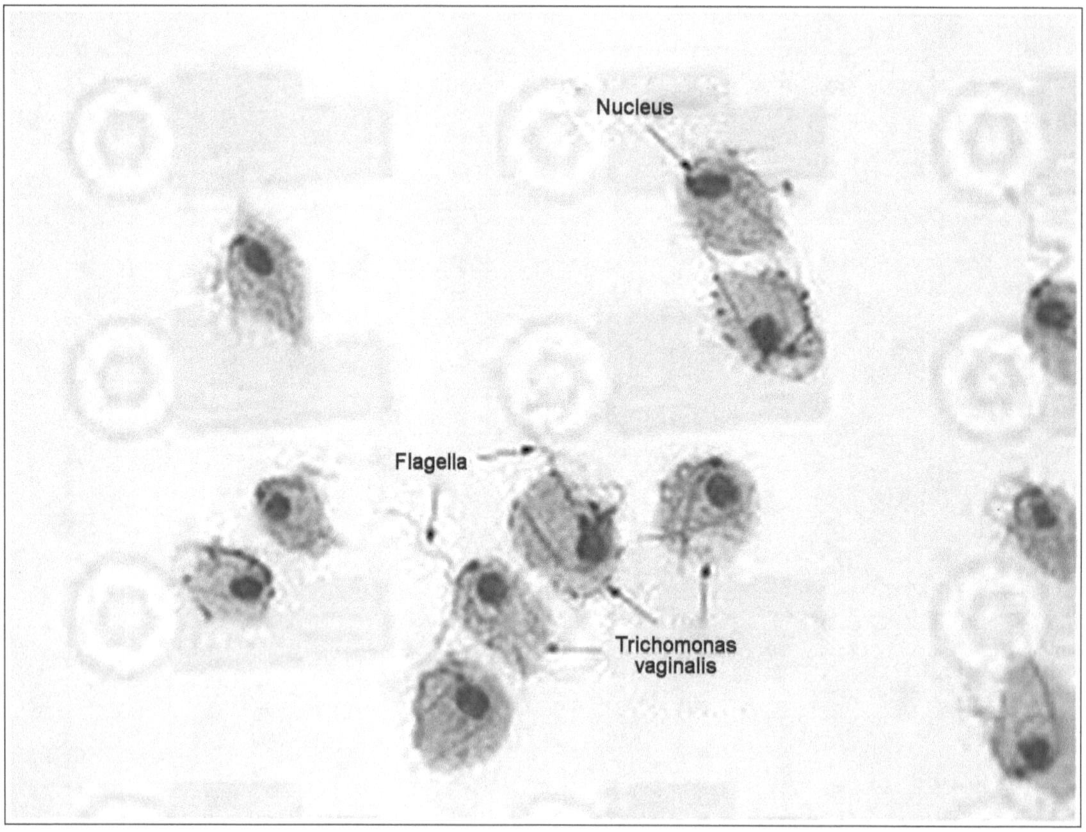

Ans : (a) H. ducreyi

Ref: *Paniker's Textbook of Medical Parasitology, 8th Edition, Page 36*

9. Which of the following is most likely to be acquired by traumatic inoculation?

(a) Blastomycosis dermatitidis
(b) Sporothrix schenckii
(c) Coccidioides immitis
(d) Paracoccidioides brasiliensis

Explanation:

Sporothrix Schenckii

- It is a **thermally dimorphic fungi** (yeast form at 36°C and mycelial form at 25°C).
- Causes Sporotrichiosis.
- Fungal infection affecting cutaneous, subcutaneous and lymphatic tissue.
- Most commonly affects gardeners. Infection by rose prick. Hence called **rose gardener's disease**.
- **Incubation period:** 1-3 weeks.
- KOH/HPE shows asteroid body. Tissue sections shows cigar-shaped bodies.
- Immunohistochemical staining shows Splendore-Hoeppli phenomenon (immune complex deposition around the organism).
- Mycelial form shows '**flower like pattern'.**
- **Skin tests: Sporotrichin** skin test and **peptido-rhamno-mannan** antigen skin test.

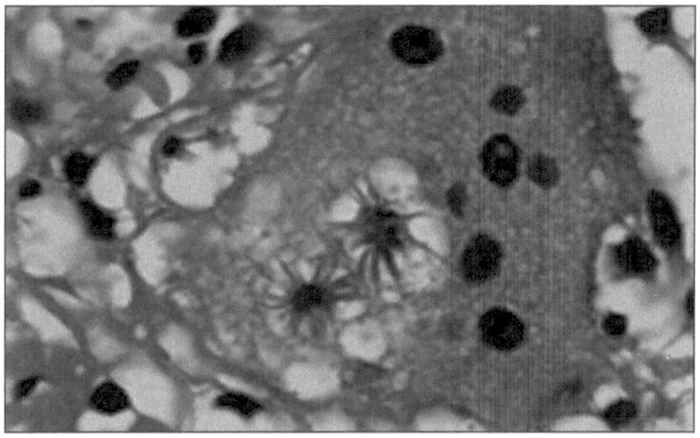

Asteroid body

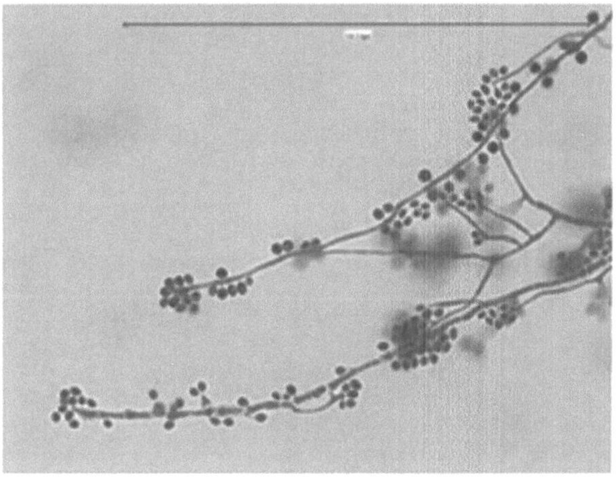

Mycelial form showing flower like pattern

Blastomycosis Dermatitidis

- Thermally dimorphic fungi.
- Causes a systemic mycosis called Blastomycosis. Also called '**Chicago's disease**' or '**North American Blastomycosis').**
- Mode of infection is inhalation of spores from soil.
- Most common presentation is Pulmonary blastomycosis. Also causes cutaneous and disseminated infection.
- Shows **broad-based budding** in yeast form (figure of eight appearance).
- Skin test – Using **blastomycin** antigen. (mycelial form antigen).

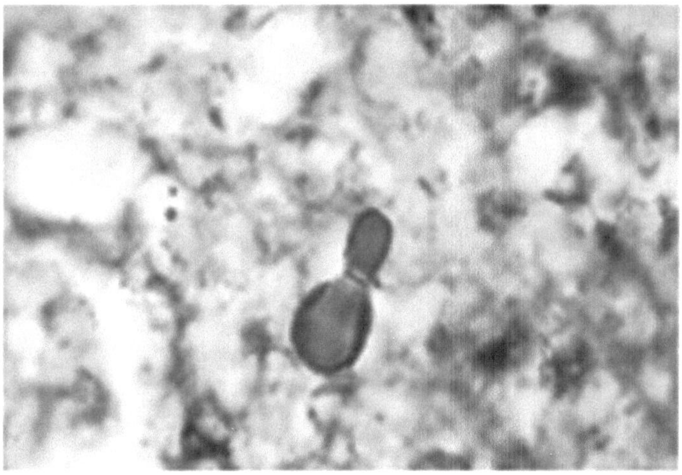

Broad-based budding (figure of eight appearance)

Coccidioides Immitis

- Thermally dimorphic fungi, causing Coccidioidomycosis. Also called **'Rift valley fever or desert rheumatism'.**
- Mode of infection is through **inhalation of arthroconidia** from soil.
- Biosafety level 3 agent.
- Yeast form – spherules with endospores.
- Mycelial form – branched septate hyphae with thick walled rectangular arthroconidia.
- Skin tests use:
  - **Coccidioidin:** Mycelial phase antigen.
  - **Spherulin:** Yeast phase antigen.

Paracoccidioides Brasiliensis

- Thermally dimorphic.
- Causes paracoccidioidomycosis or Lutz's mycosis or 'South American Blastomycosis'.
- Mode of infection is inhalation of spores from soil.
- Yeast phase – **Mariner's or Pilot's wheel appearance.**

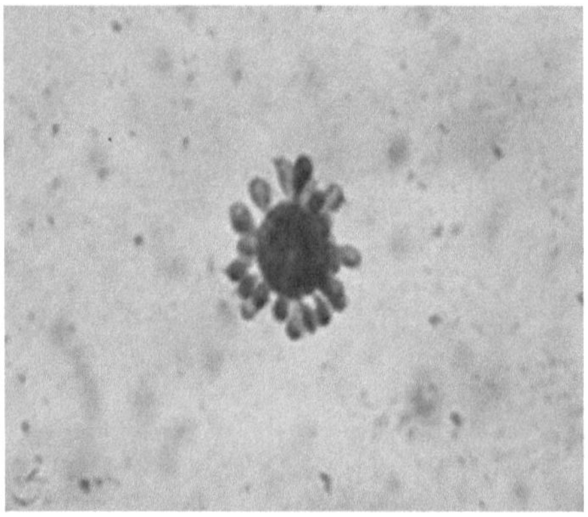

Pilot's or Mariner's wheel appearance

Ans : (b) Sporothrix schenckii

Ref: *Textbook of Medical Mycology by Jagdish Chander, 4th Edition, Page 229*

10. All of the following are correct for JE *except*:

(a) Humans are reservoir
(b) Main vector is culex tritaeniorhynchus
(c) Birds are maintenance host
(d) It has seasonal transmission

Explanation:

Japanese Encephalitis (JE)

- It is an arthropod-borne viral infection affecting the central nervous system.
- **Family: Flaviviridae**. **Genus: Flavivirus.**
- Spherical virus with single stranded positive sense **RNA.**
- **Vector: Culex tritaeniorhynchus** and **Culex vishnui** (second common vector in India).
- **Reservoir host: Andreid birds** (herons, ergets, ducks).
- **Amplifier host: Pigs** (JE virus multiplies exponentially without causing any symptoms).

- **Accidental dead end host: Humans.**
- JE is endemic in Uttar Pradesh, Assam, West Bengal, Bihar,Tamilnadu and Karnataka in India.
- Disease transmission is more in **rainy season**.

Encephalitis A or Von Economo disease or Encephalitis lethargica is a disease seen in Japan.

Natural Cycle of JE

Andreid birds	Culex mosquito	Andreid birds
Pigs	Culex mosquito	Pigs

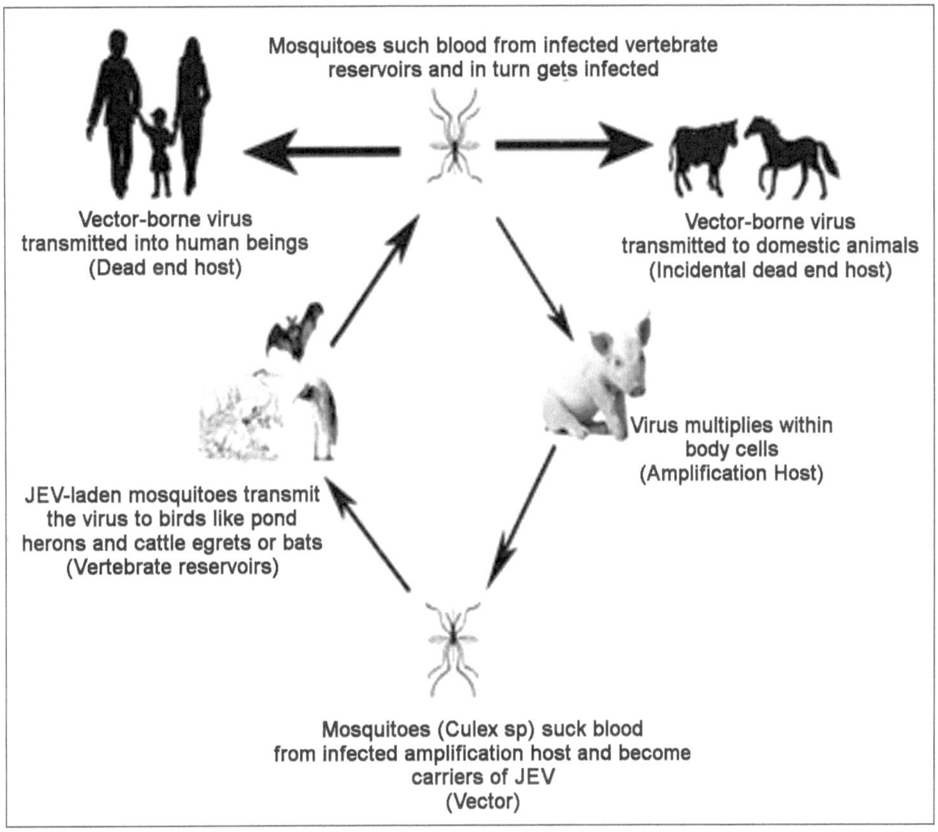

Clinical Manifestation

- **Incubation period: 5-15 days.**
- JE shows **Iceberg Phenomenon** (subclinical infection is more common than cases).
- **3 stages:**
  - **Prodromal stage** (1-6 days)–Fever, headache, vomiting.
  - **Acute encephalitic stage**–Convulsions, nuchal rigidity, altered sensorium, coma.
- **Sequelae** – Mental retardation, paralysis, aphasia, cerebellar changes.

Lab Diagnosis

- **Sample:** Blood and CSF.
- **Virus isolation:**
  - Intracerebral inoculation of suckling mice.
  - Cell lines (Vero, BHK, HeLa, MRC5).
  - Immunofluorescence with virus-specific monoclonal antibody.

Serology

- ELISA – detection of IgM and IgG in serum/CSF.
- Hemagglutination inhibition test.
- Immunochromatographic test.
- Molecular–RT-PCR.

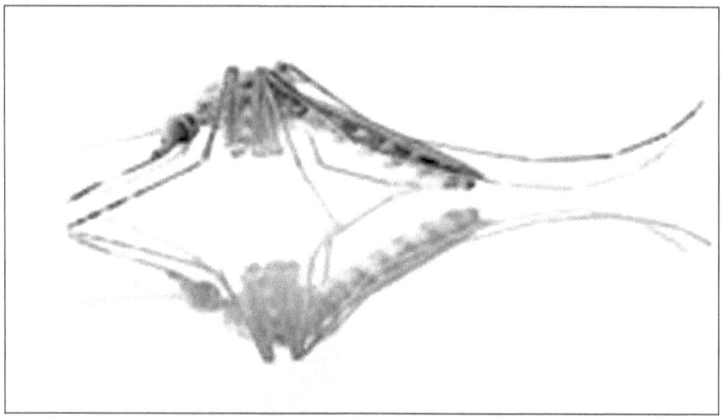

Culex tritaeniorhynchus

JE PROPHYLAXIS

- **Live attenuated vaccine**
  - Strain SA 14-14-2.
  - Derived from Primary Hamster Kidney cell line.
  - Single dose S/C to children <15 years. Booster dose 1 year later.
- **Formalin Inactivated Vaccine**
  - Nakayama strain and Beijing strain.

Note:

- In Indian national immunization schedule, JE vaccine is given in 2 doses, at 9th month and at 16-24 months, in endemic states.

Ans: (a) Humans are the reservoir

Ref: *Jawetz, Melnick and Adelerg's Medical Microbiology, 26th Edition*

11. An HIV positive patient with CD4 count 300/mm^3 presents with mucosal lesion in the mouth as shown in the figure. On microscopy budding yeast cells and pseudo hyphae are seen. What is the likely diagnosis?

(a) Oral hairy leukoplakia (b) Lichen planus

(c) Candidiasis (d) Diphtheria

Explanation:

- The image has differential diagnosis of all the options given. But the presence of budding yeast cells and pseudo hyphae confirms the diagnosis of candidiasis.

Candidiasis

- Most common fungal infection affecting humans, causing cutaneous, subcutaneous and systemic manifestations.
- Oropharyngeal candidiasis is characterized by painless, whitish, adherent patches in the oral cavity. Also called as **'oral thrush'**.

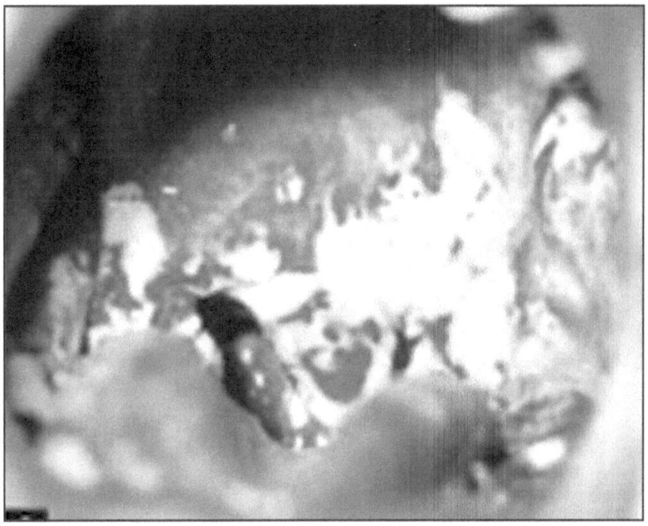

Lab Diagnosis

- Microscopy.
- Sample collected from active lesion yields gram positive oval budding yeasts and pseudohyphae.
- Culture on Sabouraud dextrose agar – white, creamy, moist colonies.
- Differentiation of Candida species is by:

  Glucose fermentation and assimilation.
- Chlamydospore formation and Germ tube test (Reynolds Braude phenomenon) is confirmative for C. albicans.
- **Serology:** b-(1,3)-D-glucan.

Treatment

- Topical clotrimazole is the drug of choice.
- Nystatin, fluconazole, itraconazole are used alternatively.

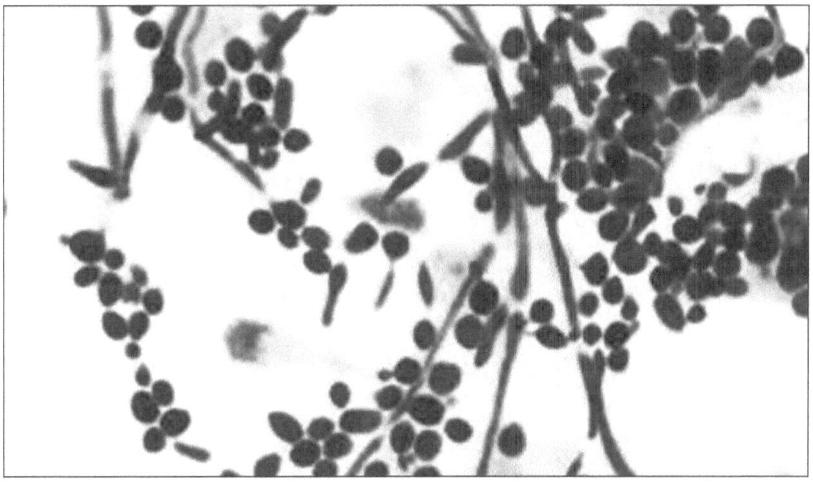

Budding yeasts and pseudohyphae

Oral Hairy Leukoplakia

- Caused by **Ebstein-Barr virus** (EBV) in immunocompromised patients.
- It is commonly associated with HIV patients with low CD4 count and transplant patients.
- It is a wart-like epithelial cell hyperplasia in the tongue.

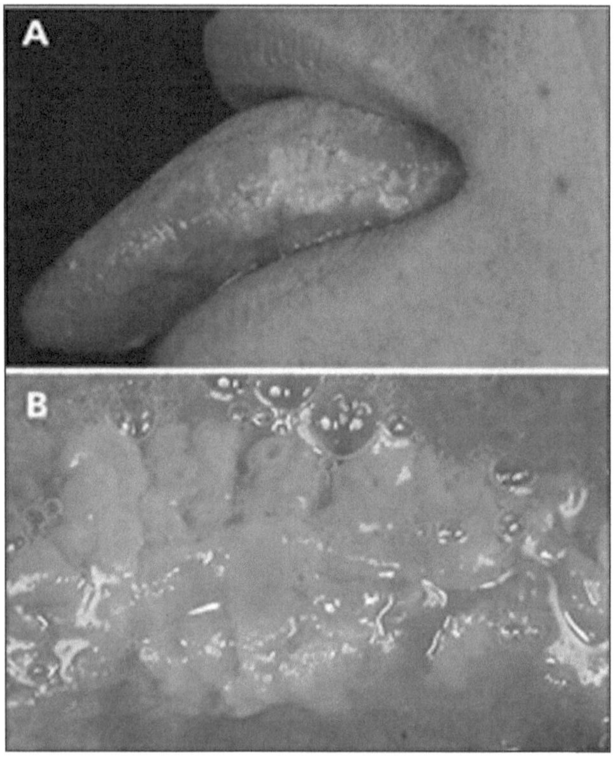

Oral hairy leukoplakia

EBV/Human Herpes Virus 4

- Belongs to family Herpesviridae, subfamily gamma. Genus Lymphocryptoviral.
- Infections caused by EBV are:
  - Infectious mononucleosis.
  - Nasopharyngeal carcinoma.
  - Burkitt's lymphoma.
  - Hodgkin's lymphoma.
  - B cell lymphoma.
  - Oral hairy leukoplakia.

Lichen Planus

- Oral lichen planus (OLP) is a chronic mucocutaneous immune related disorder of stratified squamous epithelium that affects oral and genital mucous membranes, skin, nails and scalp.
- It is a T-cell mediated autoimmune disease in which the CD8 + T cells trigger apoptosis of the basal cells of the oral epithelium.
- They are purple, polygonal, pruritic papules and plaques. The center of the papule may be slightly umbilicated and its surface is covered by very fine grayish white lines, called **Wickham striae**.

Diphtheria

- Caused by **Corynebacterium diphtheriae**.
- Respiratory diphtheria is characterized by mucosal ulcers, lined by a tough leathery pseudomembrane.
- It bleeds on removal.
- Common sites are tonsils, pharynx, nose and larynx.
- Pseudomembrane is often accompanied by tonsillar swelling and neck edema (bulls neck appearance).

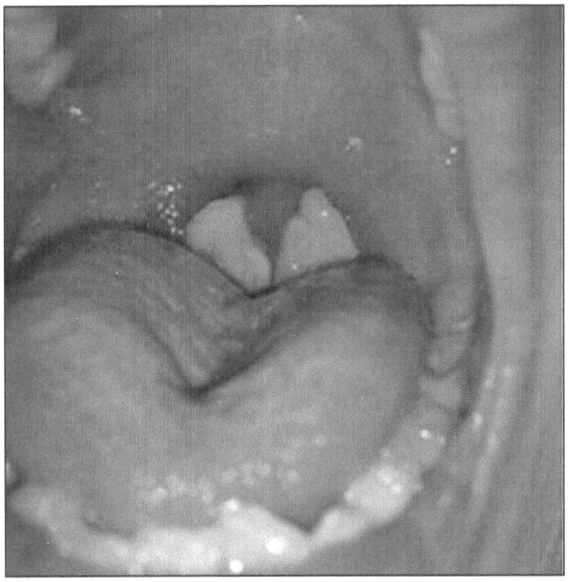

Diphtheria

Ans: (c) Candidiasis

Ref: *Jawetz, Melnick and Adelerg's Medical Microbiology, 26th Edition, Page 484*

12. Which strain of the influenza was declared recently as pandemic?

(a) H1N1 (b) H5N1

(c) H7N7 (d) H3N2

Explanation:

- Influenza viruses belong to family Orthomyxoviridae.
- **Morphololgy:** Spherical, enveloped virus with a helical nucleocapsid, containing **8-segmented negative sense RNA.**
- **Types A, B and C influenza viruses** have been classified based on the ribonucleoprotein (RNP) and Matrix (M) proteins.
- Influenza A and B have 8 segmented RNA. Influenza C has only 7 segmented RNA.
- **Hemagglutinin (HA) and Neuraminidase (NA)** are glycoproteins embedded in the lipid envelope.
- Influenza A has **16 H subtypes and 9 N subtypes**, depending on HA and NA glycoproteins.
- **Antigenic Drift**
  - Minor change in the virus due to point mutations in HA/NA genes.
  - Results in minor periodic epidemics.
  - Seen in influenza A and B.
- **Antigenic Shift**
  - Abrupt, major discontinuous variation in the HA/NA genes.
  - Results in genetic reassortment, leading to new virus strain.
  - Seen in influenza A only.
  - Causes major epidemics and pandemics.
- Primary reservoir for influenza–Birds.
- Reassortment vessel for influenza–Pigs.

Years	Subtype	Extent of Outbreak
1889-1890	H2N8	Severe pandemic
1900-1903	H3N8	Moderate epidemic
1918-1919	H1N1[a] (HswN1) (Spanish flu)	Severe pandemic
1933-1935	H1N1[a] (H0N1)	Mild epidemic
1946-1947	H1N1	Mild epidemic
1957-1958	H2N2 (Asian flu)	Severe pandemic
1968-1969	H3N2 (Hong Kong flu)	Moderate pandemic
1977-1978[b]	H1N1 (Russian flu)	Mild pandemic
2009-2010	H1N1	Pandemic

- Most recent influenza pandemic was caused by H1N1, which emerged in California in March 2009.
- It was declared as a pandemic by the WHO on June 11, 2009.
- It was found to be a quadruple-reassortant virus (1 human strain + 2 swine strains + 1 avian strain). The reassortment happened in pigs.
- Transmission was from human to human.
- An outbreak appeared in 2015 in India affecting more than 33,000 people, killing more than 2000 people and it was controlled by mid of 2015.

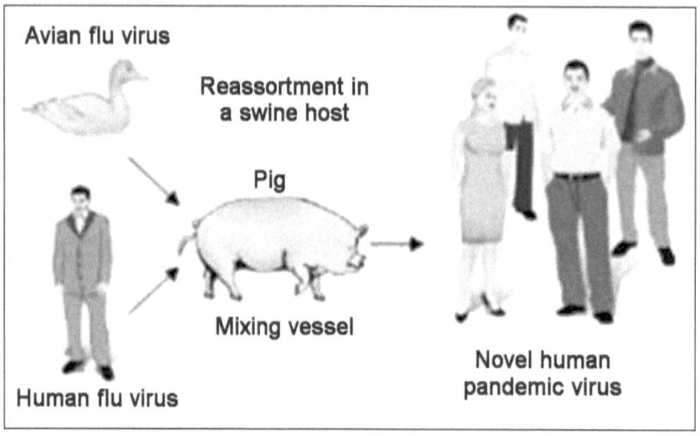

Lab Diagnosis

- **Sample:** Nasopharyngeal swab.
- **Virus isolation:** Amniotic cavity inoculation.
- **Serology:** Antigen detection by immunofluorescence.
- **Molecular:** Real time and multiplex PCR.

Treatment:

- Neuraminidase inhibitors.
  - Oseltamavir tablet 75 mg twice a day for 5 days.
  - Zanamavir 10 mg (inhalational form).
  - Peramivir (IV form).
- Matrix protein M2 inhibitor.
  - Amantadine and rimantadine.
  - A/H1N1 flu and A/H5N1 flu are resistant to amantadine.

Ans: (a) H1N1

Ref: *Jawetz, Melnick and Adelerg's Medical Microbiology, 26th Edition, Page 577*

13. Which of the following helps in bacterial adhesion:

(a) Cytoplasmic membrane (b) Mesosomes

(c) Fimbriae (d) LPS

Explanation:

- Many gram-negative and few gram-positive bacteria have short, fine, hair-like appendages called fimbriae or pili, which are organs of adhesion.
- Pili are made up of protein called **'pilin'.**
- They are antigenic, which acts as a virulence factor for bacteria but antibodies against fimbriae are not protective.
- Certain fimbriae called '**sex pili'** helps in **bacterial gene transfer** (conjugation).

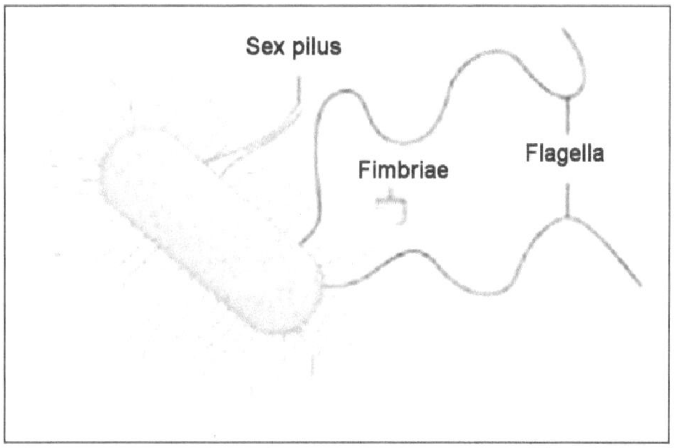

Organ of locomotion – **Flagella.**

Organ of adhesion – **Fimbria.**

Cytoplasmic Membrane

- It is a phospholipid bilayer, with integral and peripheral proteins.
- It is a semi-permeable membrane acting as an osmotic barrier for the bacterial cell.
- It helps in nutrition uptake and waste excretion.
- It is the site of bacterial respiration, synthesis of lipids and cell wall and chromosome segregation.

Mesosomes

- They are invaginations of plasma membrane in the shape of vesicles, tubules or lamellae.
- More prominent in gram-positive bacteria.
- It is involved in bacterial respiration, cell wall synthesis and chromosome replication.

Lipopolysaccharide (LPS)

- It is present only in gram-negative bacteria.
- It has 3 parts:
  - **Lipid A or Endotoxin:** Bacterial virulence factor.
  - Core polysaccharide.
  - **'O' antigen:** Major surface antigen. Also called somatic antigen. Induces antibody formation. used for serotyping.

Ans : (c) Fimbriae

Ref: *Jawetz, Melnick and Adelerg's Medical Microbiology, 26th Edition*

14. Which of the following is a type A bioterrorism agent?

(a) Nipah virus
(b) Coxiella burnetii
(c) Clostridium perfringens
(d) Bacillus anthracis

Explanation:

- **Bioterrorism** is a form of terrorism, where there is intentional and deliberate release of biological agents to cause mass illness or death of people, animals or plants.
- From October to November, 2001, 10 confirmed cases of inhalational anthrax caused by intentional release of Bacillus anthracis spores were identified in the United States.
- **Nipah virus**, a novel paramyxovirus, closely related to Hendra virus emerged in northern part of Peninsular Malaysia in 1998. The virus caused an outbreak of severe febrile encephalitis in humans with a high mortality rate. In India, there was an outbreak in May-June, 2018, in Kerala.

Category A: These agents are the highest priority pathogens which pose the greatest risk to national security	
• These agents can be easily disseminated or transmitted from person to person • Result in high mortality and have the potential for major public health impact • Might cause public panic and social disruption • Require special action for public health preparedness	• Anthrax *(Bacillus anthracis)* • Botulism (*Clostridium* botulinum toxin) • Plague *(Yersinia pestis)* • Tularemia *(Francisella tularensis)* • Smallpox (Variola major) • Hemorrhagic viruses – Arenaviruses: Lassavirus – Bunyaviridae: Crimean-Congo virus – Filoviridae: Ebola, Marburg virus
Category B: These agents are the second highest priority pathogens	
• Moderately easy to disseminate • Result in moderate morbidity rates and low mortality rates • Require specifically enhanced diagnostic capacity	• Melioidosis *(Burkholderia pseudomallei)* • Glanders *(Burkholderia mallei)* • Brucellosis *(Brucella* species*)* • Psittacosis *(Chlamydophila psittaci)* • Q fever *(Coxiella burnetii)* • Typhus fever *(Rickettsia prowazekii)* • Toxin: Ricin, *S. auerus* Enterotoxin B, Epsilon toxin of *Clostridium perfringens* • Viral encephalitis [alphaviruses (e.g., Venezuelan, eastern and western equine encephalitis)] • Food threats: *Salmonella, Shigella, E.coli* 0157 • Water threats: *Vibrio cholerae, Cryptosporidium*
Category C: These agents are the third highest priority pathogens. They are the emerging pathogens, to which the general population lacks immunity	
• These agents could be engineered for mass dissemination in the future because of availability, ease of production, and ease of dissemination • They have a potential for high morbidity and mortality rates	• Nipah virus • Hantavirus • SARS coronavirus • Pandemic influenza virus • MDR - TB • Yellow fever virus

Ans: (d) Bacillus anthracis

Ref: *Jernigan JA at al. Bioterrorism-related Inhalational Anthrax: The First 10 Cases Reported in the United States, Emerging Infectious Diseases 7(6),933-944, https://doi.org/10.3201/eid0706.010604*

15. Super antigen is produced by which of the following?

(a) Streptococcus pyogenes

(b) Clostridium perfringens

(c) Vibrio cholerae

(d) Staphylococcus epidermidis

Explanation:

- Superantigens are a class of antigens, which can activate T cells without being processed by Antigen presenting cells (APC).
- Variable ß region of T cell receptor is the receptor for superantigens.

Activation of T cells by superantigens

↓

Massive release of cytokines

↓

Polyclonal B cell activation

↓

Increased secretion of non-specific antibodies (hypergammaglobulinemia)

- Streptococcal pyrogenic exotoxin (SPE) induces fever (pyrogenic). It is responsible for streptococcal infections like scarlet fever, necrotising fascitis and toxic shock syndrome.
- It is classfied into 3 antigenic types: SPE A, B and C.
- **SPE A and C are superantigens**.
- **Dick test** – Hypersensitivity skin test to determine susceptibility to scarlet fever by detecting exposure to SPE.

Bacterial Superantigens	Viral Superantigens	Fungal Superantigens
Staphylococcal toxins Toxic shock syndrome toxin (TSST-1) Exfoliative toxin Enterotoxin	Epstein-Barr virus associated superantigen	Malassezia furfur
Streptococcal pyrogenic exotoxin A and C	Cytomegalovirus associated superantigen	
Mycoplasma arthritidis mitogen-1 Yersinia enterocolitica Yersinia pseudotuberculosis	Rabies nucleocapsid	
	HIV encoded superantigen	

Ans: (c) Streptococcus pyogenes

Ref: *Greenwood Medical Microbiology, 16th Edition, Page 92*

16. Immunoglobulin structure (dimer) given in the figure belongs to which class of antibody?

(a) IgE (b) IgA
(c) IgM (d) IgG

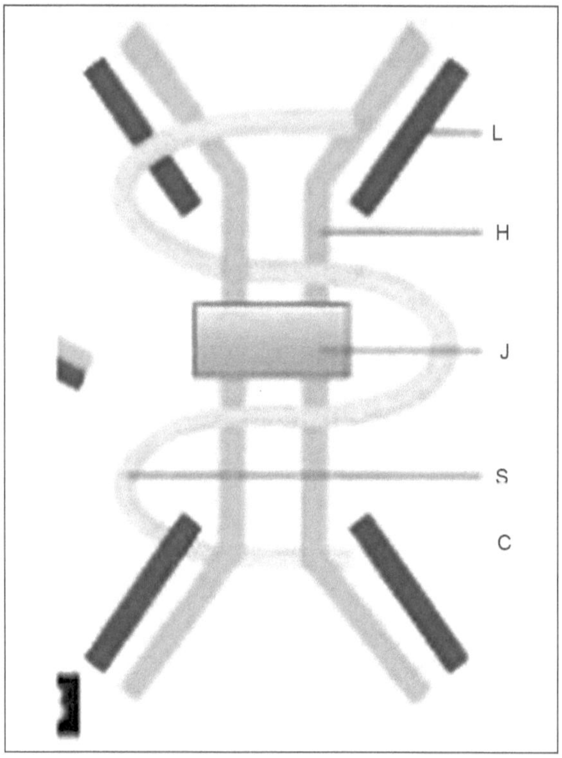

Explanation:

Antibodies or Immunoglobulins

- Igs are glycoprotein molecules that recognize a particular antigen or epitope, bind specifically to it and facilitate its clearance.
- They constitute 20-25% of total serum proteins.
- 5 classes of immunoglobulins are found: IgG, IgM, IgA, IgD, IgE.
- Each immunoglobulin (Ig) has 2 heavy chains and 2 light chains.
- Heavy chains are antigenically distinct and are designated as:
  - Alpha (α).
  - Gamma (γ).
  - Delta (Δ).
  - Mu (μ).
  - Epsilon (ε).
- Light chain kappa (κ) and lambda (λ) are similar in all classes of antibodies. An Ig molecule can have either kappa (κ) or lambda (λ) chain but never both.
- Light chain and heavy chain are bound by disulphide bonds.
- Each heavy and light chain have 2 regions – constant and variable regions.
- Variable region represents the 'antigen binding site of the antibody'.

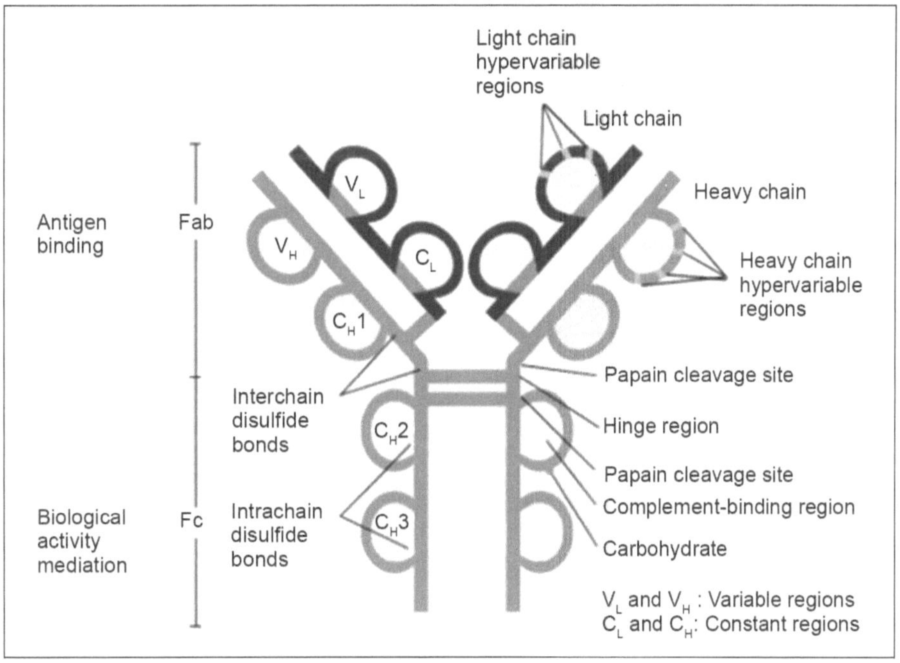

IMMUNOGLOBULIN G (IgG)

- Most abundant class of immunoglobulin.
- Has 4 subclasses: IgG1, IgG2, IgG3 and IgG4.
- **Longest half-life** (23 days).
- **Crosses the placental barrier**. Provides immunity to foetus. IgG2 has poorest ability to cross placenta.
- IgG mediates precipitation and neutralization reactions.

IMMUNOGLOBULIN M (IgM)

- Has the **highest molecular weight**.
- Present only in intravascular space.
- Exists in 2 forms: Monomeric (bound to B cell membrane) and pentameric (secreted form). Pentameric form is formed by 5 monomeric forms joined together by **J chain**.
- It is the first Ig to appear in an infection. It represents **acute infection.**
- Most potent activator of classical complement pathway.
- First Ig to be synthesized in fetal life. Presence of IgM in fetus or newborn is an indication of intrauterine infection.

IMMUNOGLOBULIN A (IgA)

- Secretory IgA is **dimeric** (2 monomers joined by J chain).
- 2 subclasses: IgA1 (predominant in serum) and IgA2 (predominant in body secretions).
- It has a secretory component.
- It is predominant in the body secretions like milk, tears, saliva, respiratory and intestinal mucosal secretions.
- It mediates **local or mucosal immunity**.

IMMUNOGLOBULIN E (IgE)

- It has lowest serum concentration and shortest half-life.
- It is the only heat labile Ig.

- Predominantly present in extravascular space.
- Exhibits **homocytotropism** (affinity for mast cells of same species).
- Mediate **type I hypersensitivity reactions**.
- Elevated in helminthic infections.

IMMUNOGLOBULIN D (IgD)

- Found as a membrane antigen on the surface of B cells.
- Has highest carbohydrate content among the Ig classes.
- Acts as a B cell receptor along with IgM.

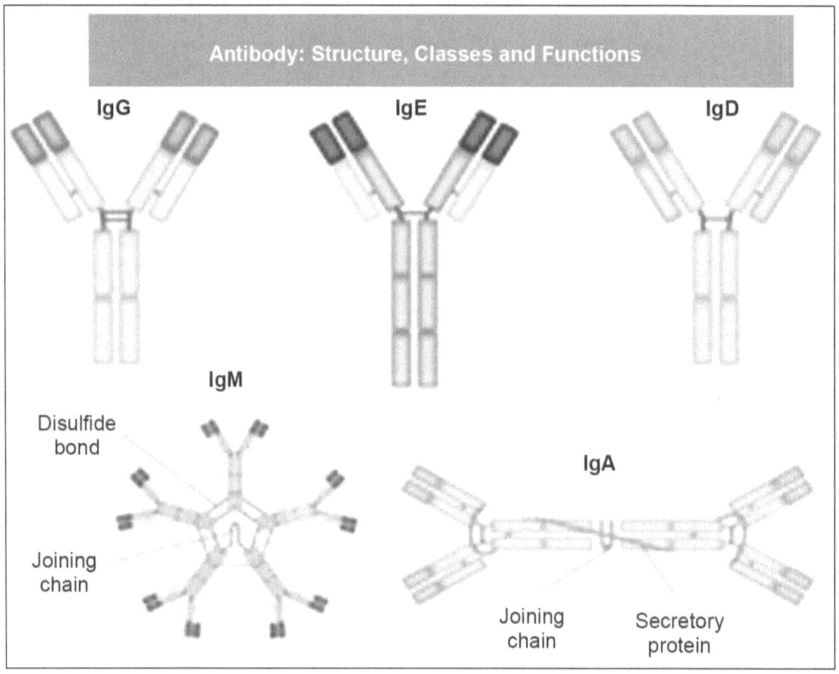

Ans : (b) IgA

Ref: *Ananthanarayanan and Panikar's Textbook of Microbiology, 9th Edition, Page 93*

17. A child develops septic shock following meningitis. On examination child has petechial rash as shown in figure. Which of the following is a gram-negative diplococcus that can be likely etiology?

(a) Pseudomonas aeruginosa (b) Streptococcus pneumoniae
(c) Neisseria meningitidis (d) E. coli

Explanation:

BACTERIAL ETIOLOGICAL AGENTS OF MENINGITIS

- **Neonates and Infants**
  - Escherichia coli.
  - Group B Streptococci–0-28 days.
  - Staphylococcus aureus.
  - Hemophilus influenzae B–3 months to 5 years.
  - Listeria monocytogenes.
  - Streptococcus pneumoniae (serotypes 6, 9, 14, 18 and 23).
  - Klebsiella spp.

- **Adults**
  - Neisseria meningitidis.
  - Streptococcus pneumoniae.
  - Hemophilus influenzae.
  - Staphylococcus aureus.
  - Listeria monocytogenes–immunocompromised.
  - Escherichia coli.
  - Proteus spp.
  - Klebsiella spp.
  - Citrobacter spp.
  - Enterobacter spp.

Meningococcal and Pneumococcal meningitis – at any age.

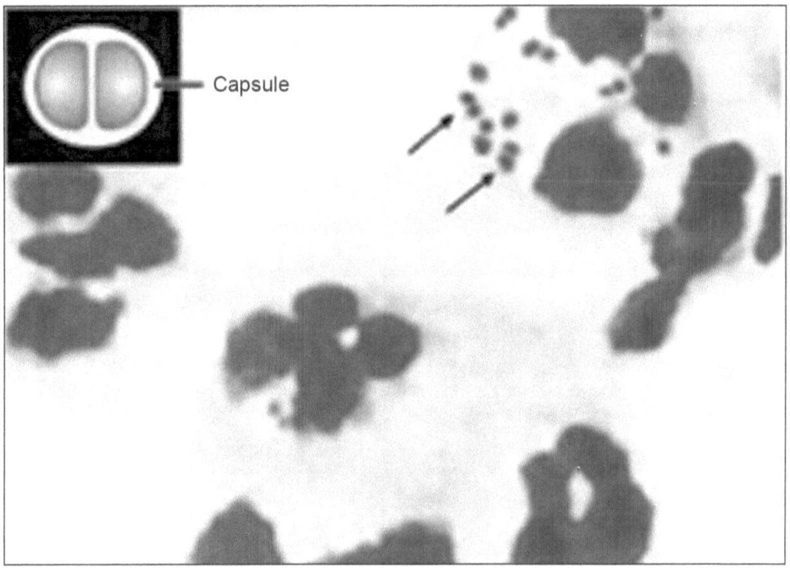

Diplococci

Neisseria Meningitidis

- Capsulated, intracellular, gram-negative diplococci (lens-shaped).
- Non-motile, non-sporing bacteria.
- Classified into 13 serogroups, based on the capsular polysaccharide. most important serogroups causing human infection are A, B, C,Y and W-135.
- Humans are the only natural host for invasive infection.
- Transmission – Droplet inhalation through nasopharynx.
- Meningococcemia – Characterized by fever, hemorrhagic rash, which may lead to disseminated intravascular coagulation and circulatory collapse **(Waterhouse-Friderichsen syndrome).**
- Post meningococcal reactive disease is characterized by fever, arthritis, rash, iritis, pericarditis and polyserositis.

Lab Diagnosis

- **Specimen** – CSF, blood, skin scrapings from the petechial rash, nasopharyngeal swabs.
- Transport medium is Stuart's medium.

- **Gram staining**–Intracellular, gram negative diplococci (lens or half-moon shaped) with abundant polymorphonuclear leucocytes.
- **Culture**–Thayer-Martin agar, New York city agar are selective media.
- **Serology**–Detection of antibodies to capsular antigens.
- **Molecular**–Multiplex PCR.

Treatment

- Drug of choice is Ceftriaxone or cefotaxime. Penicillin can also be used.
- **Chemoprophylaxis** for meningococcal infection–**Rifampicin, ciprofloxacin.**
- **Vaccine prophylaxis**–Polysaccharide vaccines, bivalent (serogroups A and C) or quadrivalent (serogroups A,C,Y, W-135).
- Pseudomonas aeruginosa and E.coli are gram negative bacilli. Streptococcus pneumoniae is a gram positive diplococci.

Ans : (c) Neisseria meningitidis

Ref: *Jawetz, Melnick and Adelerg's Medical Microbiology, 26th Edition*

18. Which of the following common soil transmitted helminthic infection in India which is characterized by eggs in stool shown in the figure?

(a) Ascaris (b) Trichuris

(c) Enterobius (d) Ancylostoma

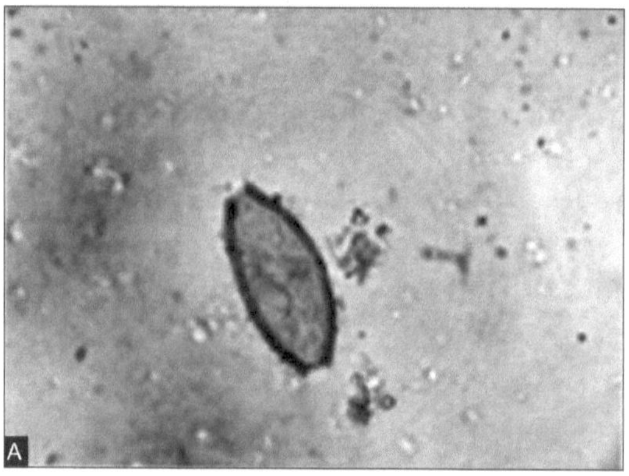

Explanation:

TRICHURIS TRICHIURA

- Commonly called 'whipworm'.
- It is a large intestinal nematode.
- **Egg of Trichuris Trichiura:**
  - Bile stained egg.
  - It is barrel shaped, 50 μm long and 25 μm wide in the middle, with mucus plug at each pole.
  - Contains unsegmented ovum.
  - The egg floats in saturated salt solution.
  - Infective form is the embryonated egg containing rhabditiform larva.

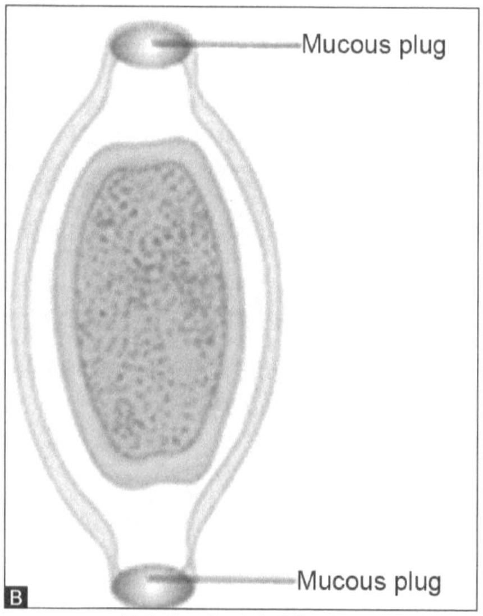

Trichuris trichiura

Ancylostoma Duodenale

- Commonly called 'hookworm'.
- Small intestinal nematode.
- Infective form is third-stage filariform larva.
- **Egg of Ancylostoma duodenale**
  - Non-bile stained.
  - Oval or elliptical, 60 μm by 40 μm.
  - Surrounded by a thin, transparent, hyaline shell membrane.
  - Contains segmented ovum with 4 or 8 blastomeres. There is a clear space between the segmented ovum and the hyaline membrane.
  - Egg floats in saturated salt solution.

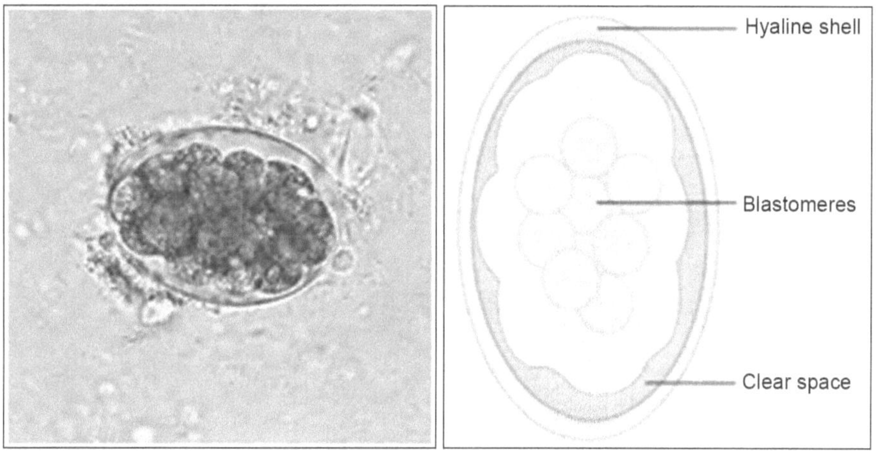

Ancylostoma duodenale

Enterobius Vermicularis

- Commonly called 'pinworm' or 'threadworm' or 'seatworm'.
- Large intestinal nematode.
- **Egg of Enterobius Vermicularis**
  - Non-bile stained.
  - Egg is elongated ovoid, planoconvex in shape, measuring 50 μm by 20 μm.
  - The outer shell is double layered and thick but transparent.
  - Egg contains tadpole shaped coiled embryo.
  - Floats in saturated salt solution.
  - Infective form is embryonated eggs.

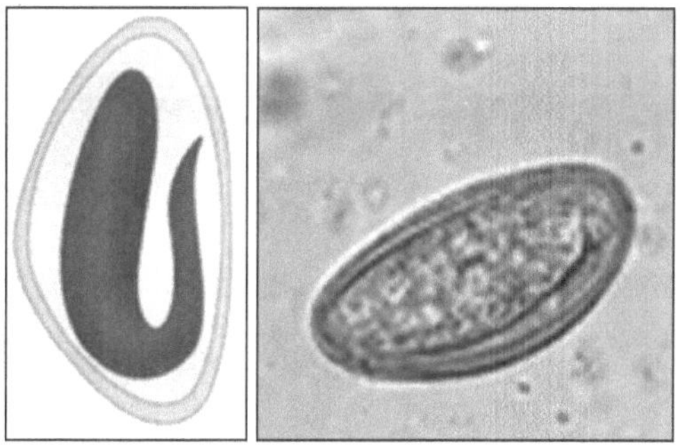

Enterobius vermicularis

Ascaris Lumbricoides

- Commonly called as 'roundworm'. It is the largest nematode.
- Small intestinal nematode.
- Infective form is the embryonated egg.
- **Egg of Ascaris Lumbricoides**
  - 2 types of eggs are passed by the adult worms: fertilised and unfertilised. Fertilised egg is embryonated and develop into infective eggs. Unfertilised eggs are not embryonated and are not infective.
  - **Fertilised egg**
    - Bile stained egg.
    - Round or oval in shape, measuring 60 μm by 40 μm.
- Surrounded by thick, smooth translucent shell with an outer coarsely mammillated albuminous coat. This is called 'corticated egg'. If the outer albuminous coat is absent, it is called 'decorticated egg'.
- It has a large unsegmented ovum, with a crescentic space at either poles.
- Floats in saturated salt solution.
  - **Unfertilised egg**
    - Elliptical in shape.
    - 80 μm by 55 μm in size.
    - Has thinner shell with irregular albuminous coat.
    - Egg has small atrophied ovum.
    - Does not float in saturated salt solution.

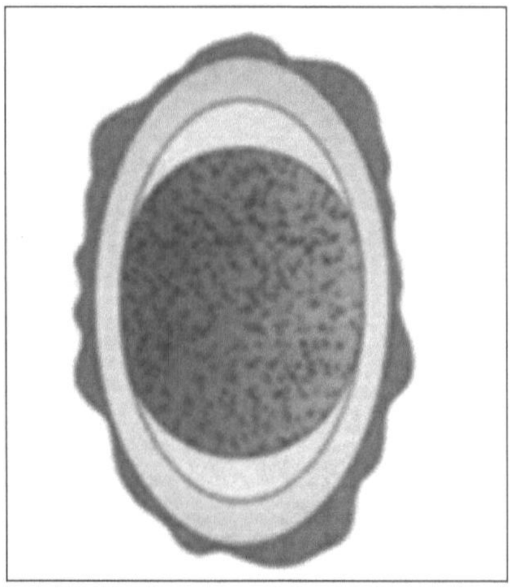

Fertilised corticated egg

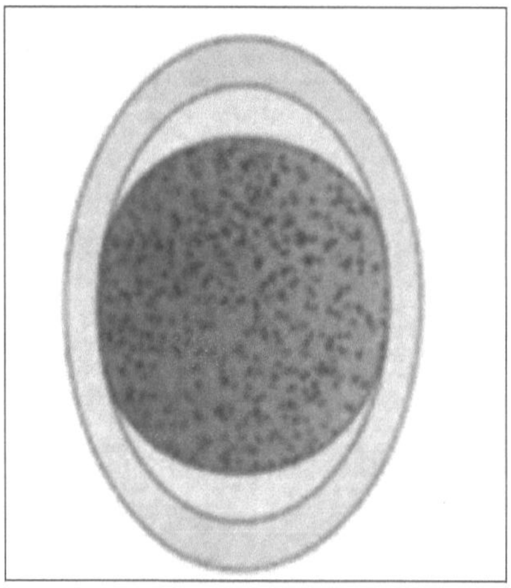

Fertilised decorticated egg

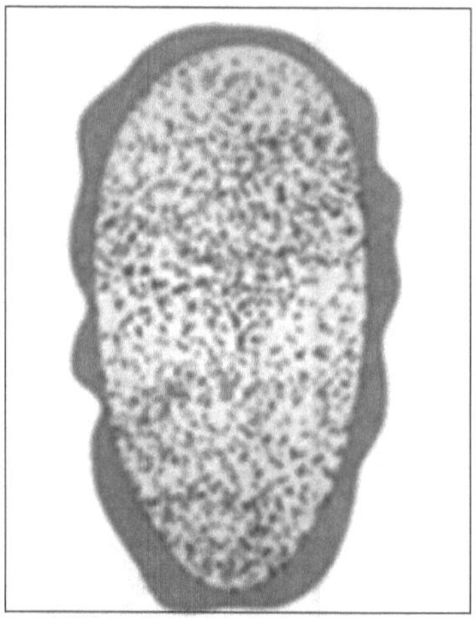

Unfertilised egg

Ans : (b) Trichuris

Ref: *Paniker's Textbook of Medical Parasitology, 8th Edition, Page 177-202*

19. The selective medium for E. coli O157: H7 is:

(a) Sorbitol MacConkey agar
(b) Xylose Lysine Deoxycholate agar
(c) Thiosulphate citrate bile salt sucrose agar
(d) Thayer Martin agar

Explanation:

- Escherichia coli (E.coli) is an actively motile, gram negative bacilli. It is the most common aerobic bacilli in the human intestine.

- **Infections** caused by E.coli are:
  - Urinary tract infection.
  - Diarrhea (6 types):
    - Enteropathogenic E.coli (EPEC).
    - Enterotoxigenic E.coli (ETEC).
    - Enteroinvasive E.coli (EIEC).
    - Enterohemorrhagic E.coli (EHEC).
    - Enteroaggregative E.coli (EAEC).
    - Diffusely adherent E.coli (DAEC).
  - Peritonitis, meningitis, pneumonia and wound infections.
- E.coli has 4 surface antigens:
  - Somatic antigen (O)–lipopolysaccharide, heat stable.
  - Flagellar antigen (H)–heat labile.
  - Capsular antigen (K).
  - Fimbrial antigen.
- Serotyping of E.coli is based on the agglutination with the specific antisera against each surface antigen.
- **TOXINS** produced by E.coli are:
  - **Enterotoxin:** Heat stable, heat labile and verocytotoxin.
  - **Hemolysin.**
  - **Cytotoxic necrotising factor 1.**
  - **Siderophores.**

157: H7 E. coli

- Most common serotype of **enterohemorrhagic E. coli**.
- Produces verocytotoxin or Shiga-like toxin. Acts by inhibiting protein synthesis, by inhibiting 28S subunit of 60S ribosome.
- Characterized by bloody diarrhea without WBCs and no fever.
- Verocytotoxin has predilection to endothelial cells, leading to hemorrhagic colitis and hemolytic uremic syndrome.
- **Diagnosis**
  - Blood agar – Non-hemolytic grey moist colonies (EPEC strains causes beta-hemolysis.
  - MacConkey agar – Circular, moist with smooth pink colonies (lactose fermenting).
- **Special medium**
  - **Sorbitol MacConkey agar**–Does not ferment sorbitol (unlike other E.coli).
  - **Rainbow agar**–Black colonies due to absence of β-glucuronidase.
  - **Xylose Lysine Deoxycholate (XLD) agar**
    - Selective medium for isolation of Salmonella and Shigella from feces.
    - Contains deoxycholate which inhibits most coliforms like E.coli and prevents spreading by Proteus.
  - **Thiosulphate citrate bile salt sucrose agar**
    - Selective medium for Vibrio cholerae.
  - **Thayer Martin agar**
    - Selective medium for Neisseria species.

Ans: (a) Sorbitol MacConkey agar

Ref: *Apurba Sastry, Essentials of Medical Microbiology, 1st Edition, Page 299*

FORENSIC MEDICINE

1. As per Protection of Children from Sexual Offences (POCSO) act, child was brought for age estimation. Wrist X-ray was taken. The maximum age of this wrist joint is:

(a) 4 years (b) 7 years

(c) 10 years (d) 13 years

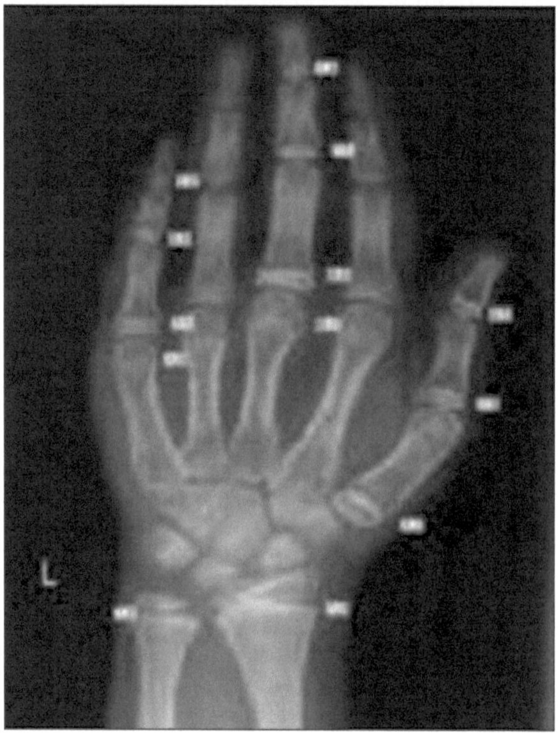

Explanation:

- The ossification centers in carpel bones appear as follows:
  - Capitates 2-3 months.
  - Hamate: 1st years.
  - Triquetrum: 3rd years.
  - Lunate: 4 years.
  - Scaphoid and Trapezoid: 5 years.
  - Trapezium: 6 years.
  - Pisiform: 9-11 years.
- All the carpal bones have appeared except the pisiform bone.
- The age between 6 years and 11 years.
- The minimum age is 7 years and maximum age is 11 years. So 10 years will be the best answer.

Ans. (c) 10 years

Ref: *Essential of Forensic Medicine and Toxicology, KSN Reddy, 33rd Edition, Page 72*

2. In a dead person with tongue swelling, bloated face was noted along with findings shown in the image. What is the probable cause?

(a) Electric burn
(b) Putrefaction
(c) Crocodile burn
(d) Scalds

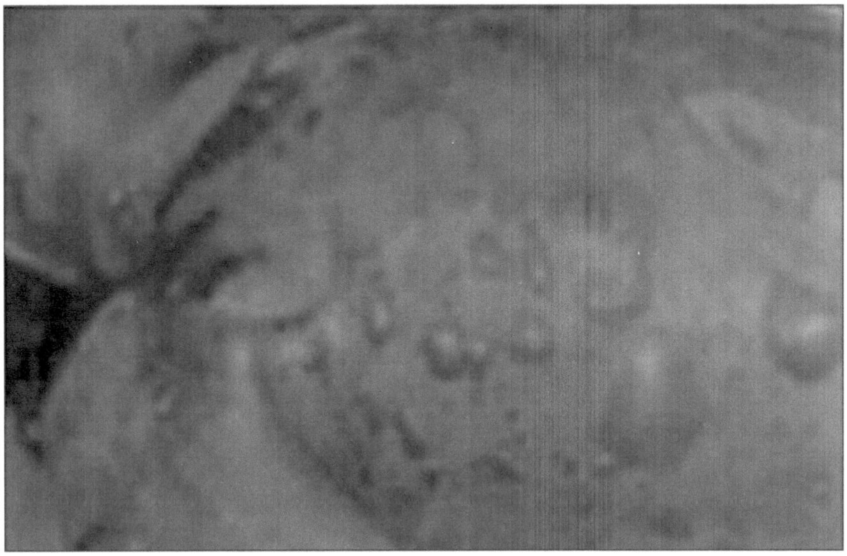

Explanation:

PUTREFACTION

- It is the process by which complex organic body tissue breaks down into simpler inorganic compounds or elements due to the action of saprophytic microorganisms or due to autolysis.
  - **Autolysis:** Without bacterial involvement.
  - **Decomposition:** With bacterial involvement.
- First external sign of putrefaction is the greenish discoloration in right iliac fossa.
- Internally, first site of discoloration in aortic intima and then the under surface of liver.
- **Marbling**: Liner branching pattern on the skin. Most commonly noted in shoulder, root of the limbs, thighs, sides of abdomen, chest and neck region.

Ans: (b) Putrefaction

Ref: *Essential of Forensic Medicine and Toxicology, KSN Reddy, 33rd Edition, Page 165*

3. In the court of law, the act of witness giving false evidence after taking oath is punishable under:

(a) 191 IPC
(b) 192 IPC
(c) 193 IPC
(d) 197 IPC

Explanation:

Perjury:

- A witness who after taking oath or making a solemn affirmation, willfully makes a false statement which he knows or believes to be the false (Sec. 191 IPC and Sec. 344 CrPC).
- Perjury is liable to be prosecuted under Sec. **193 IPC** with imprisonment **upto 7 years** and fine.

Indian Penal Code (1860)

- 191 IPC Perjury.
- 192 IPC Fabricating evidence.
- 193 IPC Punishment for **perjury** (7 years imprisonment).
- 194 IPC Punishment of perjury leading to capital punishment (life imprisonment or 10 years RI).
- 195 IPC Punishment of perjury leading non-capital punishment (life imprisonment or 7 years imprisonment).

False Certificate

- 197 IPC Issuing false certificates.
- 198 IPC Using false certificates.

Other important sections to remember

Murder	Section 300 IPC
Culpable homicide amounting to murder	Sec 299 IPC
Culpable homicide not amounting to murder	Sec 304 IPC
Rash or Negligent homicide	Sec 304-A IPC
Injury	Sec 44 IPC
Punishment of Murder by imprisonment and fine	Sec 302 IPC
Punishment of Murder by life convict (death sentence)	Sec 303 IPC
Attempt to commit suicide	Sec 309 IPC
Dowry Death	Sec 304-B IPC
Rape – Definiton	Sec 375 IPC
Punishment for rape	Sec 376 IPC
Unnatural sexual offence	Sec 377 IPC
Criminal abortion	Sec 312 IPC

Definition of grevious injury comes under section 320 of Indian Penal Code (IPC).

Ans: (c) 193 IPC

Ref: *Essential of Forensic Medicine and Toxicology, KSN Reddy, 33rd Edition, Page 13*

4. The most widely used substance-dependence drug is:

(a) Cannabis
(b) Amphetamine
(c) Heroine
(d) Cocaine

Explanation:

- Dependence causing potential is higher with heroin compared to other drugs.
- Descending order of addictive abuse potential are: Nicotine > Heroine > Cocaine > Alcohol > Cannabis.

Dependence producing drugs				
S. No.	**Drug**	**Physical dependence**	**Psychological dependence**	**Tolerance**
1.	Alcohol	Moderate	Moderate	Mild
2.	Cannabis	Little	Moderate	Mild
3.	Cocaine	Little	Moderate	None
4.	Opioids	Severe	Severe	Severe
5.	Amphetamine	Moderate	Moderate	Severe

Contd.

Contd.

6.	LSD	None	Mild	Mild
7.	Barbiturates	Moderate	Moderate	Severe
8.	Inhalants	Little	Moderate	Mild
9.	Nicotine	Mild	Moderate	Mild
10.	Caffeine	Mild	Moderate	Mild

Ans: (a) Cannabis

Ref: *World Drug Report 2018 by WHO*

5. On voluntary admission, maximum number of days for which a person can be admitted in mental hospital as per Mental Health Care Act 2017 is:

(a) 14 days
(b) 30 days
(c) 60 days
(d) 100 days

Explanation:

- The maximum number of days a person can be admitted on voluntary admission is 30 days, beyond which the approval of the board is necessary.

SALIENT FEATURES OF MHA

Advance Directive

What Does Advance Directive Specify?

- The way the person wishes to be cared for and treated for a mental illness.
- The way the person wishes not to be cared for and treated for a mental illness.
- The individual, he wants to appoint as his nominated representative.

Importance of Advance Directive

- Any person who is not a minor can write advance directive.
- It empowers the patient to choose his/her treatment and appoint a representative to take decision on behalf of patient.
- It is the duty of every psychiatrist to plan treatment, keeping advance directive in mind.
- It will not be applicable at the time of emergency.

Various Rights of Mentally Ill Person (MIP)

- An MIP must have the right of confidentiality.
- Professionals conducting research should take informed consent of mentally ill person and consent from board.
- **Right to appoint a Nominated Representative:** A person shall have the right to appoint a nominated representative to take on his/her behalf, all health related decisions.
- **Right to access mental health care:** A person shall have the right to access to mental health care, treatment by the Government which are affordable, of good quality, in sufficient quantity, available nearby and without any discrimination.
- **Right to free service:** A Person with Mental illness (PMI) living below poverty line, a destitute or a homeless, shall get free treatment at state run or funded health establishments.
- **Right to protection from cruel, inhuman and degrading treatment:** Every PMI shall be protected from cruel, inhuman or degrading treatment in any mental health establishment (MHE).

- **Right to protection:** A PMI shall have protection from all forms of physical, verbal, emotional and sexual abuse.
- **Right to legal aid:** A PMI shall be entitled to receive free legal services to exercise his/her rights available under the Act.

Prohibited Procedures/Practices and Restrictions

- No compulsion to wear uniforms.
- No discrimination.
- **Electroconvulsive Therapy (ECT):** ECT shall not be performed without the use of muscle relaxants and anesthesia. ECT shall not be performed on minors. In exceptional cases, it may be done after getting informed consent of the guardian and prior permission of the Board.
- An MIP has got the right to protect himself /herself from being sterilized.
- **Restriction on Psychosurgery:** Psychosurgery shall not be performed as a treatment for mental illness without obtaining the informed consent of the patient and approval from the Board.
- **Restriction on Physical Restraints:** Physical restrains shall be used sparingly, only when absolutely needed, and are deemed as the least restrictive method.
- Solitary confinement is totally banned.

Miscellaneous Provisions

Attempt to Commit Suicide Not An Offence

- A person who attempts to commit suicide will be presumed to be "suffering from severe stress" and shall not be punished.

Ans: (b) 30 days

Ref: *Mental Health Care Act, 2017*

6. A 5-year-old boy was presented to the OPD by his mother with complaint of pain on the perineal region. On examination of sample taken with nitric acid from his perianal region showed yellow needle-shaped crystals of spermine picrate. What is the test done?

(a) Florence test (b) Takayama's test

(c) Precipitin test (d) Barberio's test

Explanation:

BARBERIO'S TEST

- **Basis:** Detection of Spermine.
- **Procedure:** A few drops of Barberio's reagent when added to spermatic fluid produces crystals of sperm in picrate (needle shaped, rhombic and of yellow color).

Chemical Examination for Seminal Stain

- Barberio's test.
- Florence test.
- Acid Phosphate test.
- Creatine Phosphokinase.
- Immunological method.

Other options:

Test	Used for	Findings
Florence test	• Choline from seminal secretion detected in this method • Florence reagent: 8% W/V solution of Iodine in water containing 5% W/V of Potassium Iodide • Never confirmatory; maximum time false negative	• Dark brown rhombic crystals of choline iodide
Takayama's test	• Confirmatory test for blood	• Pink feathery crystals (Hemochromogen crystal)
Precipitin test	• For race determination (Differencing human blood from other animals)	• Ring of precipitation formed

Semen Characteristics

- Semen is a human body fluid present in human males.
- It is a viscid mucilaginous fluid with faint yellow colour.
- It has characteristic odour called seminal odour.
- Volume is about 3 ml per ejaculate.
- No. of Spermatozoa=**50,000 to 3,50,000** per ml.
- It is a suspension of spermatozoa in seminal plasma.

Semen Consist of the following:

1. Spermatozoa (10%).
2. Seminal Plasma (90%).
3. Epithelial Cell (< 1%).
    - The Spermatozoa is produced in the testis by the process of spermatogenesis.
    - The total length of spermatozoa is about **50 Microns.**
    - It consist of head and tail. The head is flat, oval shaped – **4.6 × 2.6 × 1.6 microns** in dimension.
    - The nucleus, which occupies major portion of the head.
    - The tail portion is responsible for the movement of sperm.
    - The seminal plasma is a mixture of secretion derived from the male accessory reproductive organs like epididymis, seminal vesicles, the prostate, vasa-deferantia, bulbourethral and urethral glands.
    - The **seminal plasma** contains Citric Acid, Ascorbic Acid, Lactic Acid, Fructose, potassium Choline Phosphate, Proteases, free Amino Acids, Ergothioniene, Zinc, Calcium, Spermine, Lipids and Enzymes.

MEDICOLEGAL SIGNIFICANCE OF DETECTION OF SPERM AND SEMEN

Rape, Sodomy (anal intercourse), bestiality (Sexual intercourse with animals), false accusation by a woman, incest (Sexual intercourse in blood relation) and sexual murders.

Methods Applied for Detection of Seminal Stains are Classified as:

1. Physical Examination.
2. Chemical Examination.
3. Microscopic Examination.

Physical Examination: Include Visual Examination. To naked eye seminal stains generally appear translucent or opaque spots, at times with yellowish tint and darker border depending on colour and thickness of substrata, which, if absorbent, also acquire stiffness due to dried semen. On good substrata seminal stains may appear to be fluorescent under ultraviolet light.

CHEMICAL EXAMINATION

Semen pH = 7.4 Alkaline.

The tests used to detect Seminal Stains are:

1. Florence Test.
2. Barberio Test.
3. Acid Phosphatase Test.
4. LDM Isoenzyme Method.
5. Acid Phosphatase Isoenzyme Test.
6. Creatinine in Phosphokinase.
7. Ammonium Molybdate Test (Phosphorus).
8. Semen Specific Glycoprotein (P30) Test.
9. Enzyme-linked immunosorbent assay (ELISA), the SEMA® assay, for a seminal vesicle-specific antigen (SVSA).

Florence Test

Basis: **Choline** is detected in this method.

- The stain is extracted by 1% hydrochloric acid and a drop is placed on a glass slide.
- A drop of Florence solution (Postassium iodine, iodine and water) is allowed to run under the cover slip.
- If semen is present, **dark-brown needle shaped crystals** of **choline iodide** appear immediately.
- They are rhombic crystals resembling haemin.

Berberio's Test

Basis: Detection of **Spermine**

- A saturated aqueous or alcoholic solution of picric acid when added to spermatic fluid, produces yellow needle shaped rhombic crystals of spermine picrate.

Acid Phosphatase Spot Test

Modified Fishman and Lerner's Method

- The prostatic secretion element of seminal fluid contains a very much higher percentage of acid phosphatase.
- This test is conclusive in the absence of demonstrable sperms or in aspermia.

LDH Isoenzyme Method

- Detection of **Spermatozoa.**
- Seminal stains are extracted with 1 ml of water. 0.25 ml of clear extract is mixed with 0.25 ml of 40% W/V of sucrose. 0.1 ml of this mixture is subjected to vertical polyacryl amide gel electrophoresis.
- Electrophoresis is carried out in refrigerators for 150 minutes using a current of 5 m A Isoenzyme bands are revealed by staining.
- This method gives a specific biochemical detection of spermatozoa in semen in the presence of Vaginal Fluid, Blood, Nasal Secretion, Saliva and Urine.

Acid Phosphatase Isoenzyme Method

- **Procedure:** Seminal stains are extracted with water and is used in polyacrylmile gel Electrphoretic method followed by staining with methyl belliferyl.
- Phosphate reagent enable the seminal acid phosphatase to be distinguished from that of other substance like vaginal secretions.

- The method is sufficiently specific and applicable to semen derived from normal, oligospermic azoospermic and vasectemized individuals.

Advantages:

1. LDH isoenzyme is stable in stains for over 4 weeks.
2. Isoenzyme pattern of human is different from that of animal.
3. Positive results are obtained in large number of cases.
4. Can differentiate from vaginal secretions on pattern of bands.

Creatinine Phosphokinase:

Basis: Detection of creatinine phosphokinase.

Normal seminal fluid contains high levels of CPK - 385 - 14000 U of CPK/W.

Diagnosis: >400V of CPK / ml.

Adv: Enzyme is stable and can be demonstrated in old stains of six months.

Ammonium Molybdate Test:

For semen stains, detect presence of phosphorous.

Glycoprotein P30: This test has replaced the quantitative analysis for acid phosphatase.

MHS-S1 is also positive and a highly reliable test for semen.

Serological typing of the semen is possible by **precipitin method**.

Microscopic Examination:

The microscopic detection of the seminal stains is based in morphology of spermatozoa.

Microscopic detection of spermatozoa. Cloth pieces from different stains are taken in 0.5 ml of 0.01 N HCL in small test tubes placed in a beaker containing water. After sonication for 5 minutes the extracts and the cloth pieces are transferred to separate microscope slides and cloth pieces delicately teased with a needle. Threads are removed and the residual liquid is gently evaporated to dryness. Residue obtained is stained hematoxylin and eosin.

Fluorescence Microscopy:

- Is also used for detection of spermatozoa.
- It is based on the principle that Y chromosome is fluorescent to quinacrine.
- With this method it is possible to detect both intact spermatozoa as well as the disconnected heads.

Ans: (d) Barberio's test

Ref: *Essential of Forensic Medicine and Toxicology, KSN Reddy, 33rd Edition, Page 434*

7. The onus of proof in civil negligence case against a doctor lies with:

(a) Doctor (b) Patient

(c) Police not below sub-inspector rank (d) Judicial Magistrate

Explanation:

- Burden of proof in **civil negligence** is on the **patient**.
- Each of the four elements (duty, dereliction, direct causation and damage) should be proved.
- Burden of proof lies on the **doctor** in case of **contributory negligence** and **Resipsa loquitur.**

Note: Resipsa Loquitur means evidence speaks for itself.

Difference Between Civil and Criminal Negligence

Trait	Civil Negligence	Criminal Negligence
Offence	No specific or clear violation of law needs to be proved	Must have specifically violated a particular criminal law in question
Negligence	Simple absence of care and skill	Gross negligence, inattention or lack of competency
Conduct of Physician	It is compared to a generally accepted simple standard of professional conduct	Not compared to a single test
Consent for act	Good defence; cannot recover damages	Not a defence; can be prosecuted
Trial by	Civil court	Criminal court
Evidence	Strong evidence is sufficient	Guilt should be proved beyond doubt
Punishment	Liable to pay damages	Imprisonment

Ans: (b) Patient

Ref: *Essential of Forensic Medicine and Toxicology, KSN Reddy, 33rd Edition, Page 35*

8. In an exhumed body which of the following poisons can be detected?

(a) Lead (b) Mercury

(c) Arsenic (d) Cadmium

Explanation:

Arsenic Poisoning

- Interferes with cellular respiration by combining with the sulphydryl groups of mitochondrial enzymes.
- Affects pyruvate oxidase and phosphatases.

Clinical Features

- Sweet metallic taste.
- Burning colicky abdominal pain.
- Purging.
- Tenesmus.
- Stools are bloody dark coloured, foul smelling.
- Stools become colourless and odourless in late stages (Rice watery stool).
- Garlicky odour of breath and feces.

Other Features

- Fatty liver.
- Nephritis.
- Increased vascular permeability.
- Ventricular tachycardia.
- Ventricular fibrillation.
- Peripheral neuropathy – **Stocking glove** distribution.
- **Fatal dose**: 0.1 – 0.2 Arsenic trioxide.
- **Fatal period**: 1 – 2 days.

Treatment

- Emetics are not recommended.
- Stomach wash with warm water and milk.
- Freshly prepared hydrated ferric oxide: Converts toxic arsenic to nontoxic ferric oxide.
- BAL.
- Penicillamine.
- DMSA.
- Castor oil or Magnesium sulphate decreases intestinal absorption.

Postmortem Appearance:

- **Raindrop** type of skin pigmentation.
- **Aldrich Mees** lines in nails.
- **Red velvety stomach** mucosa.

Mercury Poisoning:

- Acid metallic taste.
- Hoarse voice.
- Greyish white coating of tongue.
- Blood-stained stool.
- Circulatory collapse.
- Necrosis of jaw.
- Membranous.
- Colitis.
- Proximal renal tubular necrosis.
- **Acrodynia (Acro-Limbs Odynia-Pain)** is seen in mercury poisoning (also known as **Pink's Disease**).

  It is characterized by pain, swelling and parasthesia of limbs.
- **Mimimata disease**—Contamination of fish with mercury, at a place called Minimate Bay in Japan.
- **Chronic Poisoning (Hydrargyrism):**

  The symptoms are salivation, sore mouth and throat, fine tremors of the tongue, hands, arms, anemia.
- **Shaking palsy** is associated with Hg poisoning.

  Mercurial tremors are also called **Hatter's shakes or glass blower's shake or Danbury Tremors.**
- **Mercurial erethism** is seen in persons working with mercury in mirror manufacturing firms. Erethism is characterized by shyness, timidity, irritability, loss of confidence, mental depression, loss of memory and insomnia (Psychological symptoms).
- **Mercuria lentis** is a peculiar eye change due to brownish deposit of mercury through the cornea on the anterior lens capsule (**Brown-Malt Reflex**). It is bilateral and has no effect on visual acuity.

NAMED FEATURES IN METAL POISONING

- **Mercury**
  - Minamata disease.
  - Erethism.
  - Danberry tremors/Hatters shakes/Glass blower shakes.
  - Acrodynia (Pink disease).

- Mad Hatter syndrome.

- **Lead**
  - Saturnine gout.
  - Basophilic stippling.
  - Burtonian line.
  - Facial pallor.
  - Food drop (Lead palsy).
- **Copper**
  - Chalcosis.
  - Pytalism.
  - Golden hair.
  - Kayser-Fleischer ring.
- **Cadmium**
  - Bony pains due to osteomalacia (Itai-Itai disease).

Ans: (c) Arsenic

Ref: *Essential of Forensic Medicine and Toxicology, KSN Reddy, 33rd Edition, Page 541*

9. Magnan's symptoms are associated with which poisoning event?

(a) Cannabis (b) Cocaine

(c) Alcohol (d) Opium

Explanation:

- **Magnan's symptoms** also called **Cocaine bugs** (feeling of insect crawling under the skin).
- **Other features in cocaine addicts:**
  - Ulceration of nasal septum due to sniffing.
  - Cocainism → Cocaine habit.
  - **Cocainomania:** C/c abusers tolerate up to 10 gm/day.
- **Antidote for cocaine poisoning:** Aryl nitrate.

ACUTE COCAINE INTOXICATION

2 Clinical Stages:

(a) *Stage of Excitement*

- Hyperthermia (Cocaine fever).
- Intracranial bleed.
- Paresthesia.

(b) *Stage of Depression*

- Arrhythmias.
- Respiratory failure.
- Cardiac failure.

Complications

- Convulsions.

- Headache.
- Ischemic/Hemorrhagic stroke.
- Subarachnoid hemorrhage.

Cocaine Addiction / Chronic Poisoning / Cocainism

- Blackening of tongue and teeth.
- Ulceration and perforation of nasal septum.
- Magnan symptoms/formication/Cocaine bugs: Feeling of bugs/small insects creeping under the skin–a form of tactile hallucination.
- Euphoria followed by depression.
- Alcohol dependence.
- Hyperactivity.
- Loss of libido.
- Impotence in males.
- Gynecomastia.

Other Options:

- **Cannabis**: Hashish insanity, run amok.
- **Opium**: Short stage of excitement followed by stupor and coma.

Ans: (b) Cocaine

Ref: *Essential of Forensic Medicine and Toxicology, KSN Reddy, 33rd Edition, Page 603*

10. Tattoo marks were not visible during autopsy even though a relative had informed the presence of a tattoo. Which site should be checked next in this situation?

(a) Skin
(b) Blood vessel
(c) Liver
(d) Regional lymph node

Explanation:

Tattooing

- During the time of autopsy, the faded tattoo mark made visible by rubbing, UV light or burning or magnifying lens.
- The **regional lymph nodes** near a tattoo mark shows a deposit of a pigment in dead bodies.
- Infrared photography makes old tattoos readily visible.
- When tattoo marks are obscure by decomposition or mummification, they can be visualized by treating the area with 3% H_2O_2 which temporarily removes the products of decomposition.
- **Pigments/Dyes Used in Tattooing:**
  - Prussian Blue (Ferric ferrocyanide).
  - Indian Ink.
  - Chromic Acid (green).
  - Vermillion (Lead tetroxide or mercuric sulphide).
  - Indigo and Cobalt.
- Tattoo may fade if pigments are introduced in the subepithelial level, or on exposed parts of the body.

Ans: (d) Regional lymph node

Ref: *Essential of Forensic Medicine and Toxicology, KSN Reddy, 33rd Edition, Page 92*

11. In a rape incident occurred in a child of 5 years the hymen is:

(a) Ruptured, because it is thin
(b) Ruptures because it is situated superficially
(c) Don't rupture, because it is situated deeply
(d) Don't rupture, because it is thick and elastic

Explanation:

- In child, the hymen is usually intact as it is situated deep and underdeveloped.

Rape in Children:

- In young children there are few or no signs of general violence, for the child usually has no idea of what is happening.
- The hymen is deeply situated, and as the vagina is very small, it is impossible for the penetration of the adult organ to take place.
- As such, the hymen is usually intact and there may be little redness and tenderness of the labia.

SECTION 375 IN THE INDIAN PENAL CODE, 1860 DEFINES RAPE

375. Rape – A man is said to commit "rape" who, has sexual intercourse with a woman under circumstances falling under any of the six following descriptions:

(a) Against her will.

(b) Without her consent.

(c) With her consent, when her consent has been obtained by putting her or any person in whom she is interested in fear of death or of hurt.

(d) With her consent, when the man knows that he is not her husband, and that her consent is given because she believes that he is another man to whom she is or believes herself to be lawfully married.

(e) With her consent, when, at the time of giving such consent, by reason of unsoundness of mind or intoxication or the administration by him personally or through another of any stupefying or unwholesome substance, she is unable to understand the nature and consequences of that to which she gives consent.

(f) With or without her consent, when she is under sixteen years of age.

What Constitutes Rape?

Penetration is sufficient to constitute the sexual intercourse necessary to the offence of rape.

Exception – Sexual intercourse by a man with his **own wife**, the wife not being **under 15 years** of age, is not rape.

Ans: (c) Don't rupture, because it is situated deeply

Ref: *Essential of Forensic Medicine and Toxicology, KSN Reddy, 33rd Edition, Page 421*

PREVENTIVE AND SOCIAL MEDICINE

1. Mission Indradhanush is for:

(a) Non-communicable diseases
(b) Universal immunization
(c) Family planning
(d) Safe water and sanitation

Explanation:

MISSION INDRADHANUSH

- **Launched** by Ministry of Health and Family Welfare on 25th December 2014.
- **Goal:** To ensure that all children under the age of 2 years are fully immunized with eight vaccine preventable diseases (Diphtheria, Whooping cough, Tetanus, Polio, Measles, Severe form of Childhood Tuberculosis, Hepatitis B, Meningitis and Pneumonia caused by Hemophilus influenza type B) and also pregnant women are immunized against tetanus.
- **Aim:** To expand coverage of full immunization from **65% to at least 90%** children of the country and sustain the same by 2020.
- **Focussed on high risk population** with traditionally low coverage such as slum dwellers, nomadic populations and migrant families living in brick kiln and construction sites. Also targets **underserved areas** with inadequate health services, migrant populations, recent measles/diphtheria outbreaks or high drop out rates.
- It was undertaken in **4 phases**:
  - **First phase** (started on 7th April 2015): Immunization activities in 201 high focus districts in 28 states which accounted for nearly 50% of all unvaccinated or partially vaccinated children in the country.
  - **Phase II** (launched on October 2015): Immunization activities in 352 districts including 279 mid priority districts, 33 from North East states and 40 districts from phase one where large number of missed out children were detected.
  - **Phase III** (launched on 7th April 2016): Covered 216 districts, adding 41 new districts and dropping 26 districts. In addition to immunization of children under 2 years of age, it focussed on children aged 5 years for increasing DPT booster coverage.
  - **Phase IV** (launched in 2017): 254 districts were covered.

As the goal of immunization coverage of more than 90% in newborn was **not achieved, Intensified Mission Indradhanush** was started in **December 2018** to cover all left outs and drop outs in select districts and urban cities with low immunization coverage.

Ans: (b) Universal immunization

Ref: *DK Taneja's Health Policies Programmes in India, 16th Edition, Page 160*

2. Maximum work hours for person including overtime under the Factories Act:

(a) 48 hours
(b) 50 hours
(c) 60 hours
(d) 100 hours

Explanation:

Factories Act 1948

- Amended in 1976 and again in 1987 and implemented in 1990.
- Applied to whole country except Jammu and Kashmir.

- The Act defines factory as an establishment employing 10 or more workers where power is used, and 20 or more workers where power is not used.
- Make provision especially on health, safety and welfare of the workers (waste disposal, elimination of dust and fumes, spittoons, cleanliness, control of temperature, supply of drinking water and max limit of lifting weight).
- Each worker should have a minimum of 500 Cu.ft of space (350 for factories before 1948) at height more than 14 ft.
- Appointment of one Safety Officer for >1000 workers.
- Appointment of one crèche >30 women workers.
- Appointment of one Welfare Officer for >500 workers.
- Prohibits employment of children <14 years age.
- Adolescent (15-18) employee is allowed to work only between 6 am and 7 pm.
- Max hours of work 48 per week, not exceeding 9 hours/day with rest at least half hour after 5 hours (4 and half for adolescent) of continuous work.
- The total no. of hours of work in a week including overtime shall not exceed 60.
- After 1 year services, besides weekly holiday, every worker will be entitled to leave of one day for every 20 days with wages and one day for every 15 days with wages for children.

Ans: (a) 48 hours

Ref: *Park Textbook of Preventive and Social Medicine, 25th Edition, Page 876*

3. The difference between the incidence in exposed and non-exposed group is best given by:

(a) Relative risk (b) Attributable risk

(c) Population attributable risk (d) Odds ratio

Explanation:

- Attributable risk (AR) is defined as the proportion of disease incidence (or disease risk) that can be attributed to a specific exposure. For example, how much of the lung cancer risk experienced by smokers can be attributed to smoking?
- AR is important in clinical practice and public health, because it addresses a question: How much of the risk (incidence) of disease can we hope to prevent if we are able to eliminate exposure to the agent in question?

Thus, the incidence of a disease that is attributable to the exposure in the exposed group can be calculated as follows:

(Incidence in exposed group) – (Incidence in non-exposed group)

We can express the attributable risk as the proportion:

$$\frac{\textbf{(Incidence in exposed group) – (Incidence in non-exposed group)}}{\textbf{Incidence in the exposed group}}$$

Comparison Between Relative Risk and Attributable Risk:

- The relative risk (Incidence in exposed/Incidence in non-exposed) and the odds ratio (odds that a case was exposed/odds that a control was exposed = ad/bc) measures the **strength of association**, which is an important consideration in deriving a **causal inference**.
- The attributable risk is a measure of how much of the disease risk is attributable to a certain exposure. Thus, it answers the question of **how much disease can be prevented** if we have an effective means of **eliminating the exposure** in question.

Ans: (b) Attributable risk

Ref: *Book Epidemiology, Leon Gordis, 5th Edition, Page 230-237*

4. A researcher wants to prove relation between chronic obstructive pulmonary disease (COPD) and smoking. He collected patient's record from government hospital and record of cigarette sale from finance and taxation department. This is an example of which study design?

(a) Cross sectional
(b) Case control study
(c) Ecological study
(d) Operations research

Explanation:

A study that compares two groups of people: Those with the disease or condition under study (cases) and a very similar group of people who do not have the disease or condition (controls). *(National Institute of Health, USA)*

- Both exposure and outcome (disease) have occurred before the start of the study.
- The study should be conducted for chronic and rare diseases.
- The study proceeds backwards from effect to cause.
- It uses a control or comparison group to support or refute an inference.
- Design of case control study:

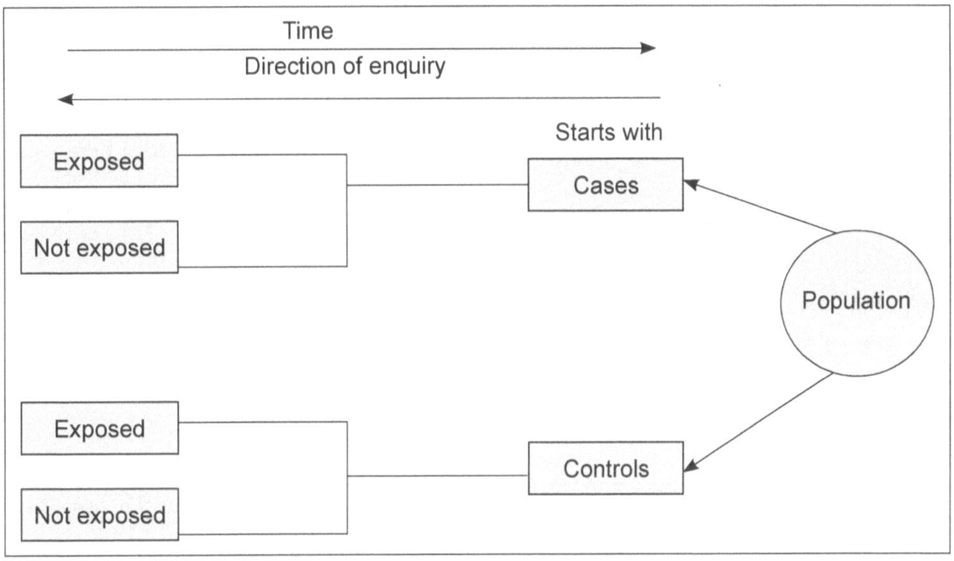

Four basic steps in conducting a case control study:

1. Selection of cases and controls.
2. Matching.
3. Measurement of exposure, and
4. Analysis and interpretation.

Selection of cases: Involve two specifications:

(i) ***Diagnostic criteria*:** The diagnostic criteria of the disease and the stage of disease must be specified before the study is undertaken.

Once the diagnostic criteria are established, they should not be altered or changed till the study is over

(ii) ***Eligibility criteria*:** It is always advisable to take the incident cases since the prevalent cases may be more related to survival with the disease rather than the development of disease.

Examples: Hospital based, population based.

Selection of Controls: Criteria

- Comparability is more important than representativeness in the selection of controls.
- The control should be at risk of the disease.

- The control should resemble the case in all respects except for the presence of disease.
- *Example:* Hospital based, population based, Neighbourhood control, best friends/sibling controls.

Number of Controls

- *Large study* – Cases: Control – 1:1.
- *Small study* – Cases: Control – 1:2, 1:3, 1:4.

  Number of controls, increases the power of study but maximum up to 4 controls.
- Use of multiple controls for generalization.

Matching: Process by which we select controls in such a way that they are similar to cases with regard to certain pertinent selected variables (e.g., age) which are known to influence the outcome of disease and which if not adequately matched for comparability, could distort or confound the results.

Two types:

- Individual matching (matched pairs).
- Group matching (frequency matching).

Advantages of Matching

- Eliminate the effect of confounding.
- Sampling convenience.
- Improves study efficiency.

Disadvantages of Matching

- Time consuming.
- Expensive.
- Matched variables cannot be examined in the study.
- Overmatching may be possible.

Measurement of Exposure

- Interviews.
- Questionnaires.
- Studying past records of cases such as hospital and employment records.
- Ruling out bias or systematic error.

Analysis

1. **Exposure rates** among cases and controls to suspected factor.
2. Estimation of disease risk associated with exposure (**Odds ratio**).

	Cases	Controls	Total
Smokers	33 (a)	55 (b)	88 (a+b)
Non-smokers	2 (c)	27 (d)	29 (c+d)
Total	35 (a+c)	82 (b+d)	N = a+b+c+d

Exposure Rates

A. Cases = a/(a+c) = 33/(33+2) = 94.2%.

B. Controls = b/(b+d) = 55/(55+27) = 67%.

Odds Ratio: Measure of strength of association between risk factors and outcome.

- Odds ratio means chance, i.e., known as the cross-products ratio.
- $$\textbf{Odds} = \frac{\textbf{the chances of something happening}}{\textbf{the chances of it } \textbf{\textit{not}} \textbf{ happening}}$$

OR = ad/bc

OR = 33 × 27/2 × 55

OR = 8.1

Interpretation: Smokers showed a risk of having lung cancer 8.1 times than that of non-smoker or smokers are 8.1 times more likely to develop lung cancer than non-smokers.

- **OR = 1 -** the odds of exposure are the same for cases and controls, implying that there was no association of exposure with diseases.
- **OR > 1 -** cases have higher odds of exposure than controls, implying that the exposure was risky.
- **OR < 1 -** cases have lower odds of exposure than controls, implying that the exposure was protective.

BIAS IN A CASE CONTROL STUDY

Definition of Bias: Any systematic error in the design, conduct, or analysis of a study that results in mistaken estimates of the effect of the exposure on disease.

- Types of bias in case control studies:
  - Selection bias.
  - Information bias.
  - Confounding bias.

SELECTION BIAS

a. **Berksonian Bias:** The probability of admission to hospital or detection of the outcome (disease) may be more among the cases simply because of the exposure.
b. **Selection of Inappropriate Cases or Controls:** Cases or controls who do not have adequate chance of exposure.
c. **Self-selection Bias:** Patients who are admitted to a particular hospital and hence taken as cases may be systematically very different from most of the patients with the disease but who are not admitted to that hospital, as regards the exposure status.
d. **Survivorship Bias:** Case control study generally takes the patients who are living. Cases who have died are generally not taken and these may be systematically very different from living case as regards the exposure status.
e. **Selection of Wrong Control Group:** Controls who are not from the same source population from where the cases have come.

INFORMATION BIAS

Occurs due to:

- Imperfect definitions of study variables, e.g.: Tonsillitis.
- Flawed data collection procedures, e.g.: If we ask about anxiety.

2 types:

1. **Recall bias:** Cases who are suffering from a disease are likely to recall much more as regards their exposure, e.g., congenital malformation with prenatal infections (Rubella infection).
2. **Interviewer bias:** When interviewer is not blinded or knows case status of subjects.

Solution: Blinding of interviewer as to case status and equal interview time for all participants.

CONFOUNDING BIAS

When a measure of the effect of an exposure on risk is distorted because of the association of exposure with other factors that influence the outcome.

Confounding Factor: Is one which is associated with both exposure and disease, and is distributed unequally in study and control groups.

- E.g.: Alcohol and Esophageal Ca; confounding factor–smoking.
- **Solution: Randomization, Restriction, Matching, Stratification, Regression.**

Advantages of Case Control Studies

- Relatively easy to carry out.
- Rapid and inexpensive (compared with cohort studies).

- Require comparatively few subjects.
- Particularly suitable to investigate rare diseases or diseases about which little is known.
- No risk to subjects.
- Allows the study of several different etiological factors (e.g., smoking, physical activity and personality characteristics in myocardial infarction).
- Risk factors can be identified. Rational prevention and control programmes can be established.
- No attrition problems, because case control studies do not require follow-up of individuals into the future.
- Ethical problems minimal.

Disadvantages of Case Control Studies

- Problem of bias relies on memory or past records, the accuracy of which may be uncertain; validation of information obtained is difficult or sometimes impossible.
- Selection of an appropriate control group may be difficult.
- Cannot measure incidence, and can only estimate the relative risk and odds ratio.
- Do not distinguish between causes and associated factors.
- Not suited to the evaluation of therapy or prophylaxis of disease.
- Representativeness of cases and controls.

Ans: (b) Case control study

Ref: *Park Textbook of Preventive and Social Medicine, 25th Edition, Page 79-82*

5. Blood bags are discarded in:

(a) Yellow category
(b) Red category
(c) White category
(d) Blue category

Explanation:

According to BMW Management Rules 2016

Schedule I, Part I: Biomedical wastes, categories and their segregation, collection, treatment, processing and disposal options:

Category	Type of bag/container used	Type of waste	Treatment/disposal options
Yellow 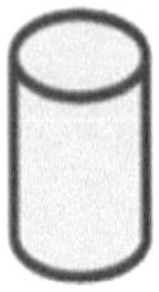	Non-chlorinated plastic bags	Human anatomical waste Animal anatomical waste Soiled waste Expired or discarded medicines Chemical waste Chemical liquid waste Discarded linen, mattresses, beddings contaminated with blood or body fluids Microbiology, biotechnology and other clinical laboratory waste	Incineration/plasma pyrolysis/ deep burial
Red 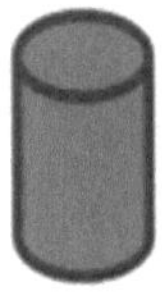	Non-chlorinated plastic bags or containers	Contaminated waste (recyclable) tubing, bottles, intravenous tubes and sets, catheters, urine bags, syringes (without needles and fixed needle syringes) and gloves	Autoclaving/microwaving/ hydroclaving and then sent for recycling. Not to be sent to landfill

Contd.

Contd.

White 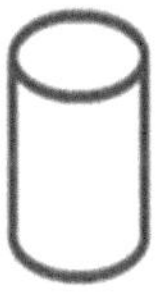	Puncture, leak, tamper proof containers (Translucent)	Waste sharps including Metals: Needles, syringes with fixed needles, needles from needle tip cutter or burner, scalpels, blades or any other contaminated sharp object that may cause puncture and cuts. This includes both used, discarded and contaminated metal sharps	Autoclaving or dry heat sterilisation followed by shredding or mutilation or encapsulation
Blue 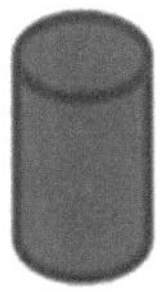	Cardboard boxes with blue coloured marking	Glassware: Broken or discarded and contaminated glass including medicine vials and ampoules except those containing cytotoxic wastes Metallic body implants	Disinfection or autoclaving/ microwaving hydroclaving and then sent for recycling

Yellow Bag:

Expired or discarded medicines: Pharmaceutical waste like antibiotics, cytotoxic drugs including all items contaminated with cytotoxic drugs along with glass or plastic ampules, vials etc.

Chemical waste: Chemicals used in production of biological and used or discarded disinfectants.

Chemical liquid waste: Liquid waste generated due to use of chemicals in production of biological and used or discarded disinfectants, silver X-ray film developing liquid, infected secretions and body fluids, liquid from floor cleaning and house-keeping activities etc.

Microbiological, biotechnology and other clinical laboratory waste: Blood bags, laboratory cultures, specimens of microorganisms, live or attenuated vaccines, residual toxins, dishes and devices used for cultures.

Schedule I, Part 2

- Non-chlorinated plastic bags shall be used for the storage and transportation of biomedical wastes, as per Bureau of Indian Standards (BIS).
- For chemical treatment 10% sodium hypochlorite having 30% residual chlorine for 20 minutes or any other equivalent chemical reagent as given in Schedule III.
- Chemical treatment before incineration is required only for microbiological and potentially infectious waste.
- Dead fetus before age of viability (as per MTP Act 1971) can be viewed as human anatomical waste and transported in yellow bag for disposal along with a copy of MTP certificate issued by competent authority.
- The hub of syringes should be cut, and needles should be either destroyed or placed in puncture proof container.
- **Schedule II: Standards for Treatment and Disposal**

Standards for:

- Incinerators.
- Waste autoclave.
- Liquid waste.
- Microwaving.
- Deep burial:
  - Waste treatment facility should be available within a distance of seventy-five kilometer.
  - Occupier shall hand over segregated waste to common biomedical waste treatment facility.
  - The biomedical waste shall be segregated into containers or bags at the point of generation.

- The Occupier or Operator of a common biomedical waste treatment facility shall maintain a record of recyclable wastes.

Schedule – IV Part A: Label for BMW Container/Bags

BIOHAZARD SYMBOL

BIOHAZARD

CYTOTOXIC HAZARD SYMBOL

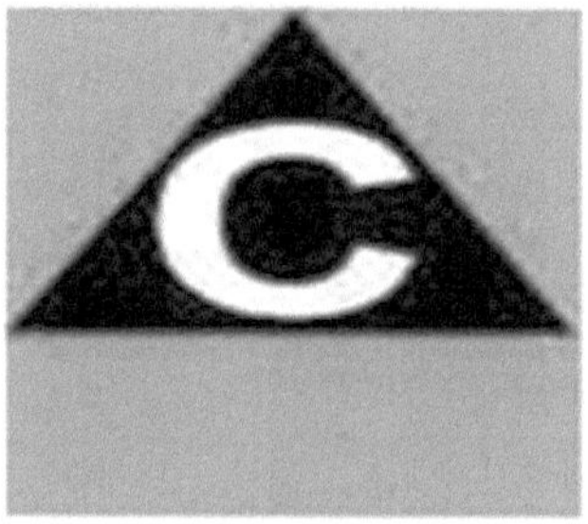

CYTOTOXIC

HANDLE WITH CARE

Note: Label shall be non-washable and prominently visible.

Ans: (a) Yellow category

Ref: *Park Textbook of Preventive and Social Medicine, 25th Edition, Page 852-854*

6. Liquid chemical waste is discarded in:

(a) Yellow category (b) Red category

(c) Blue category (d) White category

Explanation:

Same explanation as previous question.

Ans: (a) Yellow category

Ref: *Park Textbook of Preventive and Social Medicine, 25th Edition, Page 852-854*

7. Monetary benefit is measured in:

(a) Program budgeting system (b) Network analysis

(c) Cost effective analysis (d) Cost benefit analysis

Explanation:

Economic evaluation: The comparative analysis of alternative courses of action in terms of both their costs and consequences. Methods of economic evaluation are:

a. In monetary units: Cost-benefit analysis
b. In natural unit: Cost-effectiveness analysis
c. In units of cardinal utility: Cost-utility analysis
d. Only costs are compared: Cost-marginal analysis

a. Cost benefit analysis: Assesses all effects, including health effects, in monetary units.

- The main objective of cost benefit analysis is to obtain maximum benefit from the resources available.
- Benefits arising out of health programmes are the desired effects of the programme like the reduction

in mortality, morbidity, and control or eradication of a disease. Efforts have been made to estimate the cost of human morbidity and mortality.

- E.g., A cost benefit analysis of the **intensified campaign against smallpox in India** during the period July 1973 to December 1975 has been shown to give a **net benefit** of about Rs. 1058 million and **eradication** of smallpox in yearly saving of about Rs. 728 million.

Disadvantage: It is difficult to measure the clinical results in monetary terms and thus can ignore many intangible but very important benefits, e.g., Relief of anxiety.

It is expressed as "cost benefit ratio" (CBR), calculated as:

$$\text{CBR} = \frac{\text{Costs in monetary terms}}{\text{Benefits in monetary terms}}$$

For any intervention, CBR less than 1 is accepted.

Net benefit = Benefits in unit of money – Cost in units of money > 0

b. Cost effectiveness analysis (CEA):

- The costs are expressed in monetary units and the results are expressed in nonmonetary units like years of life gained, hospital days prevented.
- It is the most commonly applied form of economic analysis and is frequently used in drug therapy.

c. Cost utility analysis (CUO):

- The costs are expressed in monetary units and the benefit is measured in nonmonetary units but utility adjusted outcome, the quality-adjusted life years (QALY).
- It combines the life expectancy and quality of life. If quality of life is an important aspect of therapy, this form of analysis should be chosen.

d. Cost minimization analysis (CMA):

- It compares only the cost of different intervention assuming to provide equal benefits.
- It is a partial evaluation because only the costs are compared not the benefits, e.g., Generic drug versus branded equivalent.

	Investment	Advantage	Result
Cost benefit	Money	Money	Cost : benefit ratio
Cost effectiveness	Money	Services provided-life saved, disability avoided, blood pressure reduced, etc.	Cost per unit of advantage (e.g. cost per life saved)
Cost utility	Money	Multiple effects (quality as well as quantity) – money and/or life saved	Quality adjusted life year (QALY), Disability adjusted life year (DALY), etc.

Network Analysis:

- It is a type of Mathematical Management Technique for unraveling organizational complexity.
- It is a graphical representation of all operations and activities to be completed in order to reach an end objective.
- First, entire project or program is broken into small events or activities.
- Then all the activities are arranged into logical sequence and relation between all activities is described.
- A network consists of **nodes** that represent– agent, programs, knowledge, tasks, resources or other entities.
- Nodes are connected by **links** (lines or arrows) which shows relationship between them.
- First activity to be completed before other events is described.
- Linkage between two or more events is shown and time schedule for every event is also mentioned.

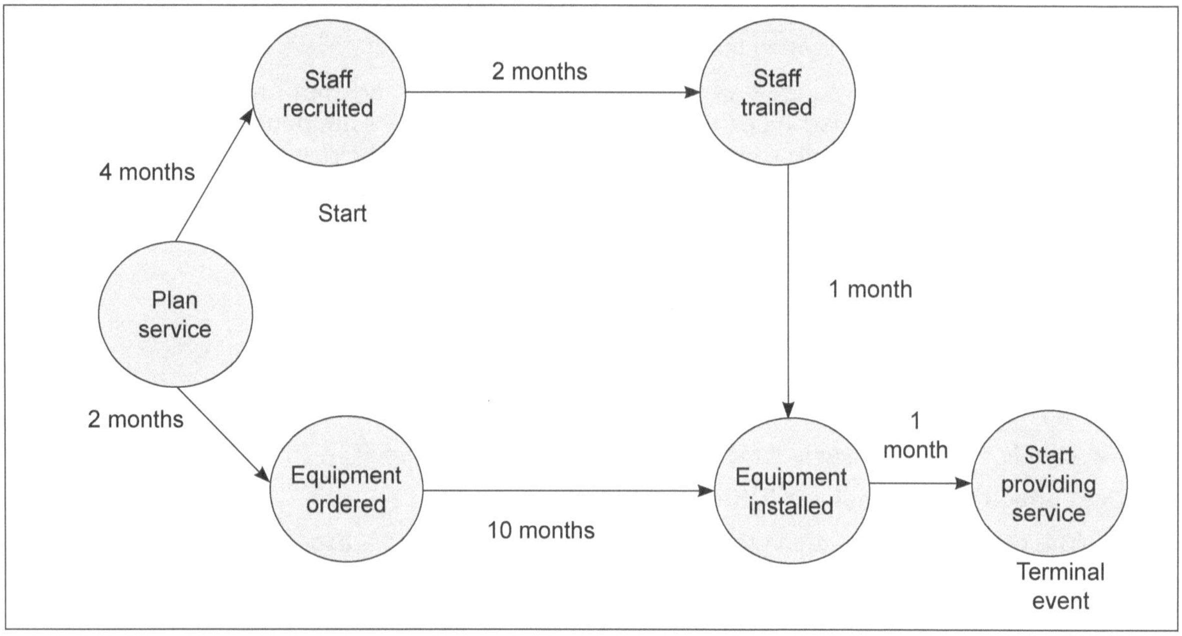

- Steps of network analysis:
  - Enlist all activities.
  - Arrange all activities in logical sequence (Flowchart).
  - Find the duration of each activity.
  - Know the dependencies between activities (by Gnatt Chart).
  - Set logical end point (milestones) or nodes for each activity.
  - Identify critical path.
  - Calculate total time.
  - Replan.
- Network analysis is done by 2 methods:
  - Program Evaluation Review Technique (PERT).
  - Critical Path Method (CPM): The "longest path" of the network.

Ans: (d) Cost benefit analysis

Ref: *IAPSM's Textbook of Community Medicine, Page 973, 1027-1028*

8. Best indicators for air pollution are:

(a) Sulphur dioxide, smoke and suspended particles

(b) Sulphur dioxide, hydrogen sulphide, carbon monoxide

(c) Carbon dioxide, hydrogen sulphide, lead

(d) Sulphur dioxide, lead and particulate matter

Explanation:

There are more than 100 substances which pollute air but the important ones are:

- **Carbon monoxide**, Carbon dioxide, **Hydrogen sulphide**, **Sulphur dioxide**, Sulphur trioxide, Nitrogen oxides, Flourine compounds, Organic compounds (e.g., hydrocarbons, aldehydes, ketones, organic acids), metallic contaminants (e.g., arsenic, zinc, iron resulting from smelting operation), radioactive compounds, photochemical oxidants (e.g., ozone).

- Others include asbestos, beryllium, mercury, benzene, fluorides, vinyl chloride, lead and radiation.

Air Quality Index: It is an indicator of air quality which can be easily communicated to the public. It converts several air quality related data into a single number, name and colour.

Seven pollutants (PM10, PM2.5, NO_2, SO_2, CO, O_3 and NH_3) are used for calculating AQI.

Categorization of AQI:

AQI Category	Value of AQI	Health impact
Good	0-50	Minimal health impact
Satisfactory	51-100	May cause minor breathing discomfort to sensitive people
Moderate	101-200	May cause breathing discomfort to people with asthma, heart disease, children and elderly
Poor	201-300	On prolonged exposure, may cause breathing difficulty to otherwise healthy individuals but even short-term exposure can result in breathing difficulty in people with heart disease
Very poor	301-400	May cause respiratory illness to healthy individuals on prolonged exposure but even short exposure can result in the same in those with lung and heart disease
Severe	401-500	May cause respiratory effects to healthy individuals and persons with underlying lung or heart disease can have severe problems. Health impact manifests even with light physical activity

Ans: (b) Sulphur dioxide, hydrogen sulphide, carbon monoxide

Ref: *Park Textbook of Preventive and Social Medicine, 25th Edition, Page 793; IAPSM's Textbook of Community Medicine, Page 847*

9. A study had a normal distribution with the median value as 200 and standard deviation 20. 68% of area will fall between:

(a) 160 and 240
(b) 170 and 230
(c) 180 and 220
(d) 190 and 210

Explanation:

To determine the chances or probability of an observation or observations being normal and also to determine the proportion of observations that lie between mean and a higher or lower observation→we represent the sample in frequency distribution table by keeping group interval small→take into account the mean or central position and dispersion or variability or variability of observations up to the extremes on either side of mean in terms of SD.

It is seen:

- Maximum number or frequencies is seen in the middle around the mean and fewer at the extremes.
- Normally almost **half observations** lie on **each side** of the **mean** in symmetrical way.
- The area under the curve between any two points depicting values of the variable, corresponds to the number of observations lying between these two values, and can be calculated in terms of mean and the standard deviation as shown below:
  - Mean **± 1 SD limits include 68.27%** or roughly 2/3rd of all observations. About 32% observations will lie outside the range, Mean ± 1 SD (16% on either side).
  - Mean **± 2 SD limits include 95.45%** of observations while 4.55% of observations will be outside these limits. Similarly mean ± 1.96 SD limits, include 95% of all observations.
  - Mean **± 3 SD limits include 99.73%.** Similarly mean ± 1.96 SD limits, include 99% of all observations.

Median = mean = mode value = 200

Standard deviation (SD) = 20

68% of area will fall between = x ± 1 SE

= 200 ± 20 = 180 – 220

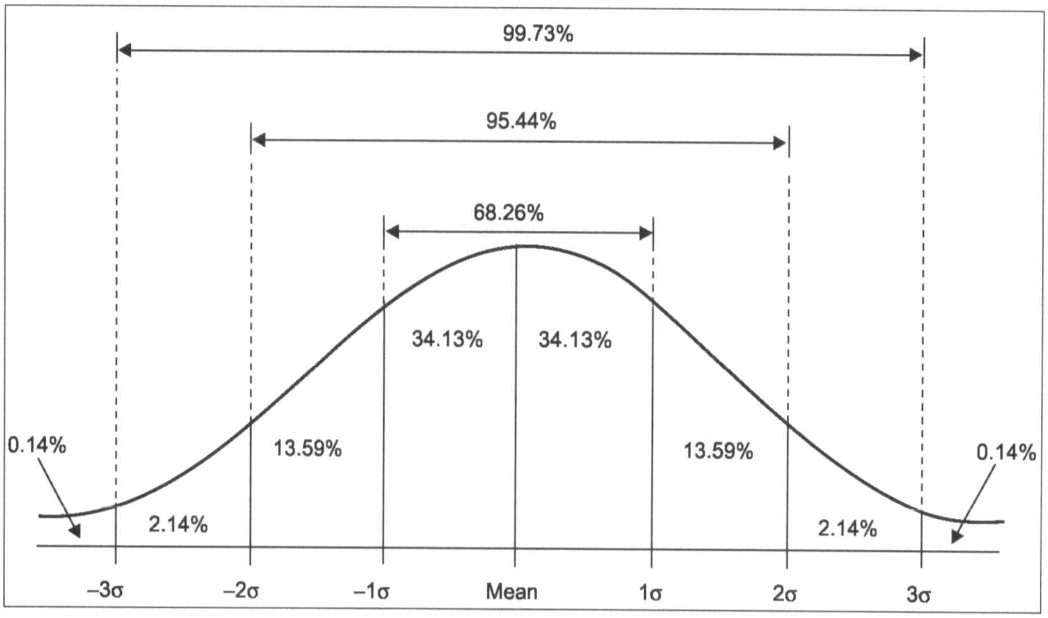

Ans: (c) 180-220

Ref: *Mahajan's Methods in Biostatistics, 9th Edition, Page100-102*

10. Extended sickness benefit for tuberculosis under Employees' State Insurance (ESI) Act is:

(a) 91 days (b) 1 year

(c) 2 years (d) 4 years

Explanation:

The Employees State Insurance Act, 1948:

- Amended in 1975, 1984, 1989 and 2010. Head Office at New Delhi.
- It is an important measure of social security and health insurance.
- It extends to all factories of whole country except seasonal factories, mines, railways and defence establishments.
- It extends to shops, hotels and restaurants, cinemas and theatre, road-motor transport establishments, newspaper establishments and can be extending to agriculture or commercial establishments.
- Applied to those who are getting pay of **Rs. 21000/- month** as per notification of ESIC on 6/9/16.
- It consists of CEO-DG, assisted by four principal officers—(1) Insurance commissioner (2) Medical commissioner (3) Financial commissioner (4) Actuary.
- The **employer contributes 4.75% of total wages** bill and **employee contributes 1.75%** of total wages bill since 1/1/97.
- **State Government share is one-eighth and ESIC share is seven-eighth** of total expenditure on medical care.
- One service dispensary with full time medical and para-medical personnel is established for >1000 employees' family units, part time for <750.
- One doctor will attend to about 80 OPD/day and makes one home visit a day.
- In case of **sickness**, the benefit is payable for a **maximum period of 91 days at 50% of average wages** and can be **extended up to 2 years for certain 34 long-term diseases** (w.e.f. 1/1/2000). This statement is according to Textbook Park.

But according to Employees State Insurance Corporation site, the statement is "In case of **sickness**, the benefit is payable for a **maximum period of 91 days at 70% of average wages** and can be **extended up to 2 years for certain 34 long-term diseases** at an enhanced rate of 80 per cent of wages". [ESI site]

I. **Infectious Diseases (Tuberculosis**, Leprosy, Chronic Empyema, AIDS).
II. **Neoplasms (**Malignant Diseases).
III. **Endocrine, Nutritional and Metabolic Disorders** (Diabetes Mellitus with proliferative retinopathy/ diabetic foot/nephropathy).
IV. **Disorders of Nervous System** (Monoplegia, Hemiplegia, Paraplegia, Hemiparesis, Intracranial Space Occupying Lesion, Spinal Cord, Compression, Parkinson's disease, Myasthenia Gravis/Neuromuscular Dystrophies).
V. **Disease of Eye** (Immature Cataract with vision 6/60 or less, Detachment of Retina, Glaucoma).
VI. **Diseases of Cardiovascular System** (Coronary Artery Disease: (a) Unstable Angina (b) Myocardial infraction with ejection less than 45%, Congestive Heart Failure–Left, Right; Cardiac Valvular Diseases with failure/complications, Cardiomyopathies, Heart disease with surgical intervention along with complications).
VII. **Chest Diseases** [Bronchiectasis, Interstitial Lung Disease, Chronic Obstructive Lung Diseases (COPD) with congestive heart failure (Cor Pulmonale)].
VIII. **Diseases of the Digestive System** (Cirrhosis of liver with ascities/chronic active hepatitis).
IX. **Orthopedic Diseases** (Dislocation of vertebra/prolapse of intervertebral disc, non union or delayed union of fracture, post traumatic surgical amputation of lower extremity, compound fracture with chronic osteomyelitis).
X. **Psychoses** [Sub-group under this head are listed for clarification: Schizophrenia, Indogenous depression, Manic Depressive Psychosis (MDP), Dementia].
XI. **Others** (More than 20% burns with infection/complication, chronic renal failure, Reynaud's disease/ Buerger's disease).

- Enhanced sickness benefit of **full wages for 14 days for tubectomy and 7 days for vasectomy**.
- **Maternity benefit** with full wages:
  - For 26 weeks in case of delivery, 6 weeks for miscarriage and 30 days in case of sickness arising out of pregnancy.
  - Delivery expenses of Rs 2,500- 5,000.
- **90% wages** as long as **temporary** disablement lasts.
- **Lifelong pension** is given in case of **permanent disability** (decided by medical board).
- In case of **death during work**, pension at the rate of **90% wages** shared by dependents in **fixed ratio on monthly basis**.
- **Funeral** expenses not exceeding **Rs 10,000/- w.e.f. 1/4/11**.
- On monthly payment of Rs. 10, the insured person and his family members continue to get medical benefit after permanent disability.
- One safety committee for every mine where >100 miners are working.
- One inspector for >500 miners.

Benefit to Employee	Benefit to Employers
• Medical benefit • Sickness benefit • Maternity benefit • Disabilities benefit • Dependent's benefits • Funeral expenses • Rehabilitation allowances	• Exemption from the applicability of Workman's Compensation Act 1923 • Exemption from Maternity Benefit Act 1961 • Exemption from payment of medical allowance to the employees and their dependents • Rebate under the Income Tax Act on contribution deposited in the ESI Account • Healthy work force

Ans: (c) 2 years

Ref: *Park Textbook of Preventive and Social Medicine, 25th Edition, Page 877-879*

11. The variation in a data is compared with another data set by:

(a) Variance
(b) Coefficient of variation
(c) Standard error of mean
(d) Standard deviation

Explanation:

- Measures of variability of observations help to find how individual observations are dispersed around the mean of a large series.
- They are also called measures of dispersion, variation or scatter as against the averages which are measure of central tendency.
- Measures of variability of individual observations (within a sample):
  - Range.
  - Interquartile range.
  - Mean deviation.
  - Standard deviation.
  - Coefficient of variation.
- Measures of variability of samples (between 2 or more samples):
  - Standard error of mean.
  - Standard error of difference between two means.
  - Standard error of proportion.
  - Standard error of difference between two proportions.
  - Standard error of correlation coefficient.
  - Standard deviation of regression coefficient.

Ans: (c) Standard error of mean

Ref: *Methods in Biostatistics by BK Mahajan, 7th Edition, Page 69-70*

12. If one variable is given then you can find another variable by:

(a) Coefficient of variation
(b) Coefficient of correlation
(c) Coefficient of regression
(d) Coefficient of determination

Explanation:

- Regression analysis is mathematical measure of average relationship between two or more variables.
- Technique concerned with predicting some variables by knowing others.

Regression Types:

1. **Simple Regression:** Single explanatory variable.
2. **Multiple Regression:** Includes any number of explanatory variables.

Another Classification:

1. **Linear Regression:** Straight-line relationship.
2. **Non-linear Regression:** Implies curved relationships.
   Logarithmic relationships.

Simple Linear Regression:

- It uses one independent variable to explain and/or predict the outcome of one dependent variable.

- General assumption: One variable generally y as dependent variable and x as independent variable.
- It tells us how values in y change as function of values of x changes.
- It determine the form of the relationship by a line which best fits the data. This line is called as '**Regression line or 'estimating line'.**

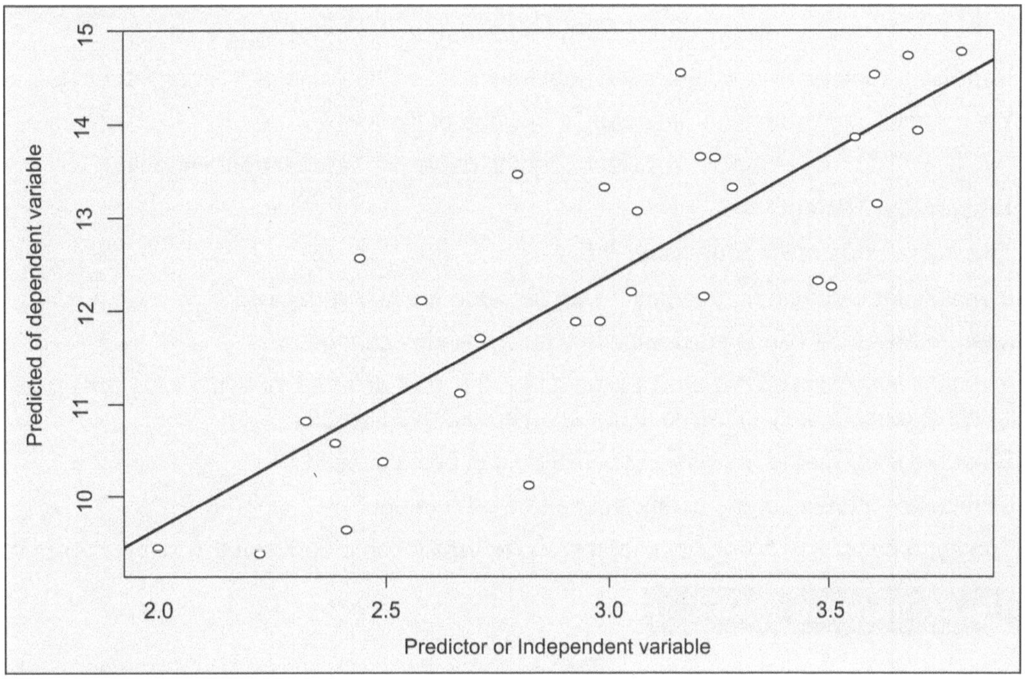

Regression Equation:

The equation of the straight line is given by regression equation.

- Population regression equation $Y = \alpha + \beta X + e$
- Sample regression equation

  $Y = a + bx$

Where '**α**' or '**a**' is the intercept.

- '**β**' or '**b**' is the slope of the line which measures the amount of change in y for unit change in x.
- '**e**' is the regression residual/error.

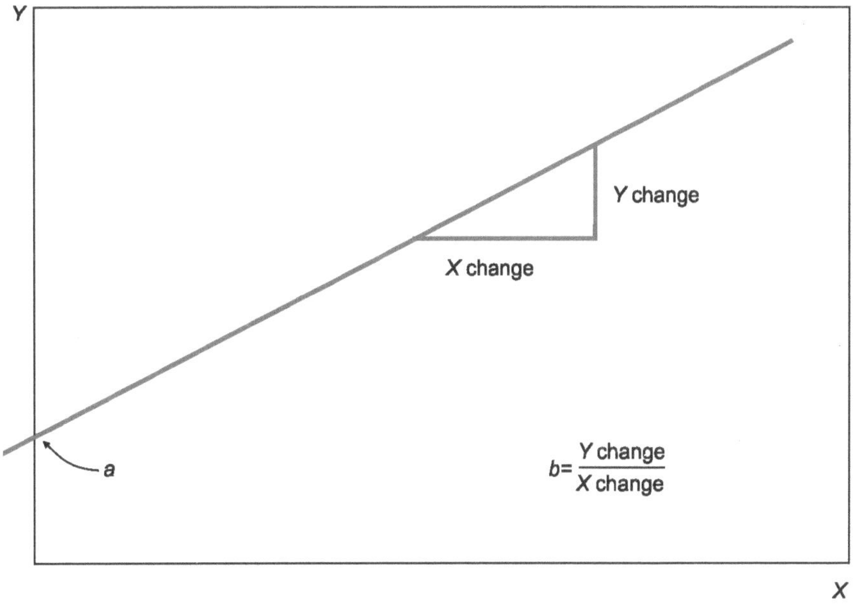

Regression Line:

- For two variables X and Y, there are always two lines of regression.
- Regression line of X on Y: gives the best estimate for the value of X for any specific given values of Y.
- **X = a + b Y** a = X – intercept, b = Slope of the line.
  X = Dependent variable, Y = Independent variable.
- Regression line of Y on X: gives the best estimate for the value of Y for any specific given values of X.
- **Y = c + dx** c = Y – intercept, b = Slope of the line.
  Y = Dependent variable, x= Independent variable.

Regression Coefficient

1. This is the slope of the regression line.
2. Indicates the strength of the relationship between the two variables.
3. Interpreted as the expected change in y for a one-unit change in x.

For example, if the beta coefficient for weight is 2.1, it indicates that for every kilogram increase in weight, the serum cholesterol is likely to increase, on an average, by 2.1 mg/dl.

4. Standard error for the regression coefficient can be calculated.
5. Confidence interval for the coefficient can be calculated.
6. The hypothesis that b = 0, i.e., that there is no relationship between the two variables can be tested.

Ans: (c) Coefficient of regression

Ref: *Methods in Biostatistics by BK Mahajan, 7th Edition, Page 260*

13. Vaccine to be given after disaster:

(a) Mass vaccination against typhoid
(b) Mass vaccination against cholera
(c) Mass vaccination against tetanus
(d) Vaccination against tetanus, typhoid and cholera to health workers

Explanation:

- Health authorities under considerable public and political pressure had begun mass vaccination programme against typhoid, cholera and tetanus.
- WHO does not recommend vaccination against typhoid and cholera following an outbreak in endemic countries rather support the provision of safe potable water and proper sanitation as the most effective strategy.
- Natural disaster does not increase the chance of tetanus significantly, thus mass vaccination against tetanus is also usually unwanted.
- Strengthening and maintenance of the existing routine immunization program along with cold chain maintenance must be given priority rather than mass vaccination programs.
- However, these vaccinations are recommended for health workers.

Ans: (d) Vaccination against tetanus, typhoid and cholera to health workers

Ref: *Park's Textbook of Preventive and Social Medicine, 25th Edition, Page 858*

14. As per the sustainable development goals (SDG) 2030, the target for Maternal Mortality Ratio (MMR) is to achieve maternal deaths of:

(a) < 7/1000 live births
(b) < 10/1000 live births
(c) < 70/lac live births
(d) < 100/lac live births

Explanation:

- On 25 September 2015, the UN General Assembly adopted the new development agenda "Transforming our world: the 2030 agenda for sustainable development".
- New development agenda integrate all **three dimensions** of sustainable development– economic, social and environmental.
- **Theme**–People, planet, prosperity, peace and partnership.
- **Assumption** – Health is a major contributor and beneficiary of sustainable development policies.
- Consists of **17 goals and 169 targets.**
- One of the goal (**goal 3**) specifically devoted to health.
- The health goal is associated with **13 targets**.

SDG Goals

1. End poverty in all its forms everywhere.
2. End hunger, achieve food security and improved nutrition and promote sustainable agriculture.
3. Ensure healthy lives and promote well-being for all at all ages.
4. Ensure inclusive and equitable quality education and promote lifelong learning opportunities for all.
5. Achieve gender equality and empower all women and girls.
6. Ensure availability and sustainable management of water and sanitation for all.
7. Ensure access to affordable, reliable, sustainable and modern energy for all.
8. Promote sustained, inclusive and sustainable economic growth, full and productive employment and decent work for all.
9. Build resilient infrastructure, promote inclusive and sustainable industrialization and foster innovation.
10. Reduce inequality within and among countries.
11. Make cities and human settlements inclusive, safe, resilient and sustainable.
12. Ensure sustainable consumption and production patterns.
13. Take urgent action to combat climate change and its impacts.
14. Conserve and sustainably use the oceans, seas and marine resources for sustainable development.
15. Protect, restore and promote sustainable use of terrestrial ecosystems, sustainably manage forests, combat desertification, and halt and reverse land degradation and halt biodiversity loss.
16. Promote peaceful and inclusive societies for sustainable development, provide access to justice for all and build effective, accountable and inclusive institutions at all levels.
17. Strengthen the means of implementation and revitalize the global partnership for sustainable development.

Goal 3: Ensure healthy lives and promote well-being for all at all ages.

Target 3.1: By 2030, reduce the Global Maternal Mortality Ratio to ***less than 70 per 100,000 live births.***

Target 3.2: By 2030, end preventable deaths of newborns and children under 5 years of age.

Target 3.3: By 2030, end the epidemics of AIDS, tuberculosis, malaria and neglected tropical diseases and combat hepatitis, water-borne diseases and other communicable diseases.

Target 3.4: By 2030, reduce by one third premature mortality from non-communicable diseases through prevention and treatment and promote mental health and well-being.

Target 3.5: Strengthen the prevention and treatment of substance abuse, including narcotic drug abuse and harmful use of alcohol.

Target 3.6: By 2020, halve the number of global deaths and injuries from road traffic accidents.

Target 3.7: By 2030, ensure universal access to sexual and reproductive health care services, including for family planning, information and education, and the integration of reproductive health into national strategies and programmes.

Target 3.8: Achieve universal health coverage, including financial risk protection, access to quality essential health care services and access to safe, effective, quality and affordable essential medicines and vaccines for all.

Target 3.9: By 2030, substantially reduce the number of deaths and illnesses from hazardous chemicals and air, water and soil pollution and contamination.

Target 3.a: Strengthen the implementation of the World Health Organization Framework Convention on Tobacco Control in all countries, as appropriate.

Target 3.b: Support the research and development of vaccines and medicines for the communicable and non-communicable diseases that primarily affect developing countries, provide access to affordable essential medicines and vaccines, in accordance with the Doha Declaration on the TRIPS Agreement and Public Health, which affirms the right of developing countries to use to the full the provisions in the Agreement on Trade- Related Aspects of Intellectual Property Rights regarding flexibilities to protect public health, and, in particular, provide access to medicines for all.

Target 3.c: Substantially increase health financing and the recruitment, development, training and retention of the health work force in developing countries, especially least developed countries and small island developing states.

Target 3.d: Strengthen the capacity of all countries, in particular developing countries, for early warning, risk reduction and management of national and global health risks.

Ans: (c) <70/lac live births

Ref: *Park's Textbook of Preventive and Social Medicine, 25th Edition, Page 523-527*

15. Prospective screening is done in case of:

(a) Neonate for thyroid diseases
(b) Immigrant screening
(c) Pap smear for 45-year-old female
(d) Diabetes mellitus for 40-year-old male

Explanation:

- Screening is defined as "the search for unrecognized disease or defect by means of rapidly applied tests, examinations or other procedures in apparently healthy individuals".

USES OF SCREENING

a. **Case detection/Prescriptive screening:**
   - Presumptive identification of unrecognized disease, which does not arise from a patient's request like neonatal screening.
   - People are screened primarily for their own benefit.

     E.g.: Bacteriuria in pregnancy, Phenyl Ketonuria, cancer screening, pulmonary tuberculosis, hemolytic disease of newborn.

b. **Control of disease/prospective screening:**
   - People are examined for the benefit of others.
   - Screening program leading to early diagnosis, permit more effective treatment and reduce the spread of infectious disease and/or mortality from the disease.

E.g.: Screening of immigrant for infectious disease like TB, syphilis to protect home population; screening for streptococcal infection to prevent rheumatic fever.

c. **Research purpose:**

Screening done to obtain more basic knowledge about natural history of chronic diseases whose natural history is not yet known, e.g., Cancer, Hypertension.

d. **Educational opportunities:**

Screening programmes (e.g., diabetes screening program) provide opportunities for creating public awareness and for educating health professionals.

	Prescriptive screening	**Prospective screening**
Definition	People screened for own benefit	People screened for others benefit
Essential purpose	Case detection	Disease control
Request for screening	No specific request	Specific request from authority
Example	Neonatal screening Cancer screening Urine for sugar	Screening of immigrant HIV screening of sex workers Screening of blood donors

Ans: (b) Immigrant screening

Ref: *Park's Textbook of Preventive and Social Medicine, 24th Edition, Page 146-147*

16. Which of the following is a technique/method based on behaviour sciences:

(a) Management by objective
(b) Network analysis
(c) Systems analysis
(d) Decision making

Explanation:

Management Techniques:

Statistical techniques	**Decision tree** Time trends and forecasting
Activity analysis	Work study Time motion studies Gantt chart
Mathematical techniques	Simulation study or model **System analysis** **Network analysis (PERT, CPM)**
Financial techniques	Cost benefit analysis Cost effective analysis Planning Programming Budgeting System (PPBS) Zero base budgeting Input output analysis
Miscellaneous	**Management by objectives** Management by exception Strength, Weakness, Opportunities, Challenges analysis

Management by Objective (MBO):

- MBO is a **personnel, participative management technique** is defined as a system wherein the superior and the subordinate managers of an organization jointly define its common goals, define each individual's major areas of responsibility in terms of the results expected of him and use these measures as guides for operating the unit and assessing the contribution of each of its members.

- Here every staff member is allotted a personal measurable objective to complete in a specified period of time. So, every individual objective works towards overall organizational goal.

Benefits:

- Employees tend to have a clear understanding of the roles and responsibilities expected of them.
- Subordinates tend to have a higher commitment to objectives.
- Better communication and coordination between superiors and subordinates.

Drawbacks:

- Setting up of targets is in reality not participatory but top management hand down targets.
- Everything else is secondary except targets.

System Analysis:

- It is a management technique of finding out the cost effectiveness of the available alternatives.
- **System analysis** is the study of inter-relationships operating in the various components within a system and also between a system and other system.
- A system is made up of independent subsystem, e.g., a huge system is made up of subsystem like out-patient department (OPD), in-patient department (IPD), medical record, hospital supply, community health services, etc.
- Through system analysis, a manager can come to know the problems across the system which may lead to unnecessary wastage of money and resources.
- Thus, it help to find alternative solutions which is comparatively cheaper, than the usual one, which is beneficial to the organization.

Decision Tree:

- It is an algorithm which is made up of all the decisions and its possible outcomes (theory of choice or decision theory).
- Best decision comes from managers of any level of the organization.
- Best example: The flowchart for diagnosis of pulmonary tuberculosis based on the algorithm.

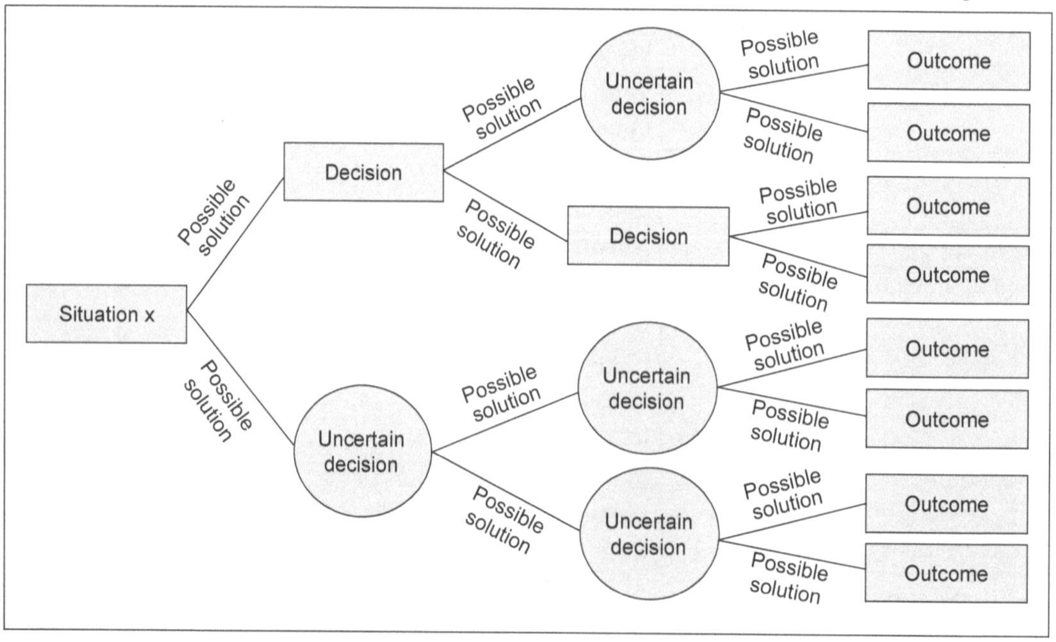

Ans: (a) Management by objective

Ref: *IAPSM's Textbook of Community Medicine, Page 971-974*

17. MONICA project is related to:

(a) Stroke
(b) Renal disorders
(c) Cardiovascular disease
(d) Diabetes

Explanation:

MONICA is the acronym for "**monitoring trends and determinants in cardiovascular disease**", and is a **WHO-coordinated international CVD surveillance research program** that began in the early 1980s **for over 10 years**.

It was population-based surveys of risk factors of CVD, carried out in **21 countries across four continents.**

MONICA **assessed trends in community rates** of hospitalized **CVD events**, their **case fatality** rate, trends in cardiovascular **risk factors** (blood pressure, cigarette smoking and serum cholesterol) in **men and women aged 25-64** in the same defined communities.

Ans: (c) Cardiovascular disease

Ref: *Article "The World Health Organization MONICA Project (Monitoring Trends and Determinants in Cardiovascular Disease): A Major International Collaboration. WHO MONICA Project Principal Investigators" J Clin Epidemiol 1988;41(2):105-114*

18. A study was done to assess the malnutrition among young children. 100 children were selected each from rural and urban areas. Out of these, 30 among rural and 20 among urban area were found to be malnourished. Which of the following statistical test is used to compare the data sets?

(a) Paired t test
(b) Chi square
(c) Standard error of mean
(d) ANOVA

Explanation:

On the basis of type of data:

If Data is Quantitative:

a. Co-efficient of variation.
b. Standard error of mean.
c. t-test if sample is small.
d. z test when sample is large.
e. Analysis of variance (ANOVA).
f. Co-relation (Karl Pearson).

If Data is Qualitative:

a. Standard error of proportion.
b. SE of difference between two proportion.
c. Chi-square test if sample is large.
d. Fisher's exact test if sample is small.
e. Spearman's rank test.

Chi-Square Test:

- Most commonly used when data are in frequencies such as the number of responses in two or more categories.
- It can be used with any data which can be reduced to proportions or percentages.
- It is used with data which is **independent, qualitative and unpaired** in nature.

Basically statistical inferences rely on the appropriate statistical tests and the type of test used has direct impact on the interpretation. **Inferential statistics** is broadly of two types:

a. Parametric test.

b. Non-parametric test.

Whether to use parametric or non-parametric test, depend on:

- **Type of data:** If data is nominal or ordinal non-parametric test is used whereas for ratio and interval data, parametric test can be applied.
- **Distribution assumption:** Parametric test is used when data is normally distributed (large sample size) and vice versa. For skewed data, non-parametric test is used.
- **Assumed variance:** Parametric test generally assume homogenous population, whereas non-parametric test do not assume this.
- **Central value:** Mean is the central measure for parametric test whereas median is used for non-parametric test.
- **Strength:** Parametric tests are considered statistically more powerful.

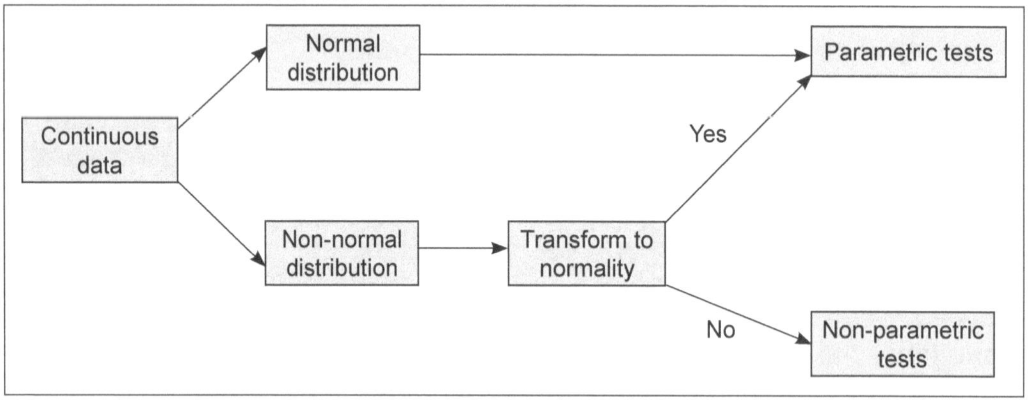

Summary of statistical tests by comparing both parametric and non-parametric tests:

Aim	Parametric test	Non-parametric test
Compare one sample to a hypothetical value	One sample t-test	Sign test
Compare 2 unpaired samples	Independent sample t test	Mann Whitney U test
Compare more than 2 unpaired samples	ANOVA	Kruskall-Wallis test
Compare 2 paired samples	Paired sample t-test	Wilcoxon signed rank test
Compare more than 2 paired samples	Repeated measures ANOVA	Friedman test
Assess linear relation between 2 variables	Pearson's correlation coefficient	Spearman and Kendall correlation coefficient

Ans: (b) Chi-square

Ref: *Biostatistics by Wayne W Daniel, 10th Edition*

19. A child diagnosed provisionally with diphtheria and on examination she has greyish white membrane patch around her tonsils. The patient reports to have another 3-year-old sibling at home, who is fully immunized as per the immunization schedule. What is the best measure to prevent diphtheria in the sibling of the diphtheria case child?

(a) Give diphtheria toxoid booster

(b) Give full course of DPT vaccine

(c) Give prophylactic erythromycin

(d) Nothing is required to be done

Explanation:

For contacts of diptheria patient:

a. Where primary immunization or booster dose was received within the previous 2 years, no further action would be needed.

b. Where primary course or booster dose of diphtheria toxoid was received more than 2 years before, only a booster dose of diphtheria toxoid need to be given.

c. Non-immunized close contact should receive prophylactic penicillin or erythromycin. They should be given 1000-2000 units of diphtheria antitoxin and actively immunized against diphtheria.

Contacts should be placed under medical surveillance and examined daily for evidence of diphtheria for at least a week after exposure.

The bacteriological surveillance of close contacts should be continued for several weeks by repeated swabbing at approximately weekly interval.

Ans: (d) Nothing is required to be done

Ref: *Park's Textbook of Preventive and Social Medicine, 25th Edition, Page 174*

20. A 3-year-old child presents to PHC with fever with cough. He had chest indrawing and respiratory rate of 38 per minute and weight of 11 kg. The next step in management based on Integrated Management of Childhood Illness (IMNCI) guideline is:

(a) Give antipyretics only

(b) Not an emergency, give oral antibiotics and follow-up

(c) Refer urgently to a tertiary care centre

(d) Give antibiotics and refer to a tertiary care centre

Explanation:

- The 3 years old child is classified as "severe pneumonia (chest indrawing present) with low weight (z score < -2)", thus after giving first dose of injectable chloramphenicol, he should be urgently referred to higher centre.

Integrated Management of Childhood Illness (IMNCI) Guideline for Children 2 months - 5 years

Check for general danger signs:

Ask:	Look:
Is the child able to drink or breast feed? Does the child vomit everything? Has the child had convulsions?	See if the child is lethargic or unconscious

Ask about main symptoms: Does the child have cough or difficult breathing?

If yes, ask: For how long?

Look, listen, feel:

- Count the breaths in one minute.
- Look for chest indrawing.
- Look and listen for stridor.

Fast Breathing:

- 2 months up to 12 months: 50 breaths per minute or more.
- 12 months up to 5 years: 40 breaths per minute or more.

Any general danger sign or Chest indrawing or Stridor in calm child	Severe Pneumonia or Very Severe Disease	Give first dose injectable chloramphenicol (if not possible give oral amoxycillin) Refer URGENTLY to hospital
Fast breathing	Pneumonia	Give Cotrimoxazole for 5 days Soothe the throat and relieve the cough with a safe remedy if child is 6 months or older Advise mother when to return immediately Follow up in 2 days
No signs of pneumonia or very severe disease	No Pneumonia: Cough or Cold	If coughing for more than 30 days, refer for assessment Soothe the throat and relieve the cough with safe home remedy if child is 6 months or older Advise mother when to return immediately Follow up in 5 days if not improving

Then check for malnutrition:

Look and feel:

- Look for visible signs of wasting.
- Look for edema of both feet.
- Determine weight for age.

Visible severe wasting or Oedema of both feet	Severe malnutrition	Give single dose of Vitamin A Prevent for low blood sugar Refer urgently to hospital While referral is being organized, warm the child Keep the child warm on the way to hospital
Very low weight for age	Very low weight	Assess and counsel for feeding Advise mother when to return immediately Follow up in 30 days
Not very low weight for age and no other signs of malnutrition	Not very low weight	If child is less than 2 years old, assess the child's feeding and counsel the mother on feeding according to the food box on the COUNSEL THE MOTHER chart Advise mother when to return immediately

Visible severe wasting: Wasting of shoulders, arms, buttocks and legs with ribs easily seen. It indicates marasmus. When wasting is extreme, there are many folds of skin on the buttocks and thigh. It looks as if the child is wearing baggy pant. The face of a child with visible wasting may still look normal. The child's abdomen may be large or distended.

Edema of both feet: May signal kwashiorkor.

Weight for age: Plotting weight for age in growth chart, based on reference population, helps to identify children with low (Z score less than -2) or very low (Z score less than -3) weight for age, those who are at increased risk of infection and poor growth and development.

(See Figure on the Next Page)

Linear Equations for Calculating Weight for Age

a. For infants < 12 months

   Expected weight (kg) = (age in months + 9)/2

b. Children aged 1-5 years:

   Expected weight (kg) = 2 × (age in years + 5)

c. Children aged 5-14 years:

   Expected weight (kg) = 4 × age in years

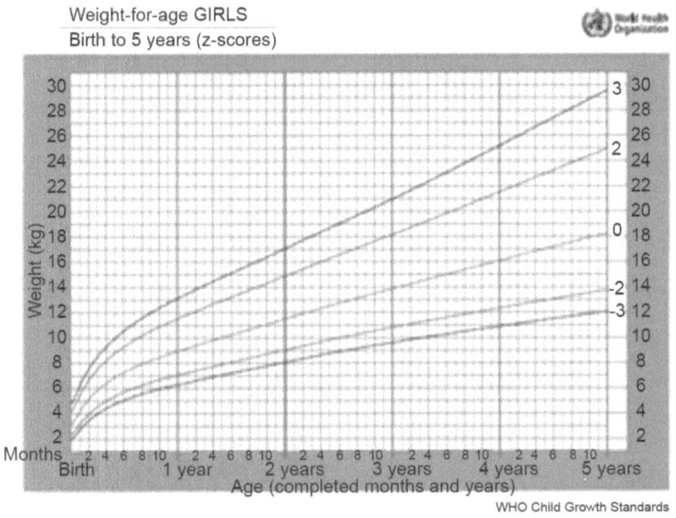

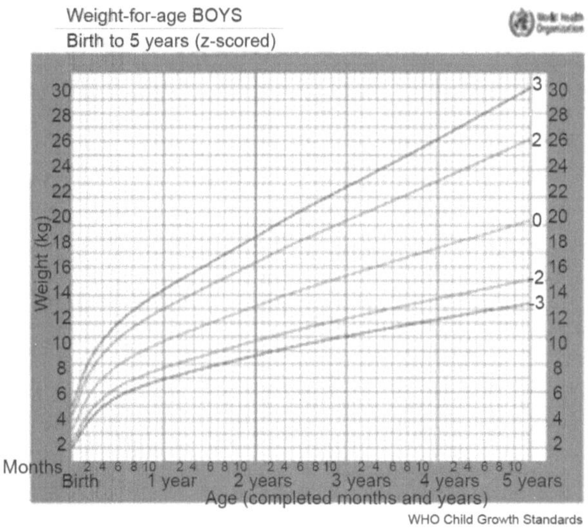

Ans: (d) Give antibiotics and refer to a tertiary care centre

Ref: *Ghai Essential Pediatrics, 7th Edition, Page 743-751*

21. Which of the following is not a specific protection method under primary level of prevention?

(a) Ribavirin to close contact meningitis patient
(b) Health education about hand washing
(c) Giving pentavalent vaccination to children
(d) Addition of iron with wheat flour

Explanation:

- Prevention – Activities designed to protect exposed and other members of the public from actual or potential health threats and their harmful consequences.
- Levels of prevention:

(See Figure on the Next Page)

Primordial Prevention

- Prevention of emergence or development of risk factors in countries, population groups or individuals, in which they have not yet appeared.
- Particularly useful for chronic diseases.
- Example: Many adult health problems (e.g., obesity, hypertension) have their early origins in childhood, because this is the time when lifestyles are formed (smoking, eating patterns, physical exercise).
- Efforts are directed towards discouraging children from adopting harmful lifestyles.
- The main intervention – is through individual and mass education.

Primary Prevention

- Action taken prior to the onset of disease which removes the possibility that disease will ever occur.
- Measures of prevention are undertaken during the pre-pathogenesis phase of disease.
- Involves two sub-steps:
  1. Health promotion.
  2. Specific protection.

A. Health promotion: Process of enabling people to increase control over, and to improve health. Interventions are:

1. Health education.

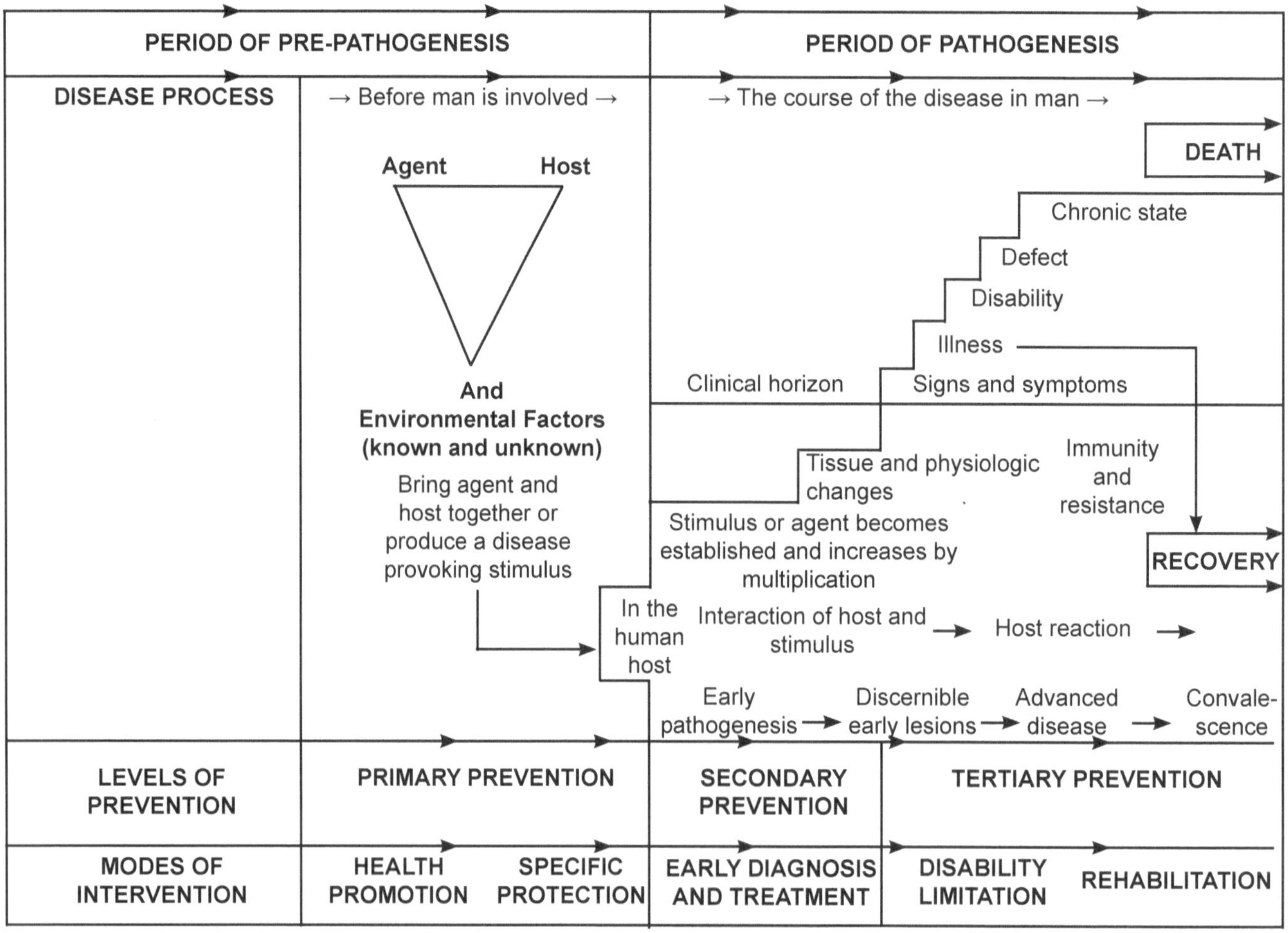

Natural history of disease

(From Preventive Medicine for the Doctor in His Community, by Leavell and Clark with permission of McGraw-Hill Book Co.)

2. Environmental modifications: Such as provision of safe water, installation of sanitary latrines, control of insects and rodents, improvement of housing, etc.
3. Nutritional interventions: Comprises food distribution and nutrition improvement of vulnerable groups; child feeding programmes; nutrition education, etc.
4. Lifestyle and behavioural changes: Involves changing of views, behavior and habits of people.

B. **Specific protection:** Includes measures to prevent the initiation of specific diseases or a group of diseases. E.g.:

- **Immunization** to protect against specific diseases.
- **Fortification of foods** with specific nutrients (as salt with iodine, wheat flour with iron).
- **Chemoprophylaxis.**
- Protection against occupational hazards, accidents (use of helmets), carcinogens, allergens.
- Control of specific hazards in general environment like air pollution, noise pollution, water pollution.
- Control of consumer product quality and safety of foods, drugs, cosmetics, etc.

APPROACHES FOR PRIMARY PREVENTION FOR CHRONIC DISEASES (WHO)

A. **Population (mass) strategy:**

- Directed at whole population irrespective of individual risk levels, e.g., towards socio-economic, behavioral and lifestyle changes.

B. High risk strategy:

- Preventive care to individuals at special risk.

Secondary Prevention

- Action which halts the progress of the disease at its incipient stage and prevents complications.
- Intervention – early pathogenesis stage.
- It is the domain of clinical medicine.

Drawback:

a. Patient already subjected to mental anguish and physical pain.
b. More expensive than primary prevention.

Modes of intervention:

a. Early diagnosis (screening tests, case finding programs).
b. Adequate/prompt treatment.

Early diagnosis and prompt treatment:

a. Earlier diagnosed – better prognosis.
b. Reduces morbidity and mortality.
c. Effective in acute conditions.
d. Reverses communicability of infectious diseases.
e. Protects community.

Tertiary Prevention

- These include all measures undertaken when the disease has become advanced, with a view to prevent or delay death, reduce or limit the impairments and disabilities, minimize suffering and to promote the subject's adjustment to conditions which are impossible to cure.
- Intervention – late pathogenesis stage.
- Tertiary prevention has two types of approaches:
  - Disability limitation.
  - Rehabilitation.

Disability Limitation

- To prevent or halt the transition of disease process from impairment to handicap.
- Disease→Impairment→Disability→Handicap.
- **Impairment:** Any loss or **abnormality** of psychological, physiological or anatomic structure or function.
- **Disability:** Any restriction or lack of **ability** to perform an activity in the manner considered normal for a human being.
- **Handicap:** Disadvantage for a given individual, resulting from impairment or disability that limits or prevents the fulfillment of a **role** that is normal for that individual.

Rehabilitation

- The combined and coordinated use of medical, educational, social and vocational measures for training and retraining the individual to the highest possible level of functional ability.
- Types of rehabilitation:
  - **Medical Rehabilitation**: Restoration of function. This is done through medical/surgical procedures to restore the anatomy, anatomical functions and physiological functions to as near normal as possible.

- **Vocational Rehabilitation:** It includes steps involving training and education so as to enable the person to earn his/her livelihood.
- **Social Rehabilitation:** This involves steps for restoration of the family and social relationships.
- **Emotional and Psychological Rehabilitation:** This involves steps to restore the self esteem, personal dignity and confidence.

Examples of Rehabilitation

- Establishing schools for blind.
- Provision of aids for crippled.
- Exercises in neurological disorders.
- Prosthetic restoration of lost tooth.

Ans: (b) Health education about hand washing

Ref: *Park's Textbook of Preventive and Social Medicine, 24th Edition, 45-49*

ENT

1. A child came to the OPD with fever and dysphagia. On examination the following is visualized. What is your most probable diagnosis?

(a) Peritonsillar abscess
(b) Parapharyngeal abscess
(c) Retropharyngeal abscess
(d) Follicular tonsillitis

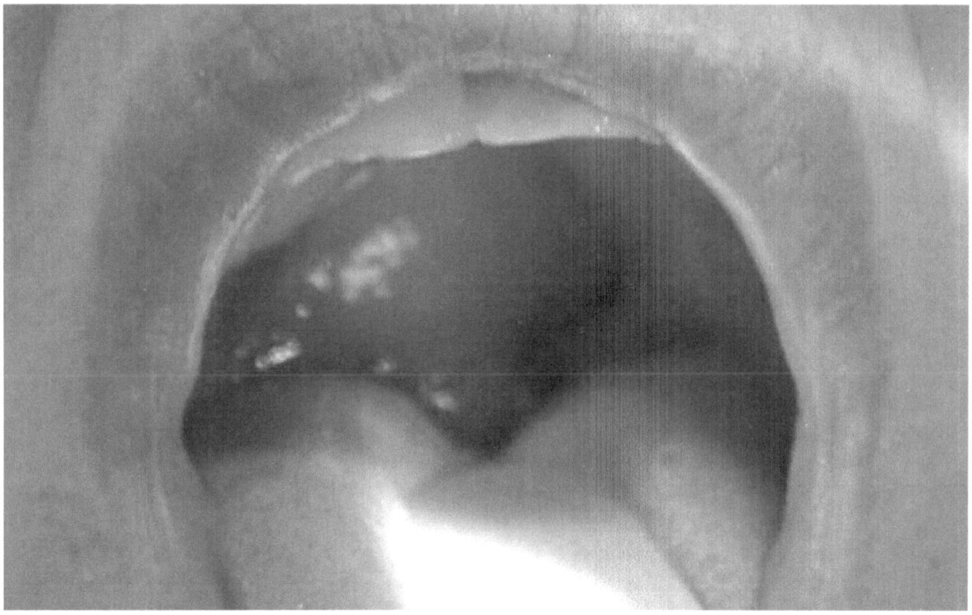

Explanation:

- The clinical scenario of fever, dysphagia and clinical picture showing asymmetric tonsillar bulge with displacement of uvula away from the affected side is diagnostic of **Peritonsillar abscess**.

Peritonsillar Abscess (Quinsy)

- Collection of pus in the peritonsillar space which lies between the **capsule of tonsil** and the **superior constrictor muscle.**
- Most common complication of **acute tonsillitis**.
- **Causative agent: Group A beta-hemolytic strep (GABHS) Streptococcus pyogenes**, S. aureus, Mixed oropharyngeal anaerobes.
- **Clinical Features:**
  - Pronounced unilateral redness and swelling of the soft palate.
  - Sore throat, fever, dysphagia, muffled speech and trismus due to spasm of pterygoid muscle which is in close proximity to superior constrictor.
- **Treatment:**
  - IV antibiotics, analgesics, oral hygiene.
  - The treatment of choice is removal or incision of the affected tonsil under antibiotic coverage.
  - Recurrent peritonsillar abscess is an indication for tonsillectomy.
- If left untreated, many Peritonsillar abscesses get resolved spontaneously by discharging into the mouth, but they may develop into a parapharyngeal abscess.

Retropharyngeal and Parapharyngeal Abscess

- Deep nodes in neck; infection from extension of localized infection of oropharynx.
- An inflammation or abscess may arise from the prevertebral or parapharyngeal lymph nodes or by hematogenous spread as the result of a minor foreign-body injury or upper respiratory inflammation.
- This abscess is called retropharyngeal or parapharyngeal abscess, depending on whether it is located between the spinal column and posterior pharyngeal wall or lateral to the pharyngeal wall.
- **Clinical Features:** Fever, severe pain on swallowing with progressive dysphagia, irritability, decreased oral intake, neck stiffness, sore throat, torticollis (due to spasm of sternocleidomastoid muscle), muffled speech, and possible trismus and dyspnea.
- **Examination:**
  - Bulging of posterior or lateral pharyngeal wall.
  - On mirror examination, pronounced swelling in the oropharynx or hypopharynx, most commonly at a prevertebral or parapharyngeal location are marked.
  - Soft tissue neck film with head extended may show increased width.
- **Treatment:**
  - Incision and drainage of the abscess under general endotracheal anesthesia.
  - Intravenous antibiotics + surgical drainage.

Ans: (a) Peritonsillar abscess

Ref: *Diseases of Ear, Nose and Throat and Head and Neck Surgery by Dhingra, 6th Edition, Page 264*

2. A person met with accident and suffers from middle cranial fossa fracture. There was blue purplish colour behind mastoid shown in the figure. What is your probable diagnosis?

(a) Bezold abscess (b) Battle sign

(c) Griesinger sign (d) Mastoiditis

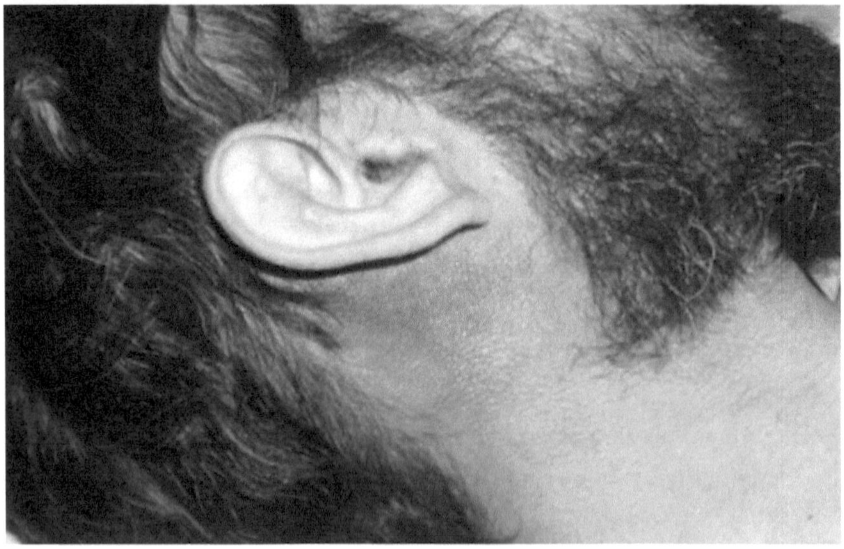

Explanation:

BATTLE SIGN

- Bruise that indicates a fracture at the bottom of the skull.
- Ecchymosis over the mastoid seen in fractures of temporal bone. Left post-auricular bruising also known as Battle's sign.

- **Findings in Temporal Bone Fractures:**
  - Blood in the external auditory canal (EAC).
  - Cerebrospinal fluid (CSF) otorrhoea.
  - Battle's sign.
  - **Hemotympanum:** Blood behind the eardrum.
  - TM perforation.
  - LMN facial nerve palsy.

Bezold Abscess

- Complication of acute otomastoiditis where the infection erodes through the cortex medial to the attachment of sternocleidomastoid.
- This is an abscess in the soft tissue medially and below the mastoid tip, extending into the neck.
- It involves the sternocleidomastoid fascial sheath.

Griesinger Sign

- It is due to thrombosis of mastoid emissary vein impeding venous drainage and thus causing edema over the mastoid.
- It is seen in lateral sinus thrombosis.

Mastoiditis

- Fluctuance and inflammation over the mastoid process roughly two weeks after the onset of otitis media.
- Ironed out appearance of the Mastoid is seen due to periostitis and subsequent inflammation.

Ans: (b) Battle sign

Ref: *Diseases of Ear, Nose and Throat and Head and Neck Surgery by Dhingra, 6th Edition, Page 446*

3. Tubercular otitis media is characterized by all *except*:

(a) Multiple perforations (b) Pale granulations
(c) Painful otorrhea (d) Foul smelling ear discharge

Explanation:

Tubercular Otitis Media

- It is most commonly following pulmonary tuberculosis.
- Patient presents with painless **foul smelling** (because of **bony erosion**) ear discharge with hearing loss (because of **ossicular necrosis**).
- **Clinical Features**
  - **Painless ear discharge:** Earache is characteristically absent in cases of tubercular otitis media.
  - **Perforation:** Multiple perforations, two or three in number, are seen in pars tensa and form a classical sign of disease. These may coalesce into a single large perforation then it becomes indistinguishable from nonspecific CSOM.
  - **Hearing loss:** There is severe hearing loss, out of proportion to symptoms. Mostly conductive, it may have sensorineural component due to involvement of labyrinth.
  - **Facial paralysis:** It is a common complication and may come unexpectedly. This may be the presenting feature in a child.

- **On examination: Multiple perforations** on the TM which may coalesce to form a single large perforation and pale granulations are seen.
- Most common complication of TB otitis media is **facial palsy**. Others include **mastoiditis**, labyrinthitis, post-auricular fistula and osteomyelitis.
- **Treatment:**
  - Medical management with anti-tubercular drugs (ATT).
  - Surgery may be required in some cases to remove sequestra and improve drainage.

Ans: (c) Painful otorrhea

Ref: *Diseases of Ear, Nose and Throat and Head and Neck Surgery by Dhingra, 6th Edition, Page 74*

4. Stimulation of external auditory canal leads to cough due to which nerve?

(a) Greater auricular nerve
(b) Auricular branch vagus
(c) Auriculotemporal nerve
(d) Jacobson's nerve

Explanation:

Auricular Branch of Vagus Nerve (Arnold's Nerve)

- It supplies the concha of pinna and also the posterior wall and floor of external meatus.
- Stimulation of vagus during probing leads to cough and even to bradycardia.
- Interestingly, sensory fibers of facial nerve also supplies posterior meatus wall and concha through the vagal fibers.
- Hence in herpes zoster oticus, vesicles are seen in concha and postauricular region.

Greater Auricular Nerve (2, 3)

- It supplies most of medial surface and only posterior part or lateral surface. It is commonly injured during parotidectomy, hence pinna sensation is lost.

Auriculotemporal nerve (V3)

- It supplies crus of helix and tragus.
- Hence its continuity also supplies the anterior wall and roof of external meatus.

Jacobson's Nerve

- Branch of glossopharyngeal nerve, which is sensory supply to middle ear.

Ans: (b) Auricular branch vagus

Ref: *Diseases of Ear, Nose and Throat and Head and Neck Surgery by Dhingra, 6th Edition, Page 4*

5. While doing parathyroid surgery, the following landmarks are used to identify the fascial nerve trunk; *except*:

(a) Tragal pointer
(b) Digastric posterior belly
(c) Dissecting from peripheral branches
(d) Inferior belly of omohyoid

Explanation:

The following methods are used to identify the facial nerve:

- **Antegrade Methods:**
  - Inferior portion of Tragal Pointer (Conley's Pointer). Facial nerve lies 1 cm deep and inferior to its tip.
  - Superior to point of insertion of posterior belly of digastric muscle.
  - Squamo-tympanic Fissure.
  - Styloid Process (Facial Nerve found Superficial to this).
  - Mastoid process can be drilled and nerve identified more proximally.
- **Retrograde Method:**
  - To identify the Buccal Branch or Cervical Branch of facial nerve and trace backwards.
  - Very useful in re-operative cases.

Ans: (d) Inferior belly of omohyoid

Ref: *Diseases of Ear, Nose and Throat and Head and Neck Surgery by Dhingra, 6th Edition, Page 327*

6. Widening of cartilaginous part of external auditory canal is called:

(a) Otoplasty (b) Myringoplasty

(c) Tympanoplasty (d) Meatoplasty

Explanation:

Meatoplasty

- It is a surgical procedure in which a **crescent of conchal cartilage** is excised to **widen the meatus.**
- This helps in epithelialization of the mastoid cavity.
- It is invariably combined with all canal walls down procedures, i.e., modified radical and radical mastoidectomies for easy access to mastoid cavity for periodic inspection and cleaning.
- It is also done as an isolated procedure in a sagging auricle seen in older people.

Otoplasty

- Done to correct prominent ears is called an **otoplasty or pinnaplasty**.
- It is a surgical technique used to correct prominent ears (For example '**bat ears'**).
- This is most commonly performed about **7 years** of age.

Myringoplasty

- In this surgery, reconstructive procedure is limited to repair of tympanic membrane perforation.
- Closure of perforation of **pars tensa** of the tympanic membrane.
- It is done in mucosal/safe **Chronic Suppurative Otitis Media (CSOM).**
- Indication: If only perforation is there, ear dry for > 6 weeks.
- Autologous temporalis fascia graft, underlay Technique preferred.

Ossiculoplasty

- Reconstruction of the ossicular chain.
- If ossicles are additionally necrosed, ossicular replacement prosthesis used either total or partial (TROP/PORP).

Tympanoplasty

- Surgery to eradicate disease in both the mastoid and middle ear cavity, and to reconstruct the hearing mechanism with or without tympanic membrane grafting.

- **Myringoplasty + Ossiculoplasty.**
- It constitutes surgical repair of the tympanic membrane, i.e., Myringoplasty along with replacement of ossicles, i.e., ossiculoplasty.

Ans. (d) Meatoplasty

Ref: *Diseases of Ear, Nose and Throat and Head and Neck Surgery by Dhingra, 6th Edition, Page 400*

7. Occipitomental X-ray view of paranasal sinuses with open mouth is called:

(a) Towne's view (b) Caldwell's view
(c) Pierre's view (d) Water's view

Explanation:

NAMED X-RAY VIEWS IN ENT

Law's View

- It is lateral oblique view of mastoid.
- Patient lies in such a way that sagittal plane of the skull is parallel to the film and X-ray beam is projected 15°cephalocaudal.
- Structures seen are:
  - (a) External auditory canal superimposed on internal auditory canal.
  - (b) Mastoid air cells.
  - (c) Tegmen.
  - (d) Lateral sinus plate.
  - (e) Temporomandibular joint.

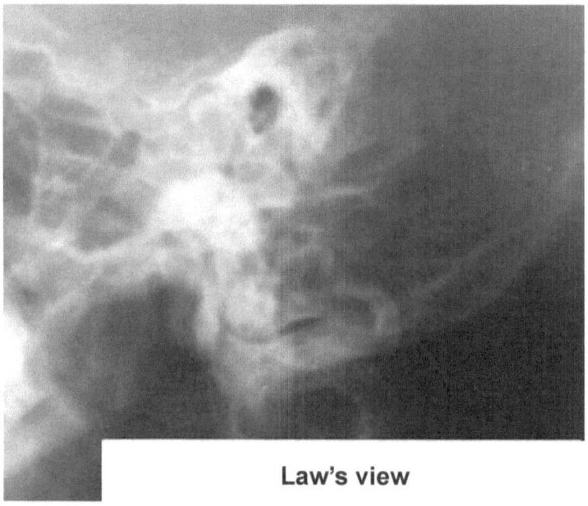

Law's view

Schuller's View

- Similar to Law's view but cephalocaudal beam makes an angle of 30° to the sagittal.
- This view is taken to see the extent of pneumatization, destruction of intercellular septa (as in mastoiditis), location of sinus plate and tegmen, cholesteatoma and longitudinal fracture of petrous pyramid.
- Structures seen are:
  - (a) External canal superimposed on internal canal.
  - (b) Mastoid air cells.
  - (c) Tegmen.
  - (d) Lateral sinus plate.
  - (e) Condyle of mandible.
  - (f) Sinodural angle.
  - (g) Antrum and upper part of attic (i.e., key area).

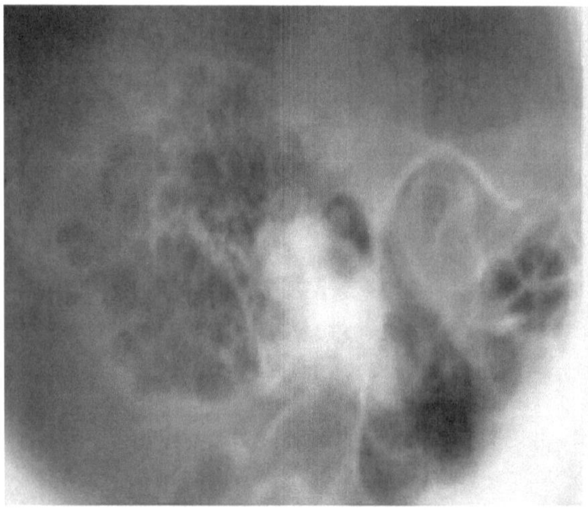

Schuller's view

Stenver's View

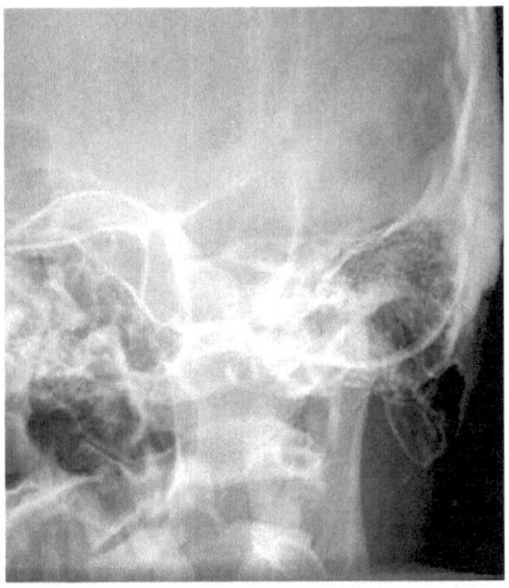

Stenver's view

- This view is taken in such a way that long axis of the petrous bone lies parallel to the film.
- Structures seen are:
  - (a) Entire petrous pyramid.
  - (b) Arcuate eminence.
  - (c) Internal auditory meatus.
  - (d) Labyrinth with its vestibule.
  - (e) Cochlea.
  - (f) Mastoid antrum.

Towne's View

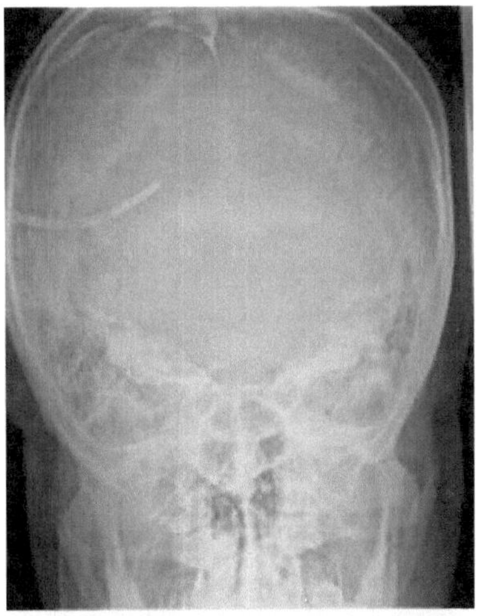

Towne's view

- It is anteroposterior view with 30° tilt from above and in front. It shows both petrous pyramids which can be compared.
- This view is usually taken for acoustic neuroma and apical petrositis.
- Structures seen are:
  - (a) Arcuate eminence and superior semicircular canal.
  - (b) Mastoid antrum.
  - (c) Internal auditory canal.
  - (d) Tympanic cavity.
  - (e) Cochlea.
  - (f) External auditory canal.

Water's View (Occipitomental view or nose-chin position)

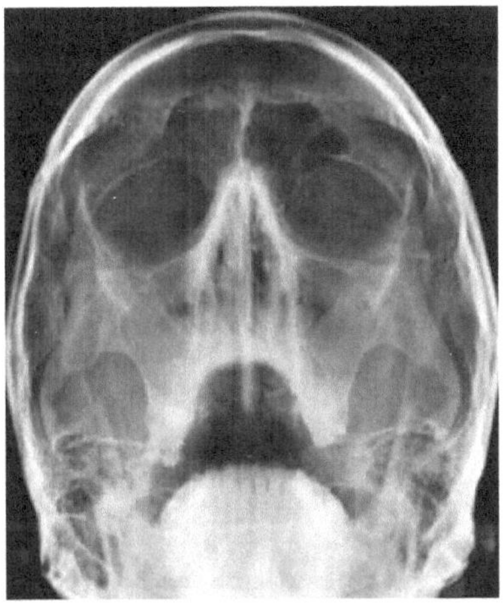

Water's view

- It is taken in such a way that nose and chin of the patient touch the film while X-ray beam is projected from behind.
- Occipitomental view (Water's view) with open mouth is **Pierre's view*** and is preferred as it also shows **sphenoid sinus**. In this view, petrous bones are projected below the maxillary antra.
- It gives end-on view of nasal arch. Fractures of right and left nasal bones and their lateral displacement can be seen.
- Structures seen are:
  - (a) Maxillary sinuses (seen best).
  - (b) Frontal sinuses.
  - (c) Sphenoid sinus (if the film is taken with open mouth).
  - (d) Zygoma.
  - (e) Zygomatic arch.
  - (f) Nasal bone.
  - (g) Frontal process of maxilla.
  - (h) Superior orbital fissure.
  - (i) Intratemporal fossa.

Caldwell View (Occipitofrontal view or nose-forehead position)

- The view is taken with nose and forehead touching the film and X-ray beam is projected 15–20° caudally. Structures seen are:
  (a) Frontal sinuses (seen best).
  (b) Ethmoid sinuses.
  (c) Maxillary sinuses.
  (d) Frontal process of zygoma and zygomatic process of frontal bone.
  (e) Superior margin of orbit and lamina papyracea.
  (f) Superior orbital fissure.
  (g) Foramen rotundum (inferolateral to superior orbital fissure).

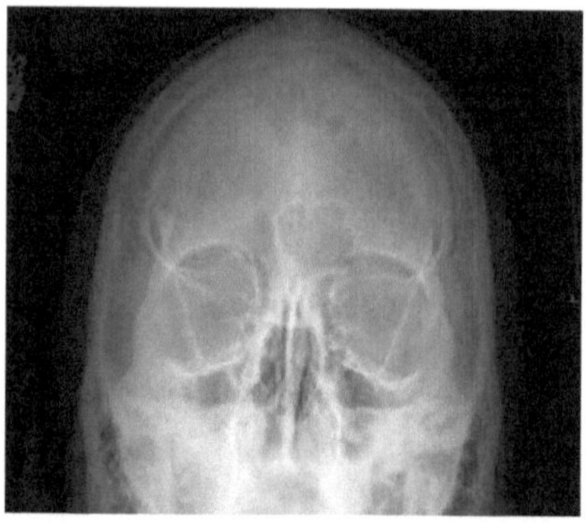

Caldwell's view

Ans: (c) Pierre's view

Ref: *Diseases of Ear, Nose and Throat and Head and Neck Surgery by Dhingra, 7th Edition, Page 207*

8. Partial and full closure of nostrils is done as management in:

(a) Atrophic rhinitis (b) Allergic rhinitis
(c) Vasomotor rhinitis (d) Occupational rhinitis

Explanation:

Atrophic Rhinitis (OZAENA)

- It is a chronic inflammation of nose characterized by **atrophy of nasal mucosa and turbinate bones**.
- Characterized by atrophy of nasal mucosa and turbinate bones and nasal cavity filled with **foul smelling crusts.** Clinical features are roomy nasal cavities, nasal obstruction (due to crusting), and **merciful anosmia**.
- **Pathology:**
  - Ciliated columnar epithelium is lost and is replaced by stratified squamous type.
  - There is atrophy of seromucinous glands, venous blood sinusoids and nerve elements.
  - Arteries in the mucosa, periosteum and bone show obliterative endarteritis.
  - The bone of turbinates undergoes resorption causing widening of nasal chambers.
  - Paranasal sinuses are small due to their arrested development.
- Medical management is the prime treatment that includes:
  - Alkaline nasal douching.
  - 25% glucose in glycerine pack.
  - Kemicetine antiozaena solution.
- **Surgical Treatment:**
  - **Young's operation:** Both the nostrils are closed by raising vestibule skin flaps and reopened after 6 months, by the time mucosae revert back to normal.
  - **Modified Young's operation:** Partial closure of nostrils, leaving 2 mm hole. It avoids the discomfort of complete nasal closure.
    - o **Lautenslager surgery:** Insertion of fat, cartilage, Teflon under mucoperiosteum of lateral wall narrows the widened airway.

- **Role of surgery in allergic rhinitis:** Turbinoplasty of hypertrophied inferior turbinate relieves nasal block.
- **Role of surgery in vasomotor rhinitis:** Vidian neurectomy is done since it decreases the parasympathetic over activity seen in vasomotor rhinitis.

Ans: (a) Atrophic rhinitis

Ref: *Diseases of Ear, Nose and Throat and Head and Neck Surgery by Dhingra, 6th Edition, Page 154*

OPHTHALMOLOGY

1. Which of the following vitamin in supraphysiologic doses is linked to macular cysts and macular edema?

(a) Vitamin D (b) Vitamin E

(c) Niacin (d) Vitamin A

Explanation:

Cystoid Macular Edema

- Cystoid macular edema (CME) is a painless disorder in which swelling develops in the macula. As the swelling increases, multiple fluid filled cysts develop in the macula, causing vision loss and distortion.
- Occurs due to accumulation of fluid in the outer plexiform and inner nuclear layers of the retina with the formation of tiny cyst-like cavities.
- **Drugs causes cystoid macular edema:**
  - Niacin: It is a cholesterol lowering agent. It causes cystoid macular edema when given in large doses. It is reversible on cessation of treatment.
  - Topical prostaglandin derivatives.
  - Epinephrine.
  - Paclitaxel.
  - Tamoxifen.
  - Timoblu.
- **Other causes of cystoid macular edema:**
  - Uveitis.
  - Diabetic retinopathy, retinal vein occlusion.
  - Retinitis pigmentosa.
  - Epiretinal membrane (conditions involving vitreomacular traction).
- **Hypervitaminosis A:** Causes papilloedema due to increased intracranial hypertension.

Ans: (c) Niacin

Ref: *Kanski's Clinical Ophthalmology, 9th Edition, Page 602*

2. Esotropia is most commonly associated with:

(a) Astigmatism (b) Hyperopia

(c) Myopia (d) Presbyopia

Explanation:

- **Hypermetropia** is defined as the parallel rays of light coming from the infinity are focused behind the retina when accommodation is at rest.
- **Complications:**
  - Recurrent stye, blepharitis, chalazion–Due to frequent rubbing to relieve fatigue and tiredness.
  - Accommodative exotropia–Excessive use of accommodation to see near vision. Along with accommodation, convergence and miosis occur.

  - Amblyopia–Hypermetropia is more amblyogenic than myopia.
  - High risk to develop primary angle closure glaucoma–The eye in hypermetropia is smell and relatively shallow anterior chamber.
- **Ocular Association of Myopia**:
  - Primary open angle glaucoma.
  - Divergent squint.
  - Retinal degeneration and retinal detachment–due to stretching of retina.
  - Posterior staphyloma.

Ans: (b) Hyperopia

Ref: *Kanski's Clinical Ophthalmology, 9th Edition, Page 727*

3. Shifting fluid is seen in:

(a) Retinal dialysis
(b) Tractional RD
(c) Rhegmatogenous RD
(d) Exudative RD

Explanation:

- **In Exudative Retinal Detachment (ERD):** An exudative retinal detachment (which is often caused by a choroidal tumour) is characterized by 'shifting' subretinal fluid.
- **Tractional Retinal Detachment:** Retinal mobility is severely reduced and shifting fluid is absent.

RETINAL DETACHMENT

- Retinal detachment is defined as **separation of inner neurosensory retina** from the outer retinal pigment epithelium.
- It is classified as rhegmatogenous, tractional and exudative.

	Rhegmatogenous RD	Tractional RD	Exudative RD
Mechanism	Due to break or hole	Fibrovascular proliferation→pulls the neurosensory retina from the RPE	Due to accumulation of fluid (exudation)
Causes	• Myopia • Old age • Trauma	• Proliferative diabetic retinopathy • CRVO • PVR	• From inflammatory process or neoplasm of retina/choroid/sclera
Pathology	• Retinal breaks present • Pigment in vitreous in 70% cases • Clear subretinal fluid	• No primary retinal breaks. May develop secondary breaks • Pigment in vitreous present in trauma cases • Clear subretinal fluid	• No retinal breaks • No pigment in vitreous • Turbid subretinal fluid which shifts rapidly to dependent location with changes in head position
Symptoms	• Sudden painless loss of vision • **3 F's** – floaters, flashes of light, field loss	• Gradual loss of vision • Field loss	• Defective vision depending on the cause
Configuration of Retina	Convex	Concave	Bullous

Contd.

Contd.

Management	**3 S** • See the hole • Seal the hole • Drain the subretinal fluid	• Vitrectomy • Endolaser photocoagulation	Treat the primary cause

Ans: (d) Exudative RD

Ref: *Kanski's Clinical Ophthalmology, 9th Edition, Page 682*

4. A 65-year-old man with history of diabetes and HTN present to OPD with complaint of diplopia and squint. On examination secondary deviation is seen to more than primary deviation. Which of the following is most probable diagnosis?

(a) Concomitant squint (b) Paralytic squint
(c) Restrictive squint (d) Pseudo squint

Explanation:

- There are two types of manifest squint:
  - Concomitant/Non-paralytic.
  - Concomitant/Paralytic squint.

Features of Non-concomitant/Paralytic squint concomitant/Non-paralytic squint

Features	Non-concomitant / Paralytic squint	Concomitant / Non-paralytic squint
Causes	Restrictive–Thyroid eye disease, myositis, orbital space occupying lesions, fibrosed muscle Paralytic–3rd, 4th and 6th nerve paralysis	Decreased vision like refractive error, cataract Central fusional reflex not formed/ broken-cerebral palsy Ocular muscle imbalance–convergence insufficiency
Diplopia	Present	Absent
Onset	Suddenly	Slow
Ocular movements	Limited in the direction of paralysed muscle	Full (No limitation)
Magnitude of squint	Varies with eye position	Same in all positions
Secondary deviation	More than primary deviation	Equal to primary deviation
False projection	It is positive: The patient cannot correctly locate the object in space when seeing in the direction of the paralyzed muscle, in early stages	Negative
Vertigo	Present	Absent
Pathological sequelae in muscles	Present	Absent
Head posture	Particular head posture depending on the muscle paralyzed, may be present	Normal

Ans: (b) Paralytic squint

Ref: *Kanski's Clinical Ophthalmology, 9th Edition, Page 704*

5. This movement is lost in:

(a) 4th nerve palsy
(b) 6th nerve palsy
(c) 7th nerve palsy
(d) 3rd nerve palsy

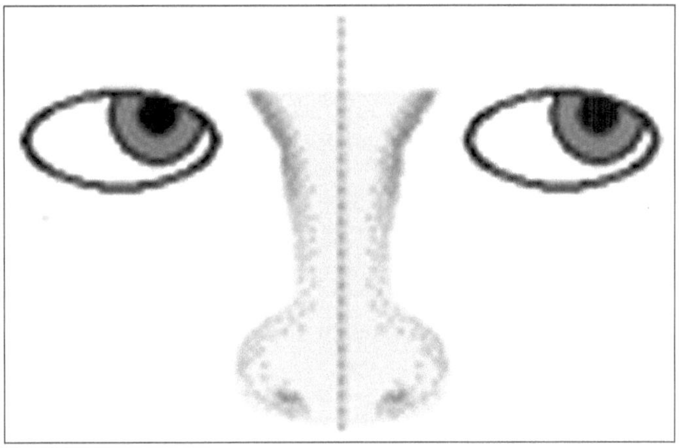

Explanation:

- Levoelevation (elevation of both eyes toward left) is shown in the illustration.
- The below figure shows the muscles in both eyes which act during binocular eye movements (versions).
- During levoversion (patient is looking toward his left side), right medial rectus and lateral rectus will be acting.
- Similarly, right inferior oblique and left superior rectus act together to bring or Levoelevation. These muscles are supplied by the third nerve. So third nerve palsy affects the Levoelevation.

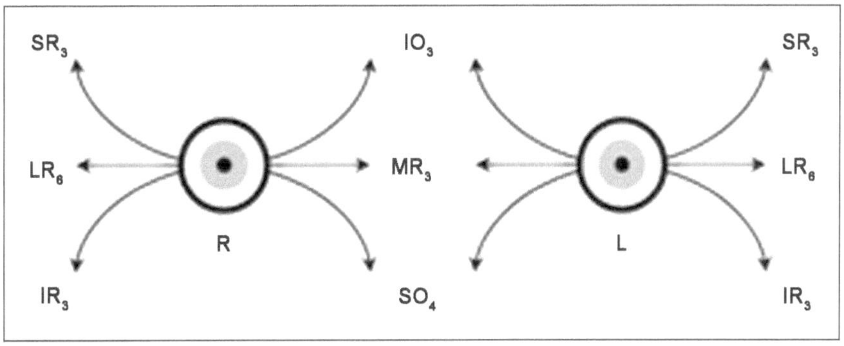

Ans: (d) 3rd nerve palsy

Ref: *Kanshki Clinical Ophthalmology, 9th Edition, Page 799*

6. A 40-year-old woman with bilateral painful proptosis, with restricted ocular movement and chemosis. She is euthyroid. What is your probable diagnosis?

(a) Orbital lymphoma
(b) Orbital cellulitis
(c) Thyroid eye disease
(d) Pseudotumor of orbit

Explanation:

- Thyroid Eye Disease (TED) is the most common causes of bilateral proptosis and it can occur with any thyroid status.

Thyroid Eye Disease (TED)

- The most common cause of unilateral and bilateral proptosis in adults is thyroid eye disease/Graves' disease.

- The major clinical risk factor for developing TED is smoking.
- Women are five times more likely to be affected by TED than men.
- It is associated with any thyroid status (hyper/hypo/euthyroid). In fact about 10-25% of cases, thyroid ophthalmopathy occurs in the absence of both clinical and biochemical evidence of thyroid dysfunction.
- Clinical features broadly can be categorized into:
  - Proptosis.
  - Soft tissue involvement.
  - Optic neuropathy; and
  - Lid retraction.
  - Restrictive myopathy.
- **Most frequent symptoms:** Pain and discomfort.
- **CT scan:** Thickening of extra ocular muscles with sparing of tendons.

Ans: (c) Thyroid eye disease

Ref: *Kanski's Clinical Ophthalmology, 9th Edition, Page 118*

7. Characteristic of fungal keratitis is:

(a) Dendrite ulcer
(b) Satellite lesion
(c) Ring abscess
(d) White hypopyon

Explanation:

Typical Features of Fungal Keratitis:

- Sudden onset of pain, photophobia, discharge and reduced vision in a patient with an inflamed eye and an opacity on the surface of the cornea suggestive of an ulcer.
- **Findings:**
  - Satellite lesions.
  - Cheesy hypopyon (So option (d) rule out).
  - Feathery margins.
  - Gritty texture while scraping.
  - Raised dry surface.
  - Endothelial plaques.

Candida Keratitis

- A rare, unilateral, insidious fungal infection which usually occurs in eyes with pre-existing chronic corneal disease or in severely debilitated patients.
- They are responsible for most cases of fungal keratitis in temperate climates.
- **Signs:** Yellow-white densely suppurative infiltrate is typical which is similar to bacterial ulcer.

Filamentous Keratitis

- A rare, unilateral, insidious fungal infection which is typically preceded by ocular trauma with wood.
- **Signs:**
  - Grey or yellow–white stromal infiltrate with indistinct fluffy margins.
  - Often surrounded by finger-like satellite stromal infiltrates.

- Penetration of an intact Descemet membrane may occur and lead to endophthalmitis without evident perforation.
- Corneal necrosis and thinning.

Acanthamoeba Keratitis

- A very rare, unilateral condition which typically affects wearers of soft contact lenses.
- Epithelial Pseudodendrites is the early sign.
- **Characteristic of this disease:** Ring infiltrate (oval shaped).

Other Signs

- Non-specific stromal infiltrates.
- Radial keratoneuritis.
- Corneal necrosis and thinning in advanced cases.

Ans: (b) Satellite lesion

Ref: *Parson's Diseases of the Eye, 23rd Edition, Page 176; Kanski's Clinical Ophthalmology, 9th Edition, Page 216*

8. Incongruous homonymous hemianopia with Wernicke's hemianopia pupil. What is the site of lesion?

(a) Optic tract (b) Optic nerve
(c) Visual cortex (d) Optic radiations

Explanation:

- Field defects in optic tract lesions are homonymous contralateral, incongruous hemianopia.
- **Visual Pathway comprises:**
  - Optic nerve.
  - Optic chiasma.
  - Optic tract (OT).
  - Lateral geniculate body (LGB).
  - Optic radiation (OR).
  - Visual cortex.
- To understand the visual pathway lesion, optic chiasma is an important anatomical landmark where the decussation of the nerve fibers.
  - Any lesion anterior to the optic chiasma (optic nerve) causes Ipsilateral Unilocular field defect.
  - Lesion involving optic chiasma causes bitemporal or Binasal hemianopia.
  - Any lesion posterior to optic chiasma (optic tract, lateral geniculate body, optic radiation, visual cortex) causes contralateral Homonymous Hemianopia.
- **Congruous:**
  - Means identical field defects in both eyes. The rule is "More posterior the lesion in the visual pathway, more congruous the field defect will be". For example:
    - OT and LGB lesions cause–incongruous contralateral hemianopia.
    - Visual cortex lesion causes congruous contralateral homonymous hemianopia.
- **Wernicke's Hemianopic Pupil:**
  - The optic tracts contain both visual and pupillomotor fibers. The visual fibers terminate in the lateral geniculate body but the pupillary fibers leave the optic tract anterior to the lateral geniculate body, projecting through the brachium of the superior colliculus to terminate in the pretectal nuclei.

- An optic tract lesion may therefore give rise to an afferent pupillary conduction defect.

Ans: (a) Optic tract

Ref: *Kanski's Clinical Ophthalmology, 9th Edition, Page 793*

9. Pre-requisite for diagnosing sympathetic ophthalmitis:

(a) Blunt ocular trauma
(b) Chemical injury
(c) Retained intra ocular iron foreign body
(d) Penetrating trauma to eye

Explanation:

Sympathetic Ophthalmitis

- Also called spared eye injury, is a diffuse granulomatous inflammation of the uveal layer of both eyes following trauma to one eye.
- Bilateral granulomatous panuveitis after penetrating trauma with prolapsed of uvea.
- **Exciting eye:** Injured eye developing the disease at a variable time after the injury.
- **Sympathizing eye:** The other eye which develops the disease synchronously or shortly afterwards.
  - Injured eye–exciting eye.
  - Normal fellow–sympathizing eye.
- It is autoimmune (T-cell mediated).
- **Causes:**
  - Penetrating injury (Most common).
  - Intraocular surgeries.
  - Cyclophotocoagulation.
  - Cyclocryotherapy.
- **Site of injury:** Involving CB, iris and lens capsule.
- **Pathogenesis:** Autoimmunity against uveal pigments (sequestered antigen).
- **Dalen Fuch's Nodules:** Granulomas between Bruch's and RPE.

CLINICAL FEATURES

- **Exciting Eye**
  - Decrease in vision and photophobia.
- **Sympathizing Eye**
  - Photophobia.
  - Lacrimation increased.
  - Visual fatigue.
  - Blurring vision.
- **Signs in Both Eyes**
  - Keratic precipitates on corneal endothelium.
  - Thickened iris.
  - Retrolental flare.
  - Clouding of vitreous.
  - Partially dilated and poorly responsive pupil.
- **Earliest Symptom:** Loss of accommodation.

- **Earliest Sign:** Retrolental flare and cells; KP's at the back of cornea.
- Enucleation of the injured eye within 10 days only in eyes with a hopeless visual prognosis.
- **Treatment:** Topical and systemic steroids.

Ans: (d) Penetrating trauma to eye

Ref: *Kanski's Clinical Ophthalmology, 9th Edition, Page 448*

10. Which layer of cornea helps in maintaining hydration of stroma of cornea?

(a) Endothelium (b) Epithelium

(c) Stroma (d) Descemet membrane

Explanation:

LAYERS OF CORNEA (FROM ANTERIOR TO POSTERIOR)

- **Epithelium**
  - Thickness 50-90 μm.
  - It is non-keratinized stratified squamous epithelium consists of 5-6 layers of cell.
- **Bowman's membrane**
  - Thickness 8-14 μm y. It is not a true membrane–PAS negative.
  - It doesn't regenerate.
- **Stroma (Substantia propria)**
  - Thickness 490 μm.
  - It constitutes 90% of the corneal thickness.
  - It contains mostly type-1 collagen and few type-5 collagen.
  - Most common ground substance is keratin sulphate.
- **Dua's layer**
  - Thickness 6.5-13.9 μm.
  - It has been recently identified. It lies between stroma and Descemet's membrane.
  - It is the toughest layer (Previously Descemet's layer considered as toughest layer).
- **Descemet's membrane**
  - Thickness 10-12 μm.
  - Its thickness varies with age (3 microns at birth and 10-12 microns in adults).
  - It is secreted by endothelial cell throughout life.
  - It can regenerate.
  - In the periphery, it ends at the anterior limit of trabecular meshwork known as Schwalbe's line.
- **Endothelium**
  - Thickness 5 μm.
  - It consists of a single layer of flat polygonal cells.
  - Most metabolically active layer, contains an "active-pump" mechanism (Na+ - K+ -ATPase) to maintain **corneal dehydration.**

Ans: (a) Endothelium

Ref: *Parson's Diseases of the Eye, 22nd Edition, Page 10*

11. Presence of extra layer of cilia posterior to grey line is:

(a) Trichiasis (b) Distichiasis
(c) Poliosis (d) Madarosis

Explanation:

DISTICHIASIS

- Extra row of cilia at the opening of the meibomian gland posterior to the grey line.
- It is also called as second row of eyelashes.
- There are two types:
  - **Acquired distichiasis (metaplastic lashes)**
    - An uncommon unilateral or bilateral condition caused by metaplasia and dedifferentiation of meibomian glands to become hair follicles in late cicatrising conjunctivitis (e.g., ocular cicatricial pemphigoid).
    - **Sign:** Crops of stunted lashes originating from meibomian gland orifices.
  - **Congenital distichiasis**
    - A rare, bilateral, hereditary condition.
    - **Sign:** Partial or complete second row of lashes originating from or slightly behind the meibomian gland orifices.

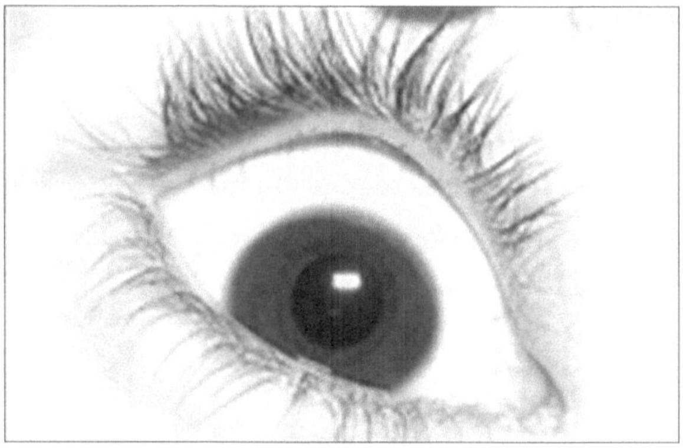
Distichiasis

ALSO NOTE:

- **Trichiasis:** Inward turning of previously normal lashes.
- **Poliosis:** Localized patch of grey or white hair due to lack of pigment in the epidermis.
- **Madarosis:** Decrease in number or complete loss of lashes.

Ans: (b) Distichiasis

Ref: *Kanski's Clinical Ophthalmology, 9th Edition, Page 62*

12. Unilateral proptosis with bilateral abducent nerve palsy is seen in:

(a) Thyroid ophthalmopathy (b) Retinoblastoma
(c) Cavernous sinus thrombosis (d) Orbital pseudotumor

Explanation:

CAVERNOUS SINUS THROMBOSIS

- The cavernous sinuses are irregularly shaped, trabeculated and consists of incompletely fused venous channels located at the base of the skull in the middle cranial fossa.
- They lie on either side of the sellaturcica, are just lateral and superior to the sphenoid sinus and are immediately posterior to the optic chiasma.
- **Nerve and blood supply of cavernous sinuses**
  - This intimate juxtaposition of veins, arteries, nerves, meninges and paranasal sinuses accounts for the characteristic etiology and presentation of cavernous sinus thrombosis.
  - The third, fourth and ophthalmic and maxillary divisions of the fifth cranial nerve are attached to the lateral wall of the sinus.

- The sixth cranial nerve and internal carotid artery with its surrounding sympathetic plexus passes through the cavernous sinus.
- So sixth cranial nerve is the first nerve to get affected in the cavernous sinus thrombosis.

- **Causes:** It occurs due to infection such as sinusitis, orbital or preseptal cellulitis or otitis.
- **Clinical Features:**
  - Headache, fever and malaise typically precede the development of ocular findings. As the infection tracks posteriorly, patients complain of orbital pain and fullness accompanied by periorbital edema and visual disturbances.
- **Ocular Signs:**
  - Proptosis rapidly.
  - Increased intraocular pressure.
  - Cranial nerve palsies (3rd, 4th and 6th). Isolated sixth nerve dysfunction may be noted before there are obvious orbital findings.
  - Edema is the mastoid region is a pathogenomic sign. It is due to back pressure in the mastoid emissary vein.
  - Fundus: Congestion of retinal veins and papilloedema.
- **Diagnosis:**
  - **MRI:** Pattern of an infarct that does not follow the distribution of an expected arterial occlusion. It may show absence of flow void in the normal venous channels.
  - **MRV:** It is an excellent method of visualizing the dural venous sinuses and larger cerebral veins.
  - **Lumbar puncture:** Systemic infection.
- **Treatment:** Intravenous antibiotics and sometimes surgical drainage. Corticosteroids: Reduce inflammation and edema.

Ans: (c) Cavernous sinus thrombosis

Ref: *Kanski's Clinical Ophthalmology, 9th Edition, Page 129*

13. Photo stress test to differentiate between pathology of which two structures?

(a) Lens and cornea
(b) Retina and vitreous
(c) Retina and optic nerve
(d) Macula and optic nerve

Explanation:

PHOTO STRESS TESTING

- **Photo stress recovery time (PSRT)** is the time taken for visual acuity to return to normal levels after the retina has been bleached by a bright light source. Photo stress recovery time measurement procedure is known as **photo stress test**. Normal recovery time is about **15-30 seconds.**
- Photo stress testing is a gross test of dark adaptation in which the visual pigments are bleached by light. This causes a temporary state of retinal insensitivity perceived by the patient as a scotoma.
- It also differentiates visual loss caused by macular disease from that caused by an optic nerve lesion.
- The PSRT is prolonged relative to the normal eye in macular disease (sometimes 50 seconds or more) but not in an optic neuropathy.

Ans: (d) Macula and optic nerve

Ref: *Kanski's Clinical Ophthalmology, 9th Edition, Page 7*

MEDICINE

1. Water hammer pulse is seen in:

(a) Mitral stenosis
(b) Aortic stenosis
(c) Aortic regurgitation
(d) Ventricular failure

Explanation:

Aortic Regurgitation

- Aortic regurgitation (AR, also called aortic insufficiency) is caused by inadequate closure of the aortic valve leaflets. It can be induced either by disease of the aortic valve leaflets or by distortion or dilation of the aortic root and ascending aorta.
- A variety of physical findings are caused by the wide pulse pressure in patients with chronic AR.
- **Corrigan pulse** – A "water hammer" or "collapsing" pulse is characterized by a rapidly rising and falling arterial pulse with a wide pulse pressure. This finding is best appreciated by palpation of the radial or brachial arteries (exaggerated by raising the arm) or the carotid pulses.
- **de Musset's sign** – A head bob occurring with each heartbeat.
- **Traube's sign** – A pistol shot pulse (systolic and diastolic sounds) heard over the femoral arteries.
- **Duroziez's sign** – A systolic and diastolic bruit heard when the femoral artery is partially compressed.
- **Quincke's pulses** – Capillary pulsations in the fingertips or lips.
- **Mueller's sign** – Systolic pulsations of the uvula.
- **Becker's sign** – Visible pulsation of the retinal arteries.
- **Landolfi's sign** – Constriction and dilation of the pupils with each heartbeat.
- **Hill's sign** – Popliteal cuff systolic pressure exceeding brachial cuff pressure by more than 20 mm Hg with patient in the recumbent position.
- **Mayne's sign** – More than a 15 mm Hg decrease in diastolic blood pressure with arm elevation from the value obtained with the arm in the standard position.
- **Rosenbach's sign** – Systolic pulsations of the liver.
- **Gerhard's sign** – Systolic pulsations of the spleen.

Ans: (c) Aortic regurgitation

Ref: *Harrison's Principles of Internal Medicine, 20th Edition, Page 1810*

2. A 65-year-old lady presents with a vascular injury to the inferior frontal gyrus. Which functional area would be mostly affected?

(a) Visual
(b) Auditory
(c) Wernicke
(d) Motor speech

Explanation:

- The **premotor area** is located just **anterior** to the **motor area.**
- It occupies the **posterior** parts of the **superior**, **middle** and **inferior frontal gyri.**
- The part of the premotor area located in the superior and middle frontal gyri corresponds to **areas 6 and 8 of Brodmann.**

- The part in the **inferior frontal gyrus** corresponds to **areas 44 and 45** and constitutes **the motor speech area (of Broca)**. Closely related to the premotor area there are two specific areas of importance. One is the motor speech area of Broca, mentioned above; and the other is the frontal eye field.

	Brodmann's Area	Name	Function	Connections
Frontal lobe	4 6 8 44,45	Primary motor cortex Premotor cortex Frontal eye field Broca's area	Voluntary muscle activation Eye movements Motor aspects of sppech	Contributes to corticospinal tract Sends projections to lateral gaze center (paramedium pontine reticular formation) Projects to Wernicke's area via arcuate fasciculus
Parietal lobe	3,1,2	Primary sensory cortex	Somatosensory	Input from VPL, VPM
Occipital lobe	17 18, 19	Striate cortex=primary visual cortex Extrastriate=visual association cortex	Processing of visual stimuli Procesing of visual stimuli	Input from lateral geniculate only Projects to areas 18,19 Input from area 17
Temporal lobe	41 42 22	Primary auditory cortex Associative auditory cortex Wernicke's area	Processing of auditory stimuli Language comprehenion	Input from medial geniculate Inputs from auditory association cortex, visual association cortex, Broca's area (via arcuate fasciculus)

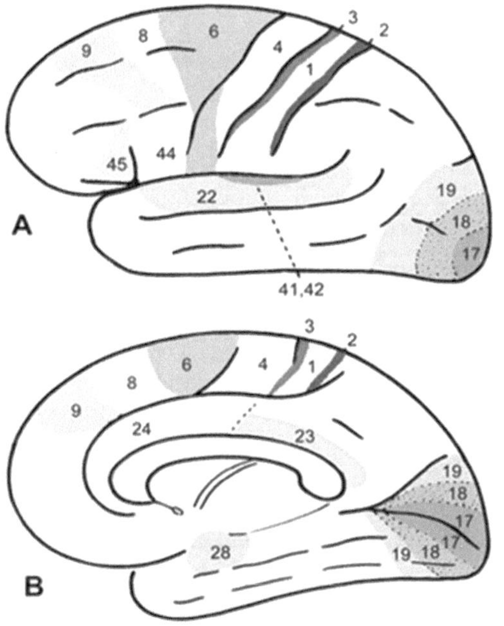

Location of some of the areas of Brodmann on the superolateral aspect (A), and on the medial aspect of the cerebral hemisphere (B)

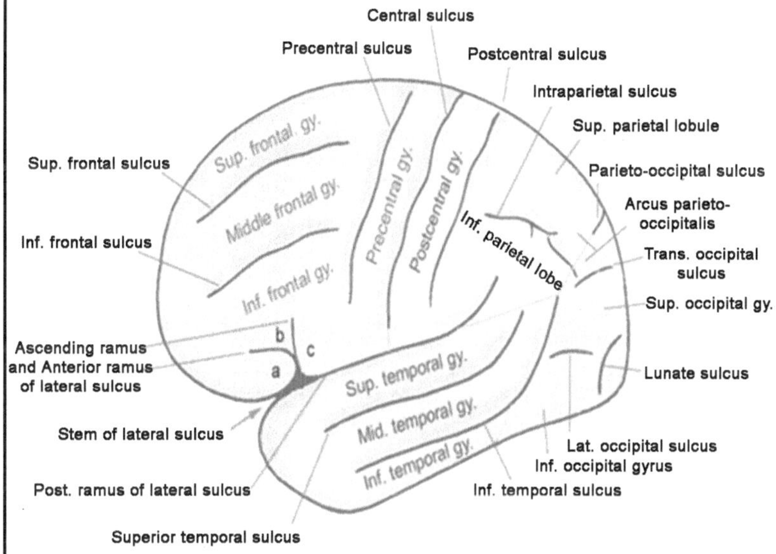

Simplified presentation of sulci and gyri on the superolateral surface of the cerebral hemisphere (a-pars orbitals; b-pars triangularis; c-pars opercularis)

Ans: (d) Motor speech

Ref: *I.B. Singh Textbook of Human Neuroanatomy, 8th Edirion, Page 86*

3. A person met with a motor bike accident. CT brain shows injury to posterior end of superior temporal gyrus. He is likely to suffer from:

(a) Fluent aphasia
(b) Non-fluent aphasia
(c) Conduction aphasia
(d) Nominal aphasia

Explanation:

Wernicke's Aphasia

- **Comprehension** is impaired for spoken and written words and sentences. **Language output is fluent** but is highly **paraphasic** and **circumlocutious**.
- The lesion site most commonly associated with **Wernicke's aphasia** caused by CVAs is the posterior portion of the language network.
- An embolus to the **inferior division** of the **middle cerebral artery** (MCA), to the **posterior temporal** or **angular branches** in particular, is the most common etiology.

Broca's Aphasia

- Speech is **nonfluent**, **labored**, **interrupted** by many word-finding pauses and usually **dysarthric.**
- The cause is most often **infarction of Broca's area** (the **inferior frontal convolution** and surrounding **anterior perisylvian** and **insular cortex** due to occlusion of the **superior division of the MCA**.

Conduction Aphasia

- **Speech output is fluent** but contains many **phonemic paraphasias**, comprehension of spoken language is intact, and **repetition is severely impaired**.
- Naming elicits phonemic paraphasias and spelling is impaired.
- Reading aloud is impaired, but reading comprehension is preserved.
- The responsible lesion, usually a CVA in the **temporoparietal** or **dorsal perisylvian region**, interferes with the function of the phonological loop interconnecting Broca's area with Wernicke's area.

Aphasia type	Lesion	Fluency	Comprehension	Repetition	Naming	Paraphasias
Broca's	Inferior frontal gyrus	Non	Intact	Impaired	Impaired	Rare
Wernicke's	Superior temporal gyrus	Fluent	Impaired	Impaired	Impaired	Common
Transcortical motor	Anterior or superior to Broca's subcortical WM	Non	Intact	Intact	Impaired	Rare
Transcortical sensory	Posterior middle temporal gyrus angular gyrus corresponding deep WM	Fluent	Impaired	Intact	Impaired	Common
Conduction	Arcuate fasciculus	Fluent	Intact	Impaired	Impaired	Variable

Ans: (a) Fluent aphasia

Ref: *Harrison's Principles of Internal Medicine, 20th Edition, Page 158*

4. All of the following are seen in Left Ventricular Failure (LVF), *except:*

(a) Pedal edema
(b) Rales
(c) Kerley B lines
(d) Pulmonary oligaemia

Explanation:

- Acute pulmonary edema usually presents with the rapid onset of dyspnea at rest, tachypnea, tachycardia and severe hypoxemia.
- Crackles and wheezing due to alveolar flooding and airway compression from peribronchial cuffing may be audible.
- Release of endogenous catecholamines often causes hypertension.

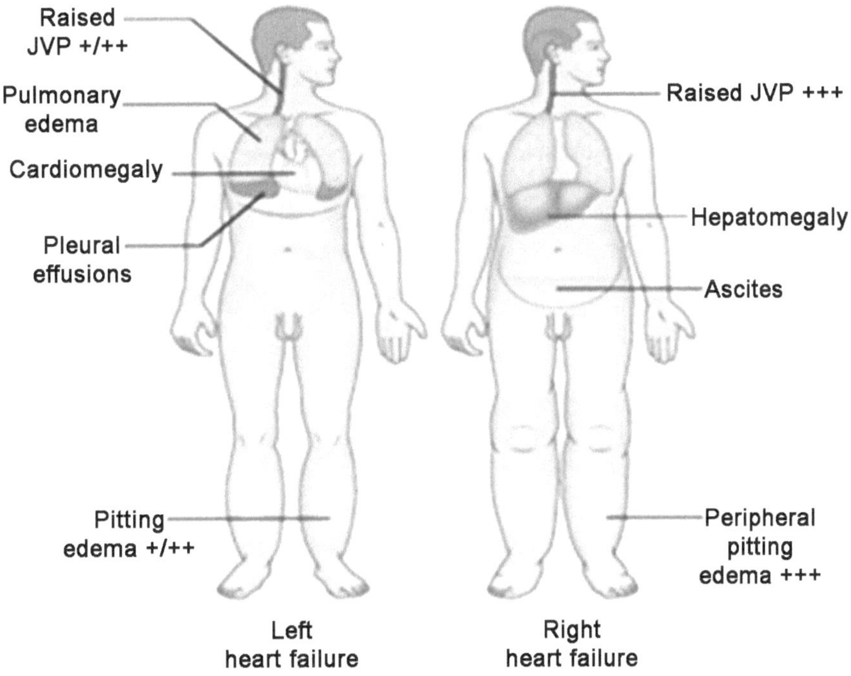

Clinical features of left and right heart failure

(JVP = Jugular venous pressure)

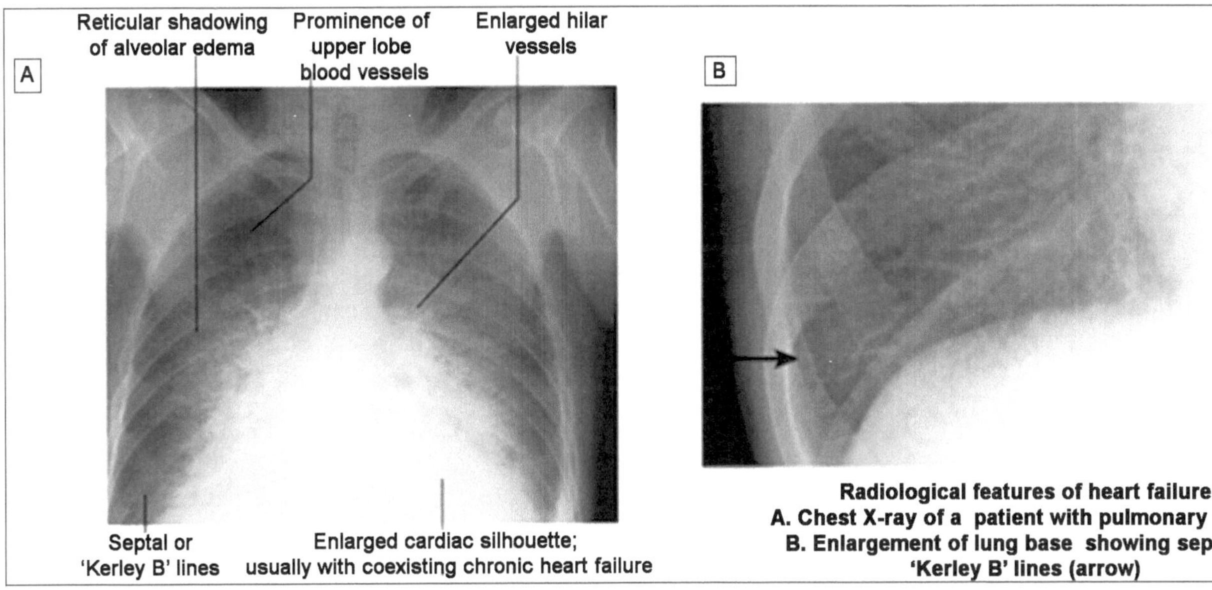

Radiological features of heart failure
A. Chest X-ray of a patient with pulmonary edema
B. Enlargement of lung base showing septal or 'Kerley B' lines (arrow)

Ans: (d) Pulmonary oligaemia

Ref: *Harrison's Principles of Internal Medicine, 20th Edition, Page 1763; Davidson's Principles and Practice of Medicine, 23rd Edition, Page 468*

5. Broad-based gait with enuresis is seen in:

(a) Normal pressure hydrocephalus
(b) Alcohol withdrawal syndrome
(c) Cerebellar lesion
(d) All of the above

Explanation:

NORMAL PRESSURE HYDROCEPHALUS (NPH)

- **Pathologically enlarged ventricular size** with **normal opening pressures** on lumbar puncture.
- NPH is a form of **communicating hydrocephalus** and is distinguished from obstructive or noncommunicating hydrocephalus, in which there is a structural blockage of the cerebrospinal fluid (CSF) circulation within the ventricular system.
- NPH is associated with a **classic triad** of:
  - **Dementia.**
  - **Gait disturbance.**
  - **Urinary incontinence.**
- **Idiopathic NPH:** When no obvious cause is identified, several possible mechanisms of NPH have been proposed.
- **Decompensated congenital hydrocephalus:** The observation that larger head sizes are more common in patients with NPH than normal controls suggests the possibility that some patients with NPH have congenital hydrocephalus that becomes symptomatic later in life.
- **Secondary NPH:** Impaired absorption of CSF is the suspected mechanism in most cases of secondary NPH.
- The most common identified underlying causes are **intraventricular or subarachnoid hemorrhage** (either from aneurysm or trauma) and prior acute or ongoing **chronic meningitis** (from infection, cancer, or inflammatory disease).
- **Paget's disease** at the skull base, **mucopolysaccharidosis** of the meninges, and **achondroplasia** are other rarely reported causes of secondary NPH.
- NPH is classically described as having three cardinal features: Gait difficulty, cognitive disturbance and urinary incontinence.
- **Gait dysfunction:**
  - Gait difficulty is the most prominent clinical feature in NPH.
  - Patients with NPH move slowly and take **small steps**, often with a **wide base**. They have difficulty turning and are most vulnerable to falls when turning. **Postural instability** demonstrated by the pull test is often present.
  - The parkinsonian gait may bear a resemblance to that of NPH but is distinguished by a narrow base and responsiveness to visual and acoustic cues.
- **Cognitive impairment:** The cognitive disturbance of NPH evolves over months to years and usually develops after the onset of gait dysfunction. Patients typically have both subcortical and frontal features, including:
  - Psychomotor slowing.
  - Decreased attention and concentration.
  - Impaired executive function.
  - Apathy.

- **Urinary incontinence:** Urinary urgency rather than incontinence may be present at early stages.

Ans: (a) Normal pressure hydrocephalus

Ref: *Harrison's Principles of Internal Medicine,20th Edition, Page 3112*

6. As per NCEP-ATP III, which of the following is not included in metabolic syndrome?

(a) Central obesity (b) High levels low-density lipoproteins (LDL)

(c) Hyperglyceridemia (d) Hypertension

Explanation:

- The metabolic syndrome (syndrome X, insulin resistance syndrome) consists of a constellation of metabolic abnormalities that confer increased risk of cardiovascular disease (CVD) and diabetes mellitus.
- The major features of the metabolic syndrome include:
  - Central obesity.
  - Hypertriglyceridemia.
  - Low levels of high-density lipoprotein (HDL) cholesterol.
  - Hyperglycemia.
  - Hypertension.

<table>
<tr><th colspan="2">NCEP: ATPIII[a] 2001 and Harmonizing Definition Criteria for the Metabolic Syndrome</th></tr>
<tr><th>NCEP: ATPIII 2001</th><th>HARMONIZING DEFINITION[b]</th></tr>
<tr><td>Three or more of the following:
• Central obesity: Waist circumfrence > 102 cm (M), >88 cm (F)
• Hypertriglyceridemia:Triglyceride level ≥ 150 mg/dl or specific medication
• Low HDL[c] cholesterol: < 40 mg/dl and < 50 mg/dl for men and women, respectively, or specific medication
• Hypertension: Blood pressure ≥ 130 mm Hg systolic or ≥ 85 mm Hg diastolic or specific medication
• Fasting plasma glucose level ≥ 100 mg/dl or specific medication or previously diagnosed type 2 diabetes</td><td>Three of the following:
Waist circumference (cm)<table><tr><th>Men</th><th>Women</th><th>Ethnicity</th></tr><tr><td>≥ 94</td><td>≥ 80</td><td>Europid, sub-Saharan African, Eastern and Middle Eastern</td></tr><tr><td>≥ 90</td><td>≥ 80</td><td>South Asian, Chinese and ethnic South and Central American</td></tr><tr><td>≥ 85</td><td>≥ 90</td><td>Japanese</td></tr></table>• Fasting triglyceride level > 150 mg/dl or specific medication
• HDL cholesterol level < 40 mg/dl and < 50 mg/dl for men and women, respectively, or specific medication
• Blood pressure > 130 mm systolic or > 85 diastolic or previous diagnosis or specific medication
• Fasting plasma glucose level ≥ 100 mg/dl alternative indication: drug treatment of elevated glucose levels)</td></tr>
<tr><td colspan="2">[a] National Cholesterol Education Program and Adult Treatment Panel III.
[b] In this analysis, the following thresholds for waist circumference were used: white men, ≥ 94 cm; African-American men, ≥ 94 cm; Mexican-American men, ≥ 90 cm; white women, ≥ 80 cm; African-American women, ≥ 80 cm; Mexican-American women, ≥ 80 cm. For participants whose designation was "other race–including multiracial", thresholds that were once based on Europid cutoffs (≥ 94 cm for men and ≥ 80 cm for women) and on South Asian cutoffs (≥ 90 cm for men and ≥ 80 cm for women) were used. For participants who were considered "other Hispanic", the International Diabetes Federation thesholds for ethnic South and Central Americans were used.
[c] High-density lipoprotein.</td></tr>
</table>

Risk Factors:

- Obesity.
- Sedentary lifestyle.
- Genetics.
- Ageing.

- Diabetes mellitus.
- Cardiovascular disease.
- Lipodystrophy.
- Metabolic syndrome has been recognized as a proinflammatory, prothrombotic state, associated with elevated levels of C-reactive protein (CRP), interleukin (IL)-6, and plasminogen activator inhibitor (PAI)-1

Therapeutic goals for management of metabolic syndrome	
	Goals
Lifestyle risk factors	
Abdominal obesity	Year 1: Reduce body weight 7 to 10 percent
	Continue weight loss thereafter with ultimate goal BMI < 25 kg/m^2
Physical inactivity	At least 30 min (and preferably $\geq$ 60 min) continuous or intermittent moderate intensity exercise 5 times per week, but preferably daily
Atherogenic diet	Reduced intake saturated fat, trans fat, cholesterol

Metabolic risk factors	
Dyslipidemia	
Primary target elevated LDL cholesterol	**High risk*:** < 100 mg/dl (2.6 mmol/> l); optional < 70 mg/dl
	Moderate risk: < 130 mg/dl (3.4 mmol/l)
	Lower risk: < 160 mg/dl (4.9 mmol/l)
Secondary target elevated non-HDL cholesterol	**High risk*:** < 130 mg/dl (3.4 mmol/l); optional < 100 mg/dl (2.6 mmol/l) very high risk
	Moderate risk: <160 mg/dl (4.1 mmol/l)
	Lower risk: < 190 mg/dl (4.9 mmol/l)
Tertiary target reduced HDL cholesterol	Raise to extent possible with weight reduction and exercise
Elevated blood pressure	Reduce to at least < 140/90 (< 130/80 if diabetic)
Elevated glucose	For IFG, encourage weight reduction and exercise
	For type 2 DM, target A1C < 7 percent
Prothrombotic state	Low-dose aspirin for high-risk patients
Proinflammatory state	Lifestyle therapies; no specific interventions

Ans: (b) High levels low-density lipoproteins (LDL)

Ref: *Harrison's Principles of Internal Medicine, 20th Edition, Page 2903*

7. Which of the following is not seen in pituitary apoplexy?

(a) Hypotension
(b) Hypertension
(c) Vomiting
(d) Headache

Explanation:

Pituitary Apoplexy

- **Sudden hemorrhage** into the pituitary gland is called **pituitary apoplexy**.
- Pituitary apoplexy may occur:
  - Spontaneously in a **preexisting adenoma.**
  - **Postpartum (Sheehan's syndrome).**
  - In association with **diabetes**, **hypertension**, **sickle cell anemia**, or **acute shock.**
- Apoplexy is an endocrine emergency that may result in severe **hypoglycemia**, **hypotension** and **shock**, **central nervous system (CNS) hemorrhage** and **death**.
- Acute symptoms may include **severe headache** with signs of **meningeal irritation, bilateral visual changes, ophthalmoplegia**, and, in severe cases, **cardiovascular collapse and loss of consciousness**.
- In its most dramatic presentation, apoplexy causes the **sudden onset of excruciating headache**, **diplopia** due to pressure on the **oculomotor nerves** and **hypopituitarism**.
- All pituitary hormonal deficiencies can occur, but the sudden onset of ACTH and therefore cortisol deficiency is the most serious because it can cause life-threatening hypotension.
- Pituitary computed tomography (CT) or MRI may reveal signs of intratumoral or sellar hemorrhage, with pituitary stalk deviation and compression of pituitary tissue.
- Patients with no evident visual loss or impaired consciousness can be observed and managed conservatively with high-dose glucocorticoids.
- Those with significant or progressive visual loss, cranial nerve palsy, or loss of consciousness require urgent surgical decompression.

Ans: (b) Hypertension

Ref: *Harrison's Principles of Internal Medicine, 20th Edition, Page 2665*

8. A patient was unable to gain weight and complaints of fatigue. On examination, body was warm. Which of the following is the expected finding?

(a) High thyroid-stimulating hormone (TSH) with normal T3 and T4
(b) High TSH with euthyroid state
(c) Increased uptake of T3 and decrease T4
(d) Low TSH with increased T3 and T4

Explanation:

- **Thyrotoxicosis** is defined as the state of thyroid hormone excess and is not synonymous with hyperthyroidism, which is the result of excessive thyroid function.

Sign and symptoms of thyrotoxicosis (Descending Order of Frequency)	
Symptoms	**Signs**[a]
Hyperactivity, irritability, dysphoria Heat intolerance and sweating Palpitations Fatigue and weakness Weight loss with increased appetite Diarrhea Polyuria Oligomenorrhea, loss of libido	Tachycardia; atrial fibrillation in the elderly Tremor Goiter Warm, moist skin Muscle weakness, proximal myopathy Lid retraction or lag Gynecomastia
[a]Excludes the signs of ophthalmopathy and dermopathy specific for Graves' disease.	

- Thyrotoxicosis may cause **unexplained weight loss**, despite an **enhanced appetite**, due to the **increased metabolic rate.**
- Other prominent features include:
  - **Hyperactivity, nervousness and irritability**, ultimately leading to a sense of easy fatigability.
  - **Fine tremor** is a frequent finding, best elicited by having patients stretch out their fingers while feeling the fingertips with the palm.
- Common neurologic manifestations include:
  - **Hyperreflexia.**
  - **Muscle wasting;** and
  - Proximal myopathy without fasciculation.
- The most common cardiovascular manifestation is **sinus tachycardia**, often associated with **palpitations**, occasionally caused by **supraventricular tachycardia**.
- The high cardiac output produces a **bounding pulse, widened pulse pressure, and an aortic systolic murmur** and can lead to worsening of angina or heart failure in the elderly or those with preexisting heart disease.
- **Atrial fibrillation** is more common in patients > 50 years of age.
- The skin is usually warm and moist, and the patient may complain of sweating and heat intolerance, particularly during warm weather.
- **Palmar erythema, onycholysis,** and, less commonly, pruritus, urticaria, and diffuse hyperpigmentation may be evident.
- **Hair texture** may become **fine**, and a **diffuse alopecia** occurs in up to 40% of patients, persisting for months after restoration of euthyroidism.
- Gastrointestinal transit time is decreased, leading to increased stool frequency, often with **diarrhea** and occasionally mild steatorrhea.
- Women frequently experience **oligomenorrhea or amenorrhea**; in men, there may be **impaired sexual function** and, rarely, **gynecomastia**.
- The direct effect of thyroid hormones on bone resorption leads to osteopenia in long-standing thyrotoxicosis; mild hypercalcemia occurs in up to 20% of patients, but hypercalciuria is more common. There is a small increase in fracture rate in patients with a previous history of thyrotoxicosis.
- Graves' disease, the TSH level is suppressed, and total and unbound thyroid hormone levels are increased. In 2–5% of patients (and more in areas of borderline iodine intake), only T3 is increased (T3 toxicosis). The converse state of T4 toxicosis, with elevated total and unbound T4 and normal T3 levels, is occasionally seen when hyperthyroidism is induced by excess iodine, providing surplus substrate for thyroid hormone synthesis.

Evaluation of Thyrotoxicosis

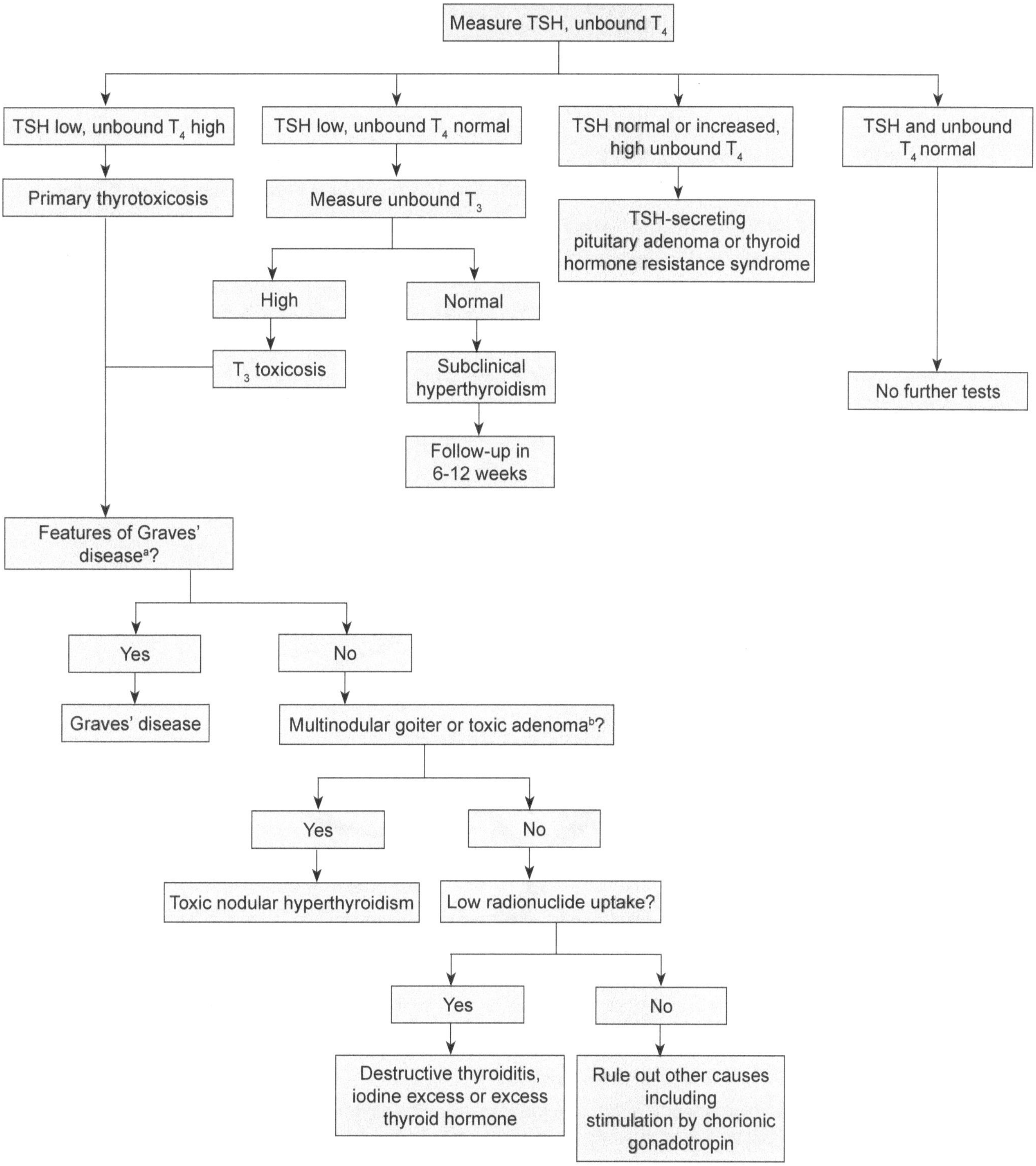

[a] Diffuse goiter, positive TPO antibodies or TRAb, ophthalmopathy, dermopathy.
[b] Can be confirmed by radionuclide scan.
TSH, thyroid-stimulating hormone.

Ans: (d) Low TSH with increased T3 and T4

Ref: *Harrison's Principles of Internal Medicine, 20th Edition, Page 2703*

9. In nystagmus, ataxia and dysdiadochokinesia which of the following artery is involved?

(a) PICA (b) AICA

(c) Vertebral artery (d) All of the above

Explanation:

- The **vertebral artery**, which arises from the **innominate artery** on the **right** and the **subclavian artery** on the left, consists of **four segments**.
  - The first (V1) extends from its origin to its entrance into the sixth or fifth transverse vertebral foramen.
  - The second segment (V2) traverses the vertebral foramina from C6 to C2.
  - The third (V3) passes through the transverse foramen and circles around the arch of the atlas to pierce the dura at the foramen magnum.
  - The fourth (V4) segment courses upward to join the other vertebral artery to form the basilar artery. Only the fourth segment gives rise to branches that supply the brainstem and cerebellum.
- The posterior inferior cerebellar artery (PICA) in its proximal segment supplies the lateral medulla and, in its distal branches, the inferior surface of the cerebellum.
- Anterior inferior cerebellar artery is a branch of basilar artery that course around pons to supply cerebellar hemispheres.

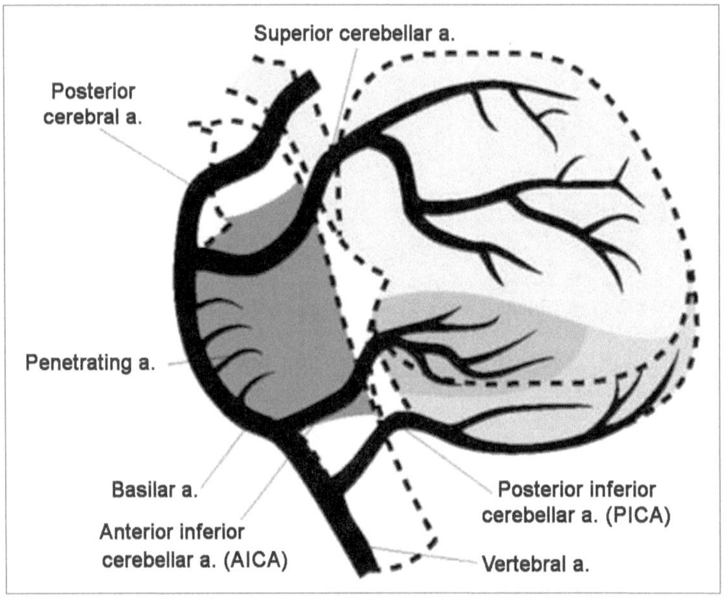

- Cerebellum has ipsilateral control over body:
  - Regulates the rate, rhythm, range and force of muscular contraction.
  - Facilitatory action on tone and reflex activity of the body.
  - Maintains posture and equilibrium.
  - Integrates the voluntary and automatic movements—'coordination'.
- Cerebellar dysfunction leads to:
  - Titubation.
  - Dysarthria.
  - Hypotonia.
  - Pendular knee jerk.
  - Intention tremor.
  - Adiadochokinesia.

- Dysmetria.
- Dyssynergia.
- Rebound phenomenon.
- Gait disturbance.

Ans: (d) All of the above

Ref: *Harrison's Principles of Internal Medicine, 20th Edition, Page 3081*

10. Which of the following differentiates between irritable bowel syndrome (IBS) and organic GI disease (IBD)?

(a) Mucus in stools (b) Stool calprotectin

(c) Abdominal pain (d) Diarrhea

Explanation:

- Irritable bowel syndrome (IBS) is a **functional bowel** disorder characterized by:
  - Abdominal pain or discomfort; and
  - Altered bowel habits in the absence of detectable structural abnormalities.
- According to the current IBS diagnostic criteria, abdominal pain is a prerequisite clinical feature of IBS.

Rome IV Diagnostic criteria for irritable bowel syndrome[a]
Recurrent abdominal pain, on average, at least 1 day per week in the last 3 months, associated with ≥ 2 of the following criteria: 1. Related to defecation 2. Associated with a change in frequency of stool 3. Associated with a change in form (appearance) of stool

[a]Criteria fulfilled for the last 3 months with symptom onset at least 6 months prior to diagnosis.

- Supportive symptoms that are not part of the diagnostic criteria include defecation straining, urgency or a feeling of incomplete bowel movement, passing mucus, and bloating.
- Inflammatory bowel disease (IBD) is an immune-mediated chronic intestinal condition. Ulcerative colitis (UC) and Crohn's disease (CD) are the two major types of IBD.

Ulcerative Colitis

- The major symptoms of UC are **diarrhea, rectal bleeding, tenesmus, passage of mucus and crampy abdominal pain.**

Ulcerative colitis: Disease presentation			
	Mild	**Moderate**	**Severe**
Bowel movements	< 4 per day	4-6 per day	> 6 per day
Blood in stool	Small	Moderate	Severe
Fever	None	< 37.5°C mean (< 99.5°F)	< 37.5°C
Tachycardia	None	< 90 mean pulse	> 90 mean pulse
Anemia	Mild	> 75% of a normal hemoglobin	≤ 75% of a normal hemoglobin
Sedimentation rate	< 30 mm		> 30 mm
Endoscopic appearance	Erythema, decreased vascular pattern, fine granularity	Marked erythema, coarse granularity, absent vascular markings, contact bleeding, no ulceration	Spontaneous bleeding, ulcerations

- Active disease can be associated with a rise in acute-phase reactants (C-reactive protein [CRP]), platelet count, and erythrocyte sedimentation rate (ESR), and a decrease in hemoglobin.
- **Fecal calprotectin** is present in neutrophils and monocytes and levels correlate well with histologic inflammation, predict relapses and detect pouchitis.
- Both fecal lactoferrin and calprotectin are becoming an integral part of IBD management and are used frequently to rule out active inflammation versus symptoms of irritable bowel or bacterial overgrowth.

Crohn's Disease

- CD usually presents as acute or **chronic bowel inflammation**, the inflammatory process evolves toward one of two patterns of disease: a fibrostenotic obstructing pattern or a penetrating fistulous pattern, each with different treatments and prognoses.
- Laboratory abnormalities include elevated ESR and CRP.
- **Fecal calprotectin** and **lactoferrin** levels have been used to distinguish **IBD** from **irritable bowel syndrome (IBS).**

Ans: (b) Stool calprotectin

Ref: *Harrison's Principles of Internal Medicine, 20th Edition, Page 2276*

11. A patient bilateral adrenalectomy in view of bilateral phaeochromocytoma. On postoperative day-1, he developed fatigue and lethargy but his BP and pulse were normal. What could be the most likely cause?

(a) Cortisol deficiency
(b) Cardiogenic shock
(c) Hypovolemic shock
(d) Septic shock

Explanation:

- **Pheochromocytomas** and **paragangliomas** are catecholamine-producing tumors derived from the **sympathetic or parasympathetic nervous system**.
- **Complete tumor removal**, the ultimate therapeutic goal, can be achieved by **partial or total adrenalectomy**.
- It is important to preserve the normal adrenal cortex in order to prevent **Addison's disease**, particularly in hereditary disorders in which bilateral pheochromocytomas are most likely.
- **Nitroprusside infusion** is useful for intraoperative hypertensive crises, and **hypotension** usually responds to volume infusion.
- Postoperatively, **catecholamine normalization** should be **documented**.
- An **ACTH test** should be used to exclude **cortisol deficiency** when bilateral adrenal cortex sparing surgery has been performed.
- Complications of surgery for pheochromocytoma are primarily due to:
  - Severe preoperative hypertension.
  - High secretion tumors; or
  - Repeat intervention for recurrence.
- The absence of adrenal glands leads to a sharp drop in cortisol, implying lifelong glucocorticoid replacement therapy and increases the risk of developing Nelson syndrome.
- **Nelson syndrome** is characterized by the enlargement of the pituitary gland and the development of pituitary gland tumors, and is estimated to occur in 15-25% of Cushing's patients who have a bilateral adrenalectomy.

Ans: (a) Cortisol deficiency

Ref: *Harrison's Principles of Internal Medicine, 20th Edition, Page 2739*

12. Nosocomial infection called after how many hours of hospital admission?

(a) 24 hours (b) 48 hours

(c) 72 hours (d) 7 days

Explanation:

- Hospital-acquired infections are caused by **viral, bacterial and fungal** pathogens; the most common types are bloodstream infection (**BSI**), pneumonia (e.g., ventilator-associated pneumonia [**VAP**]), urinary tract infection (**UTI**), and surgical site infection (**SSI**).
- **Healthcare-associated infections (HAI)** are defined as infections not present and without evidence of incubation at the time of admission to a healthcare setting.
- The term healthcare-associated infections replaced old ones such as nosocomial, hospital-acquired or hospital-onset infections.
- Most infections that become clinically evident **after 48 hours** of **hospitalization** are considered **hospital-acquired**.

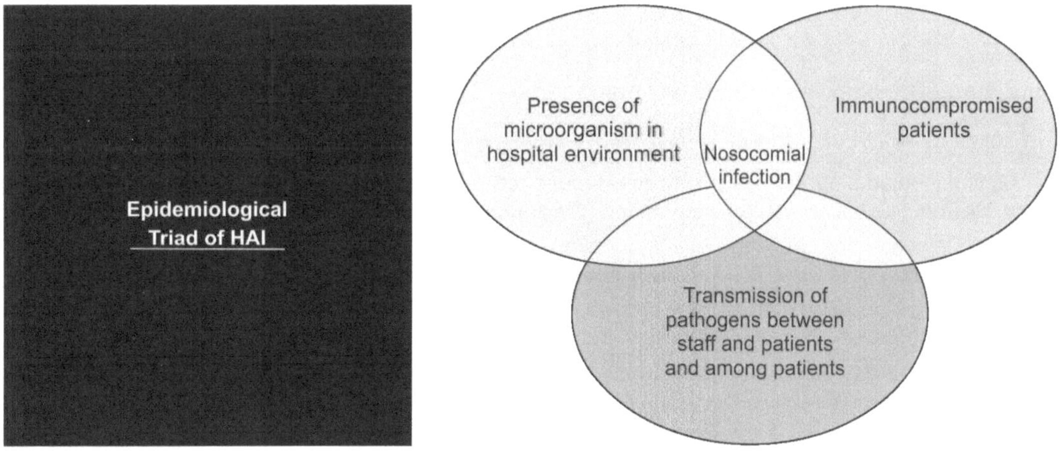

Routes of Transmission:

- Contact.
- Airborne.
- Vector borne.
- Oral.
- Parenteral.

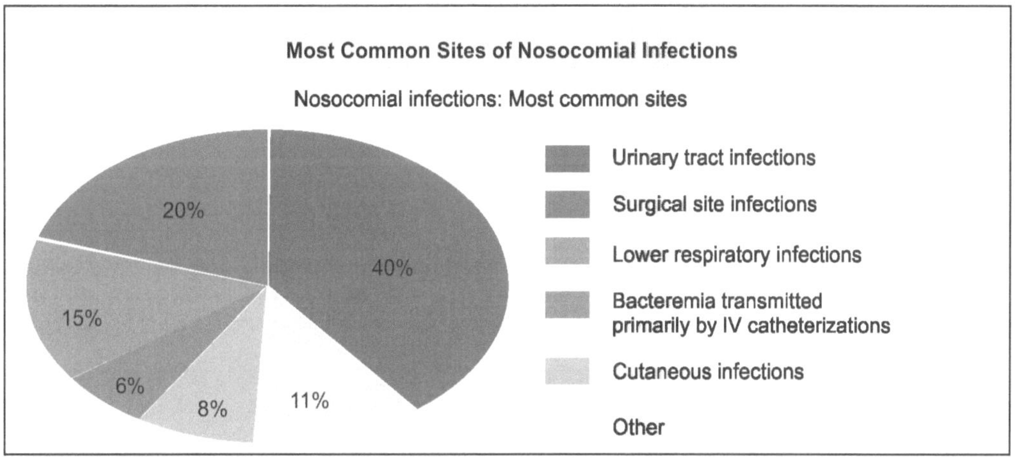

Source: Data from CDC, National Nosocomial Infection Surveillance

Ans: (b) 48 hours

Ref: *Harrison's Principles of Internal Medicine, 20th Edition, Page 1024*

13. A known case of chronic obstructive pulmonary disease (COPD) with acute exacerbation of COPD. On examination, he was conscious and alert, pulse=110/min. Which of the following is not true in management of the case?

(a) IV steroids
(b) Inhalation with salbutamol
(c) O_2 inhalation
(d) Non-invasive ventilation not indicated

Explanation:

- **Exacerbations** are episodic acute worsening of respiratory symptoms, including increased dyspnea, cough, wheezing, and/or change in the amount and character of sputum.
- They are classified as:
  - Mild-treated with short acting bronchodilators only, SABDs.
  - Moderate-treated with SABDs plus antibiotics and or oral corticosteroids.
  - Severe-patient requires hospitalization or visits the emergency room.
- More than 80% of exacerbations are managed on OP basis.

Key Points for the Management of Exacerbations
• Short-acting inhaled $beta_2$-agonists, with or without short-acting anticholinergics, are recommended as the initial bronchodilators to treat an acute exacerbation **(Evidence C).**
• Systemic corticosteroids can improve lung function (FEV_1), oxygenation and shorten recovery time and hospitalization duration. Duration of therapy should not be more than 5-7 days **(Evidence A).**
• Antibiotics, when indicated, can shorten recovery time, reduce the risk of early relapse, treatment failure and hospitalization duration. Duration of therapy should be 5-7 days **(Evidence B).**
• Methylxanthines are not recommended due to increased side effect profiles **(Evidence B).**
• Non-invasive mechanical ventilation should be the first mode of ventilation used in COPD patients with acute respiratory failure who have no absolute contraindication because it improves gas exchange, reduces work of breathing and the need for intubation, decreases hospitalization duration and improves survival **(Evidence A).**

Management of Severe But Not Life-Threatening Exacerbations*
• Assess severity of symptoms, blood gases, chest radiograph.
• Administer supplemental oxygen therapy, obtain serial arterial blood gas, venous blood gas and pulse oximetry measurements.
• **Bronchodilators:**
– Increase doses and/or frequency of short-acting bronchodilators.
– Combine short-acting $beta_2$-agonists and anticholinergics.
– Consider use of long-active bronchodilators when patient becomes stable.
– Use spacers or air-driven nebulizers when appropriate.
• Consider oral corticosteroids.
• Consider antibiotics (oral) when signs of bacterial infection are present.
• Consider noninvasive mechanical ventilation (NIV).
• **At all times:**
– Monitor fluid balance.
– Consider subcutaneous heparin or low molecular weight heparin for thromboembolism prophylaxis.
– Identify and treat associated conditions (e.g., heart failure, arrhythmias, pulmonary embolism etc.).

*Local resources need to be considered.

Ans: (d) Non-invasive ventilation not indicated

Ref: *Harrison's Principles of Internal Medicine, 20th Edition, Page 1996; Gold 2020 Guidelines*

14. A 42-year-old patient with obstructive jaundice. Alpha haptoglobin all increased. Likely reason is:

(a) Alcohol
(b) Lead
(c) Chronic renal failure
(d) None of the above

Explanation:

Haptoglobin

- Acute-phase reactant whose principal clinical utility is in defining conditions of **hemolysis**. Levels can also become elevated in **infection** and **inflammation**.
- Haptoglobin is produced by the **liver** and collects the hemoglobin from destroyed red blood cells, then transporting it back to the liver, where heme is converted to bilirubin.
- Haptoglobin is an **acute-phase reactant** whose principal clinical utility is in defining conditions of hemolysis. levels can also become elevated in infection and inflammation.
- The normal values of Haptoglobin are:
  - **Adult:** 50-220 mg/dl or 0.5-2.2 g/l (SI units).
  - **Newborn:** 0-10 mg/dl or 0-0.1 g/l (SI units).
- **Increased haptoglobin levels** are seen in the following conditions:
  - Diseases associated with elevated erythrocyte sedimentation rate (ESR) (acute-phase reactants) such as infection, trauma, inflammation, hepatitis, amyloidosis, collagen diseases, or lymphoma and leukemia.
  - Obstructive or biliary diseases.
  - Steroid use.
  - Aplastic anemia.
  - Diabetes mellitus.
  - Smoking.
  - Nephrotic syndrome.
  - Increased estrogen levels.
- **Decreased or absent haptoglobin levels** are seen in the following conditions:
  - Intravascular hemolysis (hereditary spherocytosis, pyruvate kinase deficiency, autoimmune hemolytic anemia, transfusion reactions).
  - Extravascular hemolysis (intraperitoneal hemorrhage).
  - Intramedullary hemolysis (thalassemias, sideroblastic anemias, megaloblastic anemias).
  - Genetics (haptoglobin is absent in 1% of whites and 4%-10% of blacks).
  - Cirrhosis.
  - Infancy.
  - Pregnancy.
  - Burns.

Ans: (d) None of the above

Ref: *Williams Hematology, 9th Edition, Page 499*

15. A 68-year-old male admitted to ICU for acute exacerbation of COPD develops a sudden onset of palpations. The following ECG changes are seen. What is the most likely diagnosis?

(a) AF
(b) Ventricular tachycardia
(c) AMI
(d) MAT

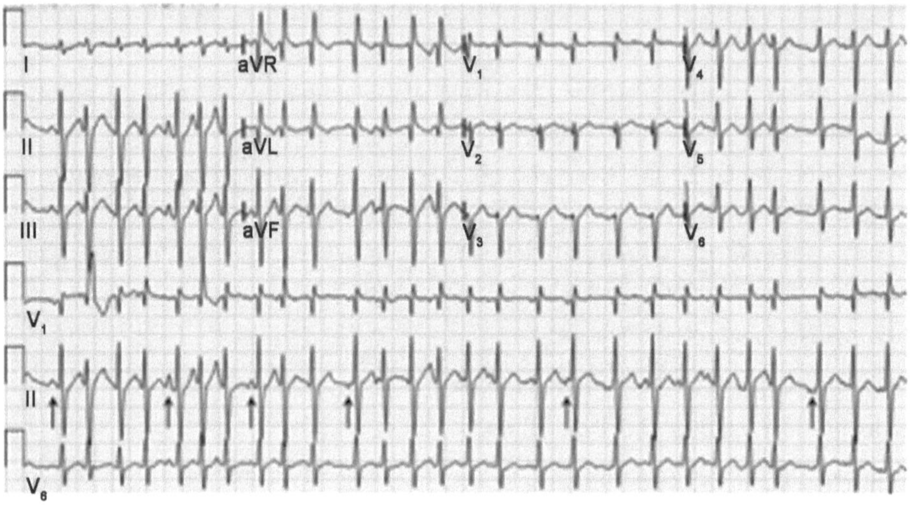

Explanation:

Multifocal Atrial Tachycardia (MAT)

- A rapid, irregular atrial rhythm arising from multiple ectopic foci within the atria.
- Most commonly seen in patients with **severe COPD or congestive heart failure**.
- It is typically a **transitional rhythm** between frequent **premature atrial complexes (PACs) and atrial flutter/fibrillation.**

Electrocardiographic Features:

- Heart rate > 100 bpm (usually 100-150 bpm; may be as high as 250 bpm).
- Irregularly irregular rhythm with varying PP, PR and RR intervals.
- At least 3 distinct P-wave morphologies in the same lead.
- Isoelectric baseline between P-waves (i.e., no flutter waves).
- Absence of a single dominant atrial pacemaker (i.e., not just sinus rhythm with frequent PACs).
- Some P waves may be nonconducted; others may be aberrantly conducted to the ventricles.
- Usually occurs in seriously ill elderly patients with respiratory failure (e.g., exacerbation of COPD/CHF).
- Tends to resolve following treatment of the underlying disorder.

Mechanism

- Arises due to a combination of factors that are present in hospitalised patients with acute-on-chronic respiratory failure:
  - Right atrial dilatation (from cor pulmonale).
  - Increased sympathetic drive.
  - Hypoxia and hypercarbia.
  - Beta-agonists.
  - Theophylline.

- **Electrolyte abnormalities:** Hypokalemia and hypomagnesemia (e.g., secondary to diuretics/beta-agonists).
- The net result is increased atrial automaticity.

Ans: (d) MAT

Ref: *Harrison's Principles of Internal Medicine, 20th Edition, Page 1745*

16. A patient present with clinical features of vertigo and nystagmus. The following condition is due to thrombosis of which artery?

(a) Posterior cerebral artery
(b) Middle cerebral artery
(c) Internal carotid artery
(d) Superior cerebellar artery

Explanation:

Stroke Within the Posterior Circulation

- The **posterior circulation** is composed of:
  - Paired vertebral arteries.
  - Basilar artery.
  - Paired PCAs.
- The vertebral arteries join to form the basilar artery at the pontomedullary junction. The basilar artery divides into two PCAs in the interpeduncular fossa.

Posterior Cerebral Artery

- Two clinical syndromes are commonly observed with occlusion of the PCA:
  - **P1 syndrome:** Midbrain, subthalamic and thalamic signs, which are due to disease of the proximal P1 segment of the PCA or its penetrating branches.
  - **P2 syndrome:** Cortical temporal and occipital lobe signs, due to occlusion of the P2 segment distal to the junction of the PCA with the posterior communicating artery.

Clinical Features of PCA Stroke

- Acute vision loss.
- Confusion.
- New onset posterior cranium headache.
- Paresthesias.
- Limb weakness.
- Dizziness.
- Nausea.
- Memory loss.

Superior Cerebellar Artery Stroke

- Superior cerebellar artery infarcts affect the:
  - Superior cerebellar hemispheres.
  - Cerebellar vermis; and
  - Parts of the midbrain.
- The superior cerebellar artery is the most constantly identified vessel arising from the **basilar artery** with its origin just below the posterior cerebral artery in the distal segment.

- Superior cerebellar artery infarction can present in two distinct patterns depending on the site of occlusion:
  - Occlusion at the origin of the artery produces the classic presentation of ipsilateral cerebellar (ataxia, dysarthria, nystagmus) and brainstem (Horner's syndrome) signs associated with a contralateral dissociated sensory impairment.
  - Peripheral occlusion presents with solely ipsilateral cerebellar signs.
- Proximal occlusions of the superior cerebellar arteries are often due to dissection or thrombosis, with peripheral occlusion typically due to embolization.

Cerebellar stroke syndromes			
Territory	**Signs and symptoms**	**Extracerebellar structures**	**Extracerebellar signs and symptoms**
Superior cerebellar artery	Ipsilesional limb and gait ataxia	Midbrain, Thalamus, occipital lobes	Top of the basilar syndrome
Posterior inferior cerebellar artery	Ipsilesional limb and gait ataxia	Dorsolateral medulla	Wallenberg's syndrome
Anterior inferior cerebellar artery	Vertigo ipsilesional deafness	Lateral pons	Contralateral facial weakness, numbness and hearing loss

Ans: (a) Posterior cerebral artery

Ref: *Harrison's Principles of Internal Medicine, 20th Edition, Page 3072*

17. A patient presented with weakness of the right side of the face with the loss of pain and temperature. Pain and temperature sensation of the left leg is lost. The lesion is most likely located at:

(a) Medial medulla (b) Lateral pons

(c) Medial pons (d) Lateral medulla

Explanation:

- **Lateral medullary infarction (Wallenberg syndrome)** is the most common and important syndrome related to intracranial vertebral artery occlusion.

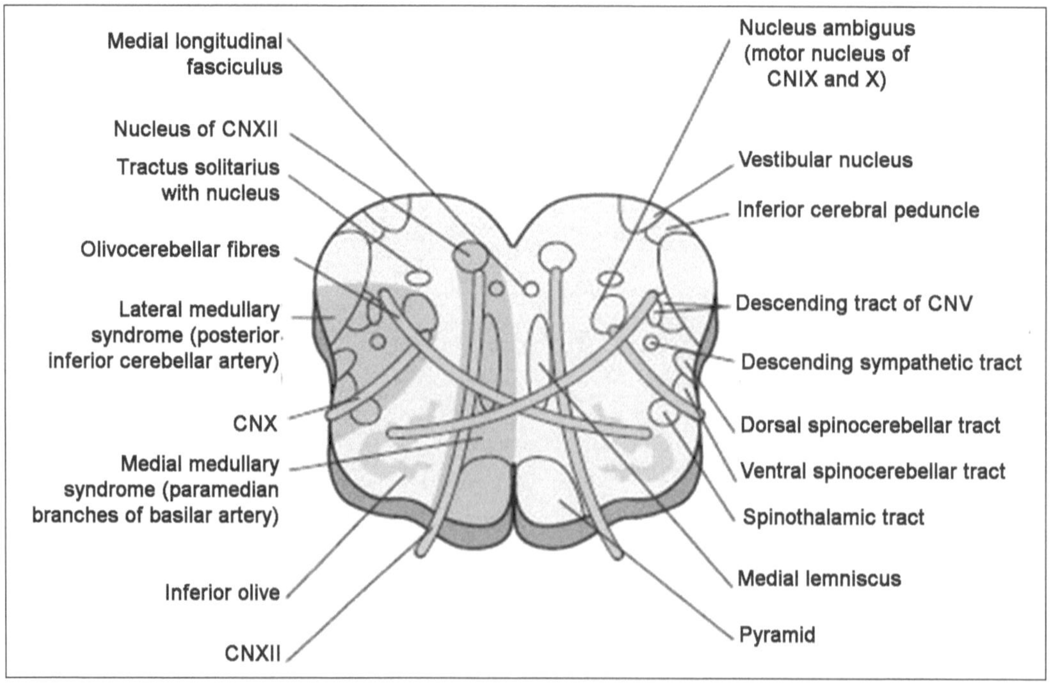

Anatomical location	Presenting symptoms
Spinothalamic tract	Contralateral loss of pain and temperature sensation
Spinal trigeminal nucleus	Ipsilateral facial loss of pain and temperature
Nucleus ambiguus	Supplies vagus and glossopharyngeal nerves; dysphagia/dysphonia/ diminished gag reflex
Inferior vestibular nucleus	Vertigo/diplopia/nystagmus/vomiting
Sympathetic fibres	Ipsilateral Horners syndrome
Central trigeminal tract	Palatal clonus
Inferior cerebellar peduncle	Ataxia

- **Medial medullary infarction**—The most consistent finding in patients with medial medullary ischemia is a **contralateral hemiparesis.**
- It is characterized by contralateral hemiplegia/hemiparesis as well as hemisensory loss with ipsilateral hypoglossal palsy (ipsilateral tongue weakness and atrophy) from involvement of CN XII nucleus.
- Other manifestations are vertigo, nausea, or contralateral limb ataxia.

Ans: (d) Lateral medulla

Ref: *Harrison's Principles of Internal Medicine, 20th Edition, Page 3072*

18. A patient with multiple sclerosis has low nerve conduction velocity. What may be the possible cause?

(a) Loss of oligodendrocytes
(b) Loss of myelin sheath
(c) Na+ channel block
(d) Defect in node of Ranvier

Explanation:

Multiple Sclerosis (MS)

- Autoimmune disease of the central nervous system (CNS) characterized by:
  - Chronic inflammation.
  - Demyelination.
  - Gliosis (plaques or scarring).
  - Neuronal loss.
- The course can be relapsing or progressive.

Physiology

- Nerve conduction in myelinated axons occurs in a **saltatory manner**, with the nerve impulse jumping from one node of Ranvier to the next without depolarization of the axonal membrane underlying the myelin sheath between nodes.
- This produces considerably **faster conduction velocities** (~70 m/s) than the slow velocities (~1 m/s) produced by continuous propagation in unmyelinated nerves.
- Conduction block occurs when the nerve impulse is unable to traverse the demyelinated segment.
- This can happen when the resting axon membrane becomes **hyperpolarized** due to the exposure of **voltage-dependent potassium channels** that are normally buried underneath the myelin sheath.
- A **temporary conduction block** often follows a **demyelinating** event before sodium channels (originally concentrated at the nodes) redistribute along the naked axon.
- This **redistribution** ultimately **allows continuous propagation** of nerve action potentials through the demyelinated segment.

Suggestive and atypical features of multiple sclerosis
Features suggestive of multiple sclerosis
Relapses and remissions
Onset between ages 15 and 50 years
Optic neuritis
Lhermitte sign
Internuclear ophthalmoplegia
Fatigue
Heat sensitivity (Uhthoff phenomenon)
Features atypical for multiple sclerosis
Steady progression
Onset before age 10 or after age 50 years
Cortical deficits such as aphasia, apraxia, alexia, or neglect
Rigidity or sustained dystonia
Convulsions
Early dementia
Deficit developing within minutes

Ans: (b) Loss of myelin sheath

Ref: *Harrison's Principles of Internal Medicine, 20th Edition, Page 3188*

19. A person presents with puffy skin and lethargy. His TSH levels are low and are improved on administration of TRH. What is the probable diagnosis?

(a) Hypothyroidism because of hypothalamus defect
(b) Diffuse thyroid enlargement
(c) Hyperthyroidism because of hypothalamus defect
(d) Hypothyroidism because of pituitary defect

Explanation:

CENTRAL HYPOTHYROIDISM

- Refers to **thyroid hormone deficiency** due to a disorder of the **pituitary**, **hypothalamus**, or **hypothalamic-pituitary portal circulation**, resulting in diminished **thyroid-stimulating hormone (TSH)**, **thyrotropin-releasing hormone (TRH)**, or both.
- **Causes of TRH deficiency: Hypothalamic diseases like:**
  - **Mass lesions** – Benign (craniopharyngiomas) and malignant tumors (metastatic from lung, breast, etc).
  - **Radiation** – For CNS and nasopharyngeal malignancies.
  - **Infiltrative lesions** – Sarcoidosis, Langerhans cell histiocytosis.
  - **Infections** – Tuberculous meningitis.
  - Other – Traumatic brain injury, stroke.

Regulation of thyroid hormone production

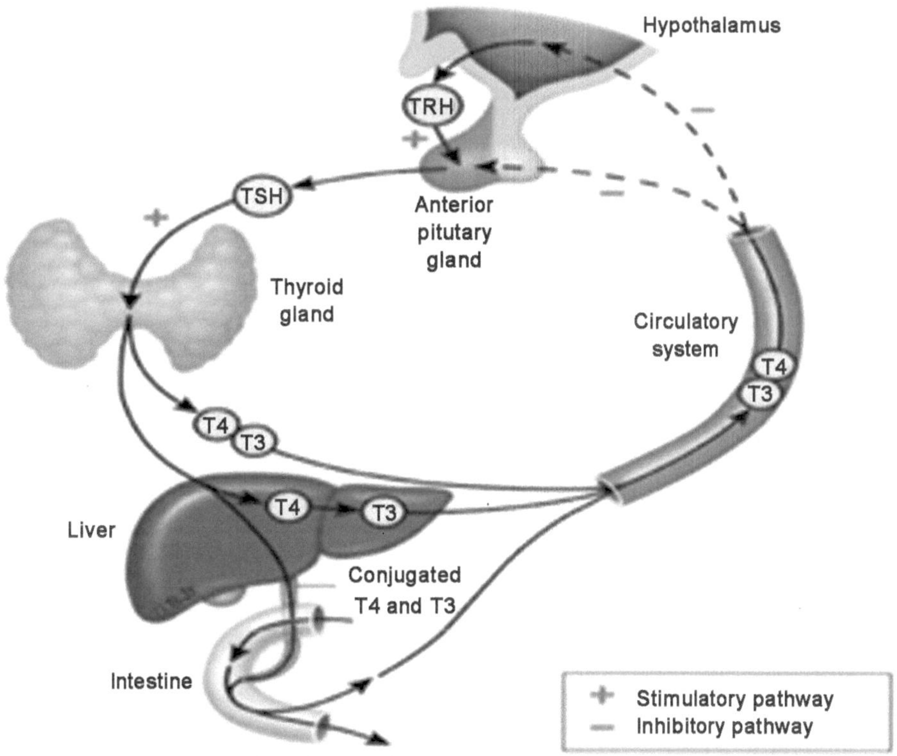

TRH increases the secretion of TSH, which stimulates the synthesis and secretion of T3 and T4 the thyroid gland. T3 and T4 inhibit the secretion of TSH, both directly and indirectly by suppressing the release of TRH. T4 is converted to T3 in the liver and many other tissues by the action of T4 monodeiodinases. Some T4 and T3 is conjugated with glucuronide and sulphate in the liver, excreted in the bile, and partially hydrolyzed in the intestine. Some T4 and T3 formed in the intestine may be reabsorbed. Drug interactions may occur at any of these sites.

TRH: Thyrotropin-releasing hormone; TSH: Thyroid-stimulating hormone; T4: Thyroxine; T3: Triiodothyronine

In Central Hypothyroidism

- Serum TSH may be low, normal, or slightly high.
- T3-low or normal.
- T4-low or low normal.

Ans: (a) Hypothyroidism because of hypothalamus defect

Ref: *Harrison's Principles of Internal Medicine, 20th Edition, Page 2698*

SURGERY

1. A 65-year-old female presented with increased SGOT, SGPT, Bilirubin, Alkaline phosphatase. She has the following findings in USG–Sclerotic Atrophic Gallbladder, large impacted stone in CBD, Distended CBD with dilated intrahepatic radicles. Which of the following is the best treatment?

(a) ERCP
(b) MRCP
(c) Cholecystectomy
(d) Observation

Explanation:

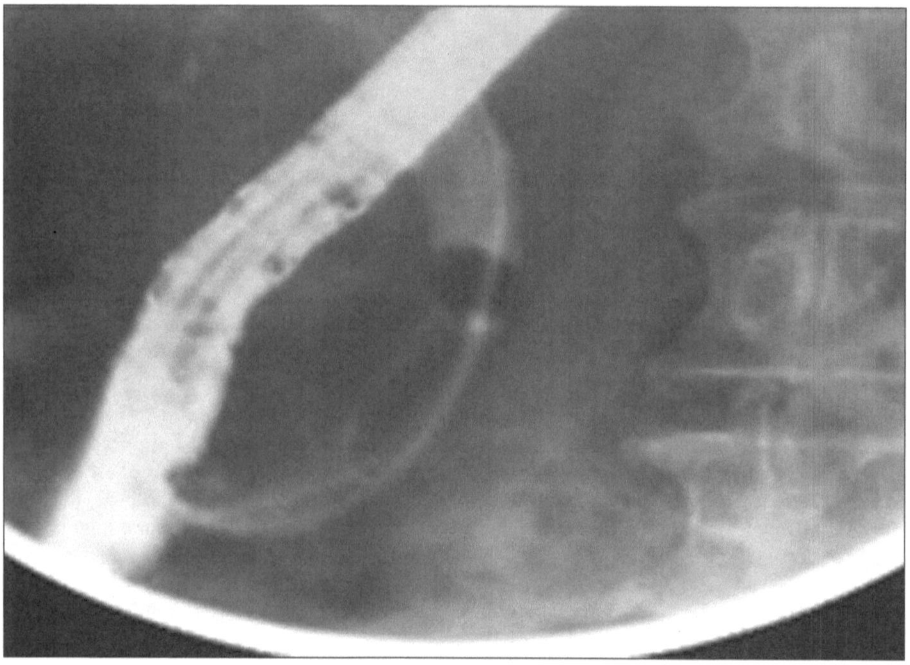

- The above scenario is a case of **Obstructive Jaundice/Surgical Jaundice –** Elevated LFT, with elevation of Alkaline phosphatase and dilated CBD on radiology.
- **Endoscopic Retrograde Cholangiopancreatogram** is both diagnostic and theraupetic.
- **ERCP sphincterotomy and retrieval of CBD calculus** is the **standard treatment of choice** for **CBD stones** and **placement of stent to relieve the obstruction.** This shall be **followed by laparoscopic cholecystectomy.**
- **MRCP:** Magnetic Resonance cholangiopancreatogram. A diagnostic study very sensitive and specific for hepatobiliary pathologies.

Ans: (a) ERCP

Ref: *Bailey and Love's Short Practice of Surgery, 27th Edition, Page 1192*

2. A patient presented in Emergency room with a stab injury in left lower chest, with low BP and Pulse rate. After resuscitation in trauma centre patient's BP became normal. X-ray chest shows clear image. What will be your next step?

(a) E-FAST
(b) CECT abdomen
(c) Immediate ICD insertion
(d) CECT chest

Explanation:

- **CECT** is the 'gold standard' for the intra-abdominal diagnosis of injury in the stable patient.
- In penetrating trauma protocol there is no role for E-FAST.

Penetrating Trauma Protocol

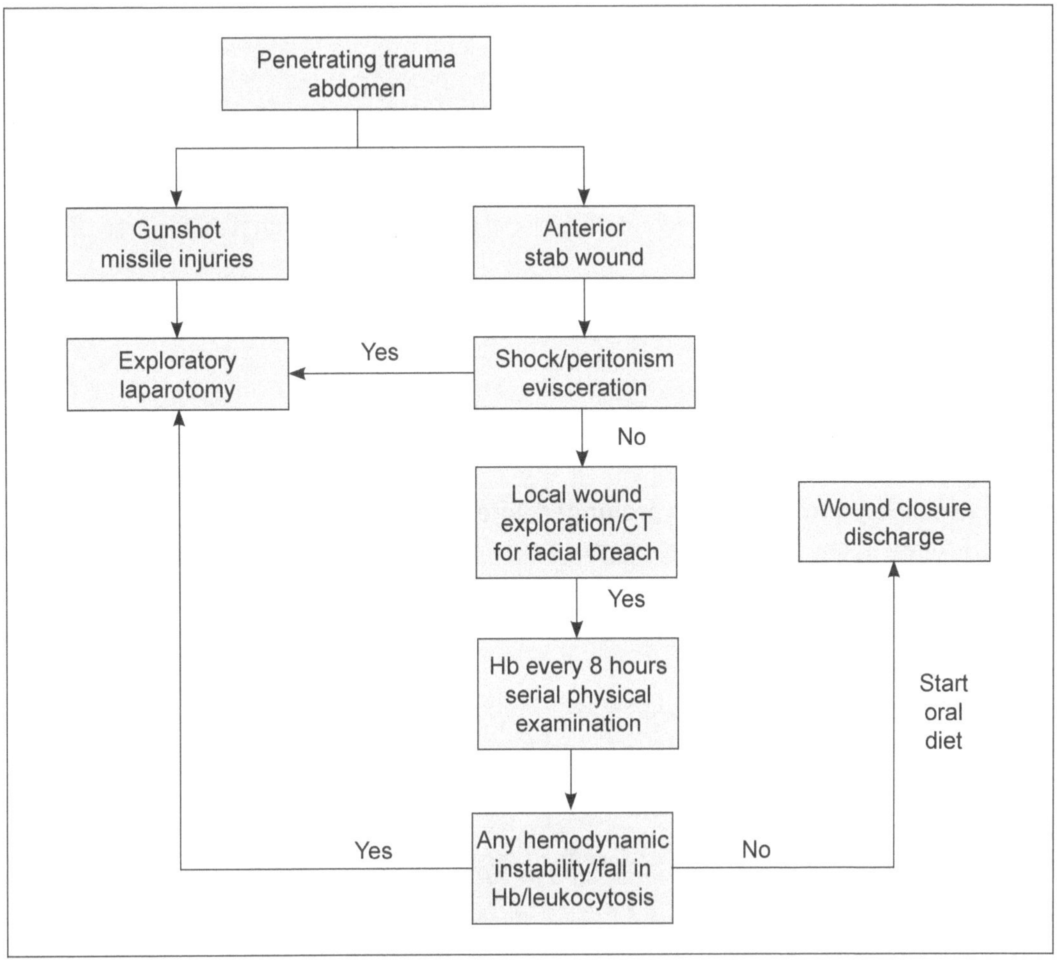

Ans: (b) CECT abdomen

Ref: *Bailey and Love's Short Practice of Surgery, 27th Edition, Page 372*

3. An elderly female with a long standing mole in face for many years presents with irregular border, enlarging size of the mole suddenly. What is the most common cause?

(a) Superficial spreading type of malignant melanoma

(b) Lentigo maligna melanoma

(c) Acral lentiginous

(d) Nodular melanoma

Explanation:

Macroscopic features in naevi suggestive of malignant melanoma

- Change in size.
- Shape.

- Colour.
- Thickness (elevation/nodularity or ulceration).
- Satellite lesions (pigment spreading into surrounding area).
- Tingling/itching /serosanguinous discharge (usually late signs).

Superficial spreading melanoma (SSM)

- This is the **most common presentation (70%),** usually **arising in a pre-existent naevus** after several years of slow change, followed by rapid growth in the preceding months before presentation.
- Nodularity within SSM heralds the onset of the vertical growth phase.

Nodular melanoma (NM)

- Nodular melanoma accounts for **15% of all MM** and tends to be more aggressive than SSM, with a shorter clinical onset.
- These lesions often **arise *de novo*** in skin and are more common in men than women, often presenting in middle age and usually on the trunk, head or neck.

Lentigo maligna melanoma LMM was previously known as Hutchinson's melanotic freckle.

- This variant presents as a **slow-growing**, variegated brown macule on the face, neck or hands of the elderly.
- They are positively **correlated with prolonged, intense sun exposure**, affecting women more than men.
- It is rare in white-skinned individuals (2–8% of MM) but **more common in the Afro-Caribbean, Hispanic and Asian population (35–60%).**
- It usually presents as a flat, irregular macule in later life. 25% are amelanotic and may mimic a fungal infection or pyogenic granuloma.

Ans: (a) Superficial spreading type of malignant melanoma

Ref: *Bailey and Love's Short Practice of Surgery, 27th Edition, Page 610*

4. Identify the cause for the swollen limb shown below:

(a) Varicose insufficiency
(b) Chronic lymphedema
(c) Congestive cardiac failure
(d) Arterial obstruction

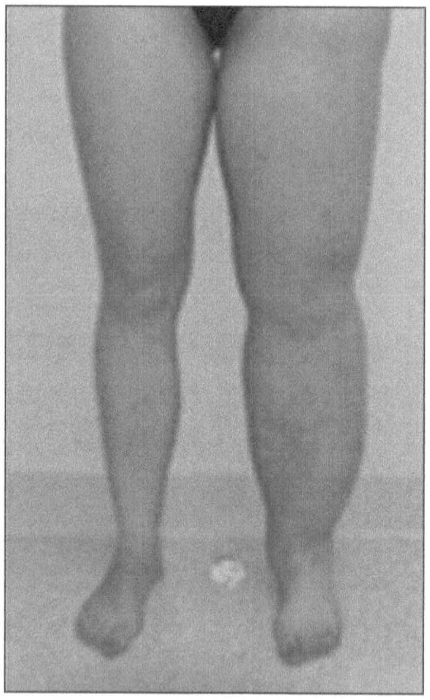

Explanation:

Dilated and tortuous veins in the lower limb associated with limb edema is a feature of varicose veins.

The descriptive CEAP (Clinical-Etiology-Anatomy-Pathophysiology) classification for chronic venous disorders.

For Clinical Classification:

- C0: No signs of venous disease.
- C1: Telangiectasia or reticular veins.
- C2: Varicose veins.
- C3: Edema.

- C4a: Pigmentation or eczema (some include malleolar flare in this category).
- C4b: Lipodermatosclerosis or atrophie blanche.
- C5: Healed venous ulcer.
- C6: Active venous ulcer.

Each clinical class is further characterised depending upon whether the patient is symptomatic (S) or asymptomatic (A), e.g., C2S.

For Etiological Classification:

- Ec: Congenital.
- Ep: Primary.
- Es: Secondary (post-thrombotic).
- En: No venous cause identified.

For Anatomical Classification:

- As: Superficial veins.
- Ap: Perforator veins.
- Ad: Deep veins.
- An: No venous location identified.

VENOUS DOPPLER IS THE INVESTIGATION OF CHOICE

The aim of the duplex scan in a patient with **varicose veins** is to establish:

- The presence of reflux in the deep and superficial venous system.
- The presence of obstruction in the deep venous system.
- Incompetency of perforators.
- The presence of thrombus within the superficial veins.
- An indication of a pelvic source of reflux or obstruction.

Congestive cardiac failure produces bilateral pitting pedal edema.

Arterial Obstruction does not produce edema, instead it produces **thinning of limbs.**

Filarial limb produces pedal edema without the presence of dilated veins and results in **chronic progressive fibrosis in subcutaneous tissue.**

Ans: (a) Varicose insufficiency

Ref: *Bailey and Love's Short Practice of Surgery, 27th Edition*

5. A 5-year-old male child is diagnosed with acute fulminant liver failure. Which one of the following criteria is not included in the King's College criteria for liver transplant?

(a) Age <10 years

(b) Prothrombin time > 50 seconds

(c) Bilirubin >300 micromol/litre

(d) Jaundice more than 7 days before development of encephalopathy

Explanation:

King's College criteria for acute liver failure
Acetaminophen group
• PH < 7.30 (Irrespective of grade of encephalopathy) Or • Prothrombin time > 100 seconds (INR > 6.5) • Serum creatinine > 3.4 mg/dl (> 300 mmol/l) in patients with grade III/IV encephalopathy
Non acetaminophen group
• Prothrombin time > 100 seconds (INR > 6.5; irrespective of grade of encephalopathy) Or Any three of following variables • Age < 10 years or > 40 years • Cause: Non-A, non-B hepatitis Drug induced Idiosyncratic reactions • Duration of jaundice before onset of encephalopathy > 7 days • Prothrombin time > 50 seconds (INR 3.5) • Serum bilirubin 17.6 mg/dl (> 300 mmol)

Ans: (b) Prothrombin time > 50 seconds

Ref: *Bailey and Love's Short Practice of Surgery, 27th Edition*

6. What is the Modified Child Pugh class for patient who has a serum bilirubin of 2.5 mg/dl, Serum albumin 3 g/dl, Prothrombin time increased 5 seconds. Moderate ascites is present but there is Grade 2 encephalopathy?

(a) CP class A
(b) CP class B
(c) CP class C
(d) CP class D

Explanation:

Child-Turcotte-Pugh Classification for Severity of Cirrhosis			
Clinical and Lab Criteria	**Points***		
	1	**2**	**3**
Encephalopathy	None	Grade 1 or 2	Grade 3 or 4
Ascites	None	Mild to moderate (diuretic responsive)	Severe (diuretic refractory)
Bilirubin (mg/dl)	< 2	2-3	> 3
Albumin (g/dl)	> 3.5	2.8-3.5	<2.8
Prothrombin time Second prolonged *or* International normalized ratio	< 4 <1.7	4-6 1.7-2.3	>6 >2.3
***Child-Turcotte-Pugh Class obtained by adding score for each parameter (total points)**			
Class A = 5 to 6 points			
Class B = 7 to 9 points			
Class C = 10 to 15 points			

Ans: (c) CP class C

Ref: *Bailey and Love's Short Practice of Surgery, 27th Edition*

7. Which of the following is not included in primary survey of a trauma patient?

(a) Airway, breathing, circulation
(b) CECT to look for bleeding
(c) Recording BP
(d) Exposure of whole body

Explanation:

The **primary survey of a trauma patient aims to identify and manage the most immediately life-threatening pathologies first and follows cABCDE.**

The cABCDE of Trauma Care

c – Control of massive external hemorrhage.

A – Airway with cervical spine protection.

B – Breathing and ventilation.

C – Circulation and hemorrhage control: Apply a pelvic binder and do not remove until a pelvic fracture is excluded.

D – Disability (neurological status).

E – Exposure (assess for other injuries).

Glasgow Coma Scale		
Behavior	**Response**	**Score**
Eye opening response	Spontaneously To speech To pain No response	4 3 2 1
Best verbal response	Oriented to time, place and person Confused Inappropriate words Incomprehensible sound No response	5 4 3 2 1
Best motor response	Obeys commands Moves to localized pain Flexion withdrawal from pain Abnormal flexion (decorticate) Abnormal extension (decerebrate) No response	6 5 4 3 2 1
Total score	*Best response* *Comatose client* *Totally unresponsive*	15 8 or less 3

'Whole Body CT' (WBCT)

- **WBCT from the head to pelvis with IV contrast** is the **gold standard investigation** of the **severely injured adult blunt trauma patient.**
- There is no role for selective scanning of body systems in these patients.
- WBCT scan is a **time-critical investigation** and should be obtained as early as possible in resuscitation of the severely injured patient.

Ans: (b) CECT to look for bleeding

Ref: *Bailey and Love's Short Practice of Surgery, 27th Edition, Page 129*

8. What is your diagnosis from the Barium enema image shown below?

(a) Intussusception (b) Sigmoid diverticulum
(c) Cancer colon (d) Polyp

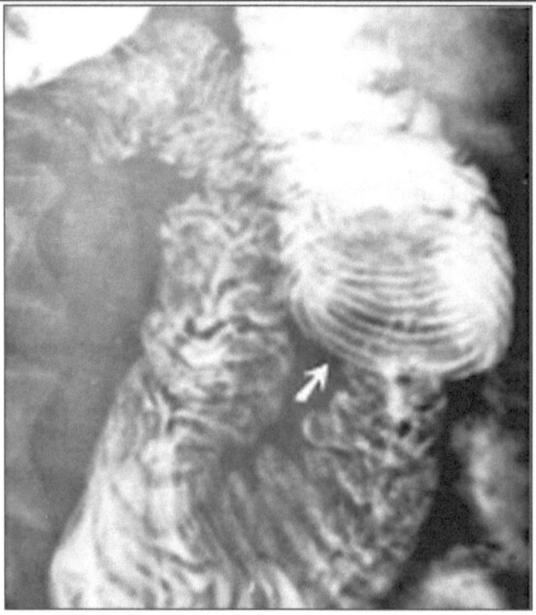

Explanation:

- The **classic signs of intussusception on barium enema** are the **meniscus sign** and **coiled spring sign.**

INTUSSUSCEPTION

- **Most common in children.**
- An intussusception is **composed of three parts:**
  - The entering or inner tube (intussusceptum).
  - The returning or middle tube.
  - The sheath or outer tube (intussuscipiens).

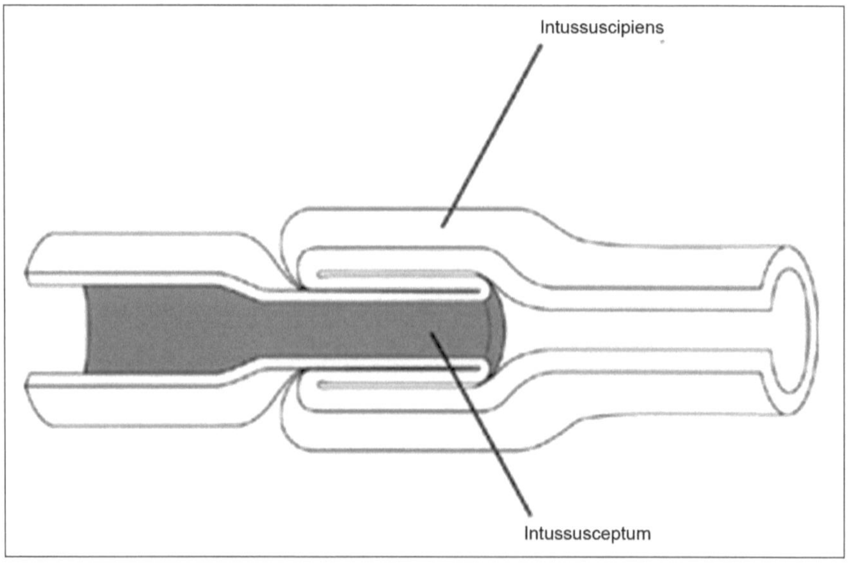

Ultrasonographic Image of Intussusception

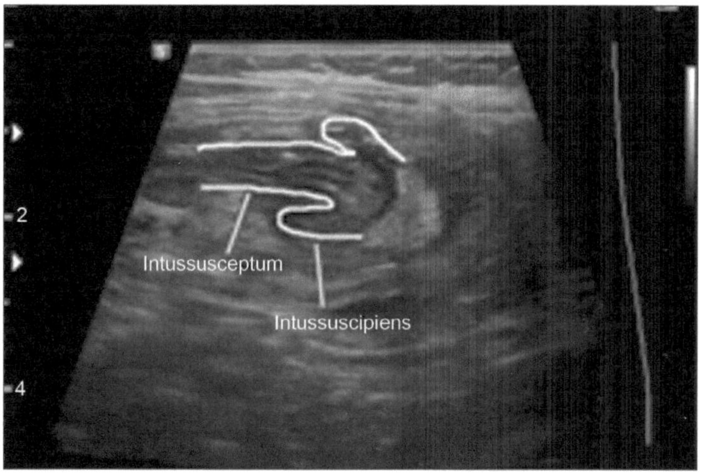

- **Intussusception on ultrasound** is seen as **doughnut or pseudo kidney appearance** composed of a **hypoechoic outer ring and a hyperechoic center.**
- Adult cases are secondary to intestinal pathology, e.g., polyp, Meckel's diverticulum.
- **Ileocolic is the most common variety.**
- Can lead to an **ischemic segment.**
- **Radiological reduction** is indicated in most **pediatric cases**; **adults require surgery.**
- Intussusception represents one of the **most common abdominal emergency** in infancy.
- The **classical clinical triad**, consisting of **abdominal colics, red jelly stools and a palpable mass,** is present only in approximately 50% of cases, 20% of patients are symptoms-free at clinical presentation.

Management Algorithm

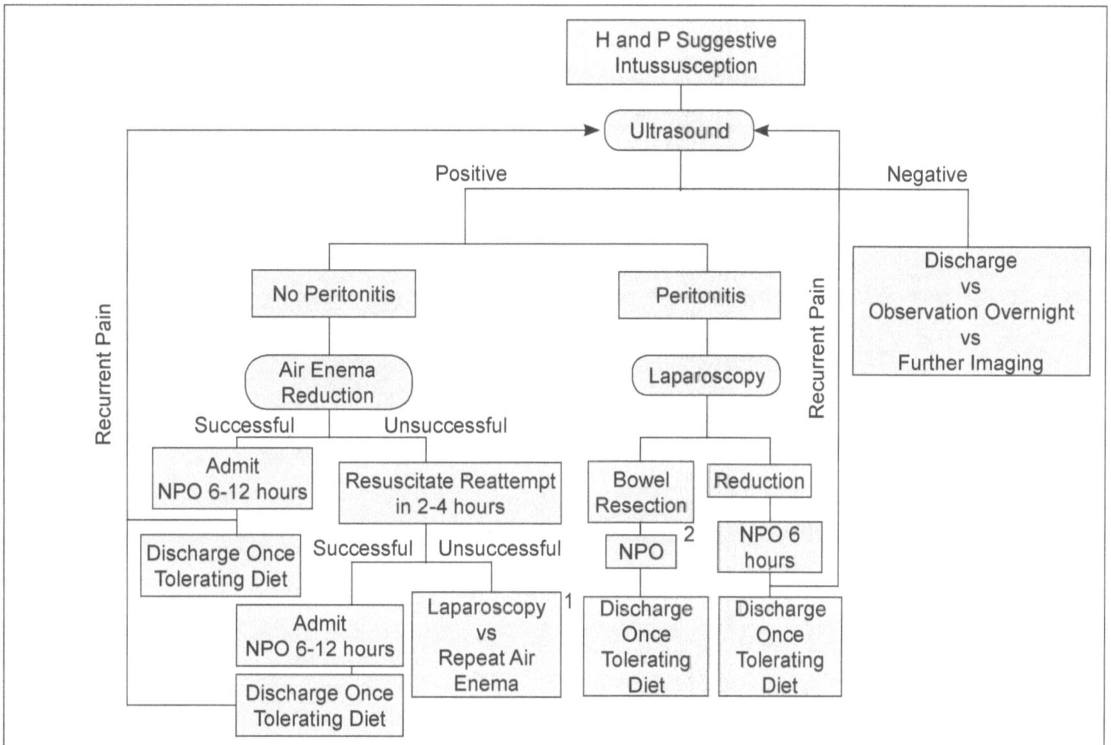

[1]Based on clinical picture and radiology resources repeat air enema may be attempted.
[2]Advance diet per surgeon preference.

Ans: (a) Intussusception

Ref: *Bailey and Love's Short Practice of Surgery, 27th Edition, Page 1091*

9. Patient underwent LSCS-post operatively patient developed abdominal distension and obstipation. Examination showed absence of bowel sounds and soft consistency on palpation. What is your diagnosis?

(a) Uterine rupture
(b) Paralytic ileus
(c) Appendicitis
(d) Amniotic fluid peritonitis

Explanation:

Intestinal obstruction with abdominal distension, obstipation and a painless soft abdomen is classically seen in functional disorders of the intestine like Paralytic ileus.

PARALYTIC ILEUS

- This is defined as a condition in which there is **failure of transmission of peristaltic waves secondary to neuromuscular failure [i.e., in the myenteric (Auerbach's) and submucous (Meissner's plexuses**)].
- The resultant stasis leads to accumulation of fluid and gas within the bowel, with associated distension, vomiting, absence of bowel sounds and obstipation.

Postoperative ileus: A degree of ileus usually occurs after any abdominal procedure and is self-limiting, with a variable duration of 24–72 hours. Postoperative ileus **may be prolonged** in the presence of **hypoproteinemia or metabolic abnormality like hypokalemia.**

Infection: Intra-abdominal sepsis may give rise to localised or generalised ileus.

Reflex ileus: This may occur following fractures of the spine or ribs, retroperitoneal hemorrhage or even the application of a plaster jacket.

Metabolic: Uremia and hypokalemia are the most common contributory factors.

Ans: (b) Paralytic ileus

Ref: *Bailey and Love's Short Practice of Surgery, 27th Edition, Page 1296*

10. Mr. Kumar, 60-year-old male with history of bladder cancer, while travelling by flight complained of leg pain and hemoptysis. On Examination–Pulse rate was 102/minute. On enquiry, he had previous history of hospitalization for pulmonary embolism. He had undergone surgical procedure 3 weeks back. What is the clinical probability of Thrombotic risk with Modified Well's Criteria?

(a) Well's score cannot be calculated as D-dimer levels are not given
(b) Low risk
(c) Moderate risk
(d) High risk

Explanation:

MODIFIED WELL'S CRITERIA

Modified Well's criteria: Clinical assessment for pulmonary embolism

Clinical symptoms of DVT (leg swelling, pain with palpation)	3.0
Other diagnosis less likely than pulmonary embolism	3.0
Heart rate > 100	1.5
Immobilization ($\geq$ 3 days) or surgery in the previous four weeks	1.5

Contd.

Contd.

Previous DVT/PE	1.5
Hemoptysis	1.0
Malignancy	1.0
Probability	**Score**
Traditional clinical probability assessment	
• High	> 6.0
• Moderate	2.0 to 6.0
• Low	< 2.0
Simplified clinical probability assessment*	
• PE likely	> 4.0
• PE unlikely	≤ 4.0

Data from van Belle, A, et al. JAMA 2006; 295:172

Ans: (d) High risk

Ref: *Bailey and Love's Short Practice of Surgery, 27th Edition, Page 981*

11. Painless cancerous lesions with inguinal nodes are seen in:

(a) Cancer of anal canal
(b) Cancer testis
(c) Cancer prostate
(d) Cancer bladder

Explanation:

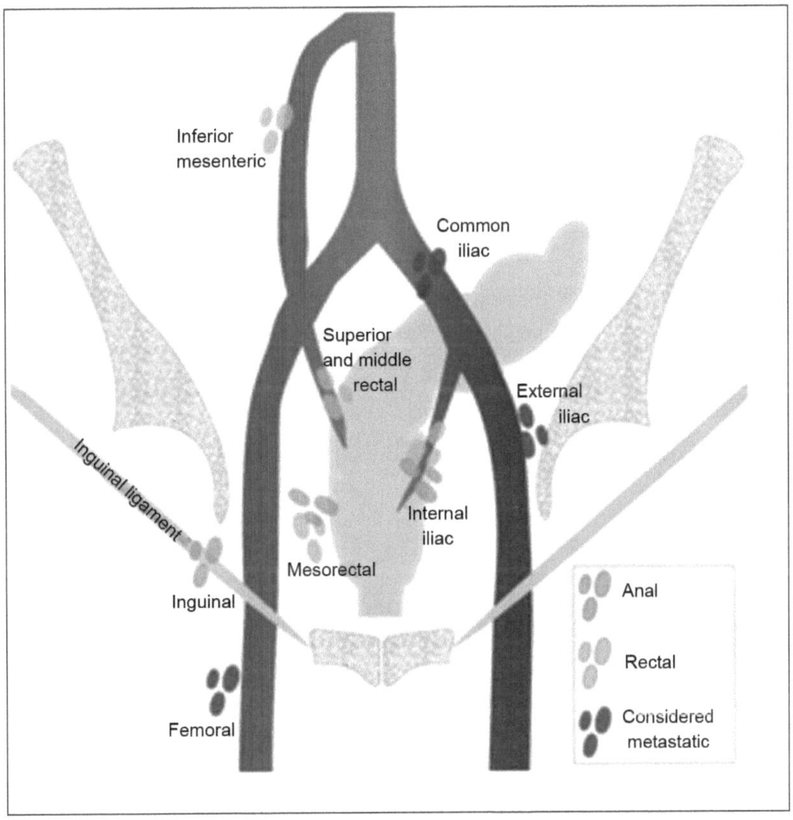

Lymph node involvement in anorectal carcinoma

Ans: (a) Cancer of anal canal

Ref: *Bailey and Love's Short Practice of Surgery, 27th Edition*

12. In a patient with Frost Bite, what is the temperature of water that must be used to recover the patient?

(a) 37-39 degrees
(b) 40-42 degrees
(c) 45-48 degrees
(d) 48-52 degrees

Explanation:

- **Frost bite** occurs when a part of the body freezes or **exposed to very low temperatures of less than 31 Fahrenheit.** The cells are disrupted and the tissue dies.
- It is a **'cold' burn** and can be **categorised according to the depth in the same way as a conventional burn**.
- It **commonly involves the fingers, toes, cheeks, the tip of the nose and the ears**. When frozen, the tissue feels hard and cannot be indented.
- Warming (temperature 42 degrees) should be gentle as the heat used may actually cause a burn.

Ans: (b) 40-42 degrees

Ref: *Bailey and Love's Short Practice of Surgery, 27th Edition, Page 423*

13. A 40 years man with diagnosis of ADPKD dependent on Tolvaptan presents with abdominal pain. What is the cause?

(a) Colonic perforation
(b) Side effects of Tolvaptan
(c) Colonic Diverticulitis
(d) Appendicitis

Explanation:

- **Tolvaptan (tolvaptan) is a vasopressin 2 receptor antagonist (vaptan)** that is used for **treatment of hyponatremia** caused by **elevated levels of arginine vasopressin (also known as antidiuretic hormone: ADH).**
- **Commonly found** in patients **with inappropriate ADH syndrome (SIADH)** or with fluid overload from heart failure or cirrhosis.
- Tolvaptan recently has been implicated in causing **serum amino transferase elevations** as well as **clinically apparent acute liver injury on long-term use.**

Most Common Side Effects of Tolvaptan from a Published Case Series

Side effects	***N=40 (%)***
Thirst	12 (30
Dry mouth	16 (40)
Hypernatremia	4 (10)
Renal dysfunction	6 (15)
Nausea/vomiting	14 (35)
Abdominal pain	8 (20)
Muscle cramp	6 (15)

Ans: (b) Side effects of Tolvaptan

Ref: *Bailey and Love's Short Practice of Surgery, 27th Edition*

14. A 20-year-old male is admitted in emergency room with respiratory distress and hypotension. He has subcutaneous emphysema and absence of air entry into right side of lungs. What is the next immediate step?

(a) Start IV fluids and resuscitate with wide bore cannulas

(b) Needle inserted in 5th ICS in Midaxillary line

(c) Shift to ICU to intubate

(d) Positive pressure ventilation connected

Explanation:

PRIMARY SPONTANEOUS PNEUMOTHORAX

This is a common condition seen in young people usually in the 20's.

SECONDARY SPONTANEOUS PNEUMOTHORAX

- This occurs when there is a **leak in the visceral pluera** due to any underlying disease like **tuberculosis, degenerative or cavitating lung disease and necrosing tumors.**
- **Tension pneumothorax** should be immediately **relieved by inserting a cannula into the affected hemithorax** in as safe a position.
- The **safest site for insertion of a drain** is in the triangle that lies: anterior to the mid axillary line; above the level of the nipple; below and lateral to the pectoralis major muscle and this **triangle is referred to as Triangle of Safety** and **usually lie in the 5th intercoastal space.**

Safe Triangle

- A "safe triangle" has been described as the preferred site of insertion. This is the triangle bordered of the latissimus dorsi, the lateral border of the pectoralis major muscle, a line superior to the horizontal level of the nipple, and an apex below the axilla

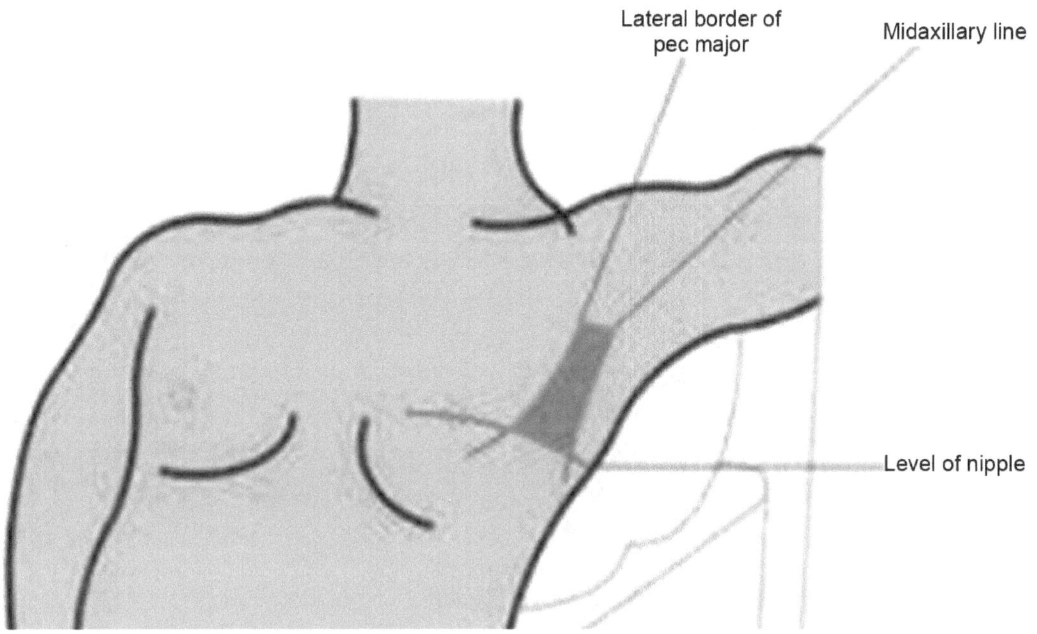

MANAGEMENT OF SPONTANEOUS PNEUMOTHORAX

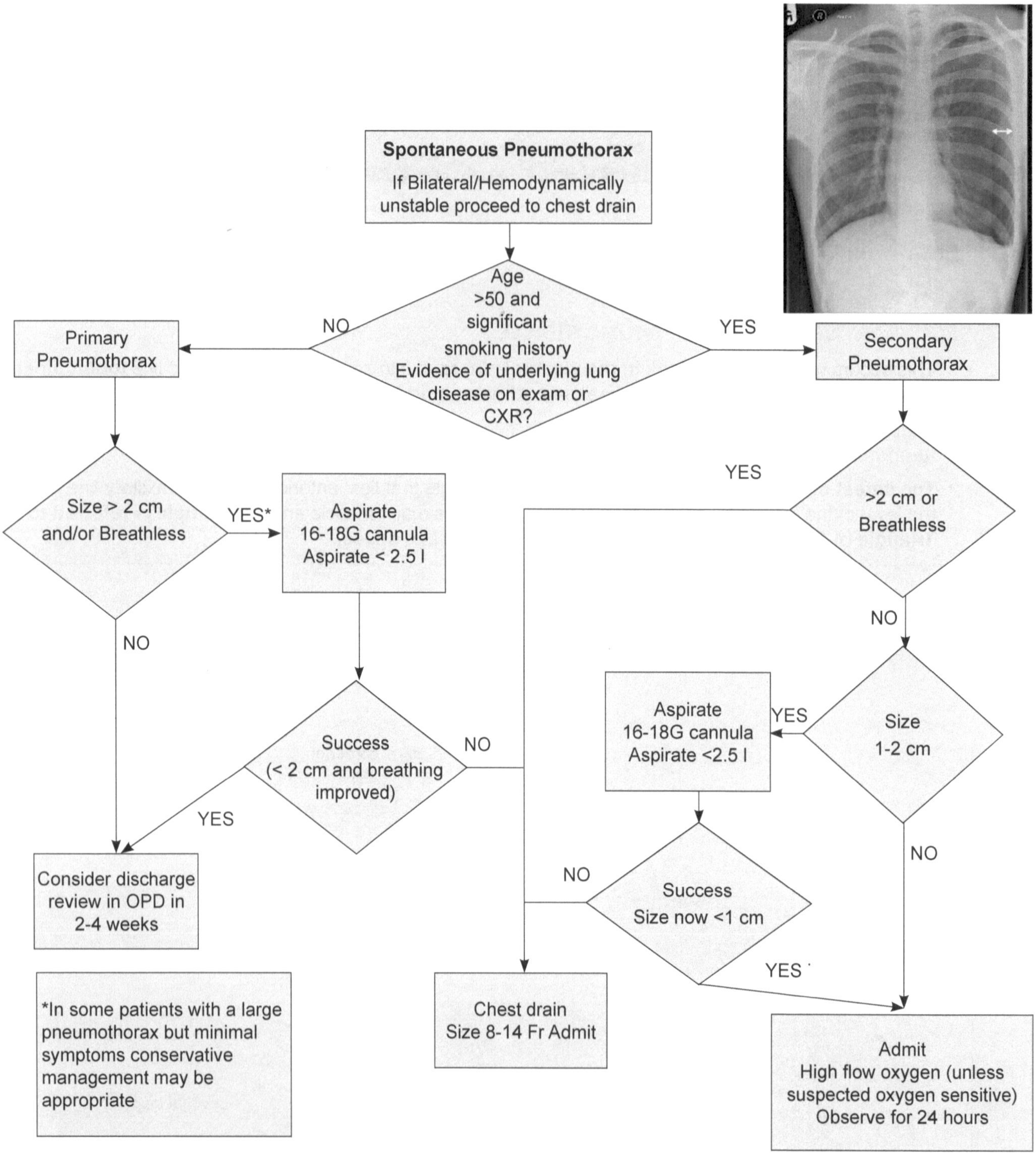

Ans: (b) Needle inserted in 5th ICS in Midaxillary line

Ref: *Bailey and Love's Short Practice of Surgery, 27th Edition, British Thoracic Society Guidelines 2010*

15. Patient presents with peritonitis and during surgery a diverticular perforation is seen with fecal peritonitis. What is the Hinchey's stage?

(a) Stage 1
(b) Stage 2
(c) Stage 3
(d) Stage 4

Explanation:

Hinchey classification	Features of disease	Risk of death
Stage 1 disease	Diverticulitis with pericolic abscess or phlegmon	5%
Stage 2 disease	Diverticulitis with walled off pelvic, intra-abdominal or retroperitoneal abscess	5%
Stage 3 disease	Generalized purulent peritonitis	13%
Stage 4 disease	Generalized fecal peritonitis	43%

Complications of Diverticular Disease

- Diverticulitis.
- Abscess.
- Peritonitis.
- Intestinal obstruction.
- Hemorrhage.
- Fistula formation.
- Plain X-ray can reveal a **pneumoperitoneum.**
- **Spiral CT has excellent sensitivity and specificity** for identifying **bowel wall thickening, abscess formation and extra luminal disease** and has revolutionised the assessment of complicated diverticular disease.
- **Laparotomy and thorough peritoneal lavage** is done and then a choice has to be made between a **Hartmann's procedure and primary anastomosis with defunctioning loop ileostomy.**
- **Hartmann's procedure:** Refers to sigmoid resection with formation of left iliac fossa colostomy and closure of the rectal stump
- **Primary anastomosis** should be used selectively in young fit patient without gross contamination or overwhelming sepsis.
- There may be a role for emergency laparoscopy in diverticular disease with washout if there is no fecal contamination, i.e., Hinchey grade III or less, allowing sigmoid resection to be avoided.

Ans: (d) Stage 4

Ref: *Bailey and Love's Short Practice of Surgery, 27th Edition, Page 1274*

16. In a patient with parathyroid adenoma, to confirm the removal of the correct gland after surgery Miami Criteria is used. Regarding Miami Criteria which is correct?

(a) 50% reduction in PTH within 10 mins of gland removal
(b) 50% reduction in PTH within 5 mins of gland removal
(c) 25% reduction in PTH within 10 mins of gland removal
(d) 25% reduction in PTH within 5 mins of gland removal

Explanation:

- The **half life of circulating PTH is 3–5 minutes** and there **should be a significant drop detected in**

the plasma PTH following resection of a single adenoma. If **no such drop** is detected, then **multiple gland disease** may be suspected and conversion to a bilateral neck exploration should be considered.

- The **Miami Criteria** were developed **to determine the extent of resection**. A **drop in the PTH to the normal range** and **to less than half the maximum preoperative PTH at 10 minutes accurately predicts** single-gland disease.

IOPTH results using the Miami Criterion	
True-positive	IOPTH adequately decreases by > 50% from either preincision or pre-excision levels at 10 minutes after removing abnormal parathyroid gland(s) and the patient remains normocalcemic at 6 months
False-positive	IOPTH decreases by > 50% from either pre-incision or pre-excision levels at 10 minutes despite all abnormal glands not being removed
True-negative	IOPTH fails to decrease by > 50% from either pre-incision or pre-excision levels at 10 minutes after removing parathyroid gland(s), indicating an incomplete resection
False-negative	IOPTH fails to fall > 50% from either pre-incision or pre-excision levels at 10 minutes despite adequately removing the abnormal parathyroid gland(s)

IOPTH–Intra Operative Parathormone Assay

- All symptomatic patients should be offered surgery.
- An expert panel recently published recommendations on which asymptomatic patients should be considered for surgical intervention (Bilezikian *et al.*, 2014).
- When criteria has been met and where a single adenoma has been confidently identified by radiological means, a **minimally invasive parathyroidectomy** may be offered.
- Conversely, where there is **discordant imaging** or where imaging fails to identify any parathyroid abnormalities, then a **bilateral neck exploration and three and a half-gland parathyroidectomy or a four gland parathyroidectomy and autotransplantation of small portion of the gland** should be performed.

Ans: (a) 50% reduction in PTH within 10 mins of gland removal

Ref: *Bailey and Love's Short Practice of Surgery, 27th Edition*

17. A patient aged 30 years presents with dysphagia. High resolution manometry was done for that patient showed the following findings. There was pan esophageal pressurization with distal contractile integrity as > 450 mm Hg cm. What is the diagnosis?

(a) Type 1 Achalasia
(b) Type 2 Achalasia
(c) Type 3 Achalasia
(d) Diffuse esophageal spasm

Explanation:

Esophageal motility diagnoses and criteria proposed for the Chicago Classification v3.0	
Disorders with EGJ outflow obstruction	**Criteria**
Type I achalasia (classic achalasia)	• Increased median IRP (> 15 mm Hg[a]), 100% failed peristalsis (DCI < 100 mm Hg) • Premature contractions with DCI values < 450 mm HG s cm meet criteria for failed peristalsis
Type II achalasia (with esophageal compression)	• Increased median IRP (> 15 mm HG[a]), 100% failed peristalsis, panesophageal pressurization with ≥ 20% of swallows • Contractions may be masked by esophageal pressurization and DCI should be calculated
Type III achalasia (spastic achalasia)	• Increased median IRP (> 15 mm Hg[a]), no normal peristalsis, premature (spastic) contractions with DCI > 450 mm Hg s cm with ≥ 20% of swallows • May be mixed with panesophageal pressurization

Contd.

Contd.

EGJ outflow obstruction	• Increased median IRP (> 15 mm Hg[a]), sufficient evidence of peristalsis such that criteria for type I-III achalasia not met[b]
Major disorder of peristalsis	• Not encountered in normal subjects
Aperistalsis	• Normal median IRP, 100% failed peristalsis • Should consider achalasia with borderline IRP values when there is evidence of esophageal pressurization • Premature contractions with DCI values < 450 mm Hg s cm meet criteria for failed peristalsis
Distal esophageal spasm	• Normal median IRP, ≥20 premature contractions with DCI > 450 mm Hg s cm[a]. Some normal peristalsis may be present
Hypercontractile esophagus (jackhammer)	• At least 2 swallows with DCI > 8000 mm Hg s cm[a,c] • Hypercontractility may be localized to the LES and may be missed using DCI criteria
Minor disorders of peristalsis	• Characterized by vigor, pattern and MRS response
IEM	• > 50% ineffective swallows • Ineffective swallows can be failed or weak • Multiple repetitive swallow assessment may be helpful in determining peristaltic reserve
Fragmented peristalsis	• > 50% fragmented contractions not meeting IEM criteria
Normal esophageal motility	• Not fulfilling any of the classifications listed earlier

Ans: (c) Type 3 Achalasia

Ref: *Bailey and Love's Short Practice of Surgery, 27th Edition, Page 1096*

18. What is the name of the Flap reconstruction shown in the image below?

(a) PMMC flap

(b) DIEP flap

(c) LD flap

(d) DP flap

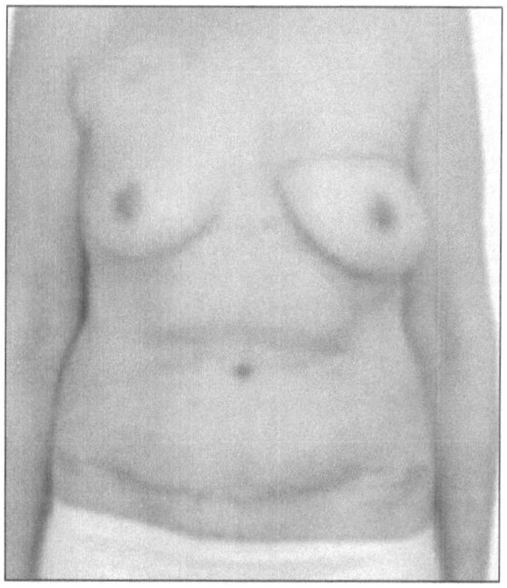

Explanation:

- If the skin at the mastectomy site is poor (e.g., following radiotherapy) or if a larger volume of tissue is required, a **musculocutaneous flap** can be constructed either from the **latissimus dorsi muscle (an LD flap) or using the transversus abdominis muscle (a TRAM flap).** The latter gives an excellent cosmetic result in experienced hands but is a lengthy procedure and requires careful patient selection. It is now usually performed as a free transfer using microvascular anastomosis, although the pedicled TRAM from the contralateral side is still used.
- Variations on the TRAM flap requiring less muscle harvesting, such as the **DIEP flap (based on deep inferior epigastric vessels)**, are increasingly being used.

Ans: (b) DIEP flap

Ref: *Bailey and Love's Short Practice of Surgery, 27th Edition*

19. All of the following are part of the ASEPSIS wound grading *except:*

(a) Serous discharge

(b) Purulent exudate

(c) Induration

(d) Erythema

Explanation:

The ASEPSIS wound score						
	Proportion of wound affected (%)					
Wound characteristics	**0**	**< 20**	**20-39**	**40-50**	**60-79**	**> 80**
Serous exudates	0	1	2	3	4	5
Erythema	0	1	2	3	4	5
Purulent exudates	0	2	4	6	8	10
Separation of deep tissues	0	2	4	6	8	10

Criteria	**Points**
Additional treatment	
• Antibiotics	10
• Drainage of pus under local anesthesia	5
• Debridement of wound (general anesthesia)	10
Serous discharge	Daily 0-5
Erythema	Daily 0-5
Purulent exudates	Daily 0-10
Separation of deep tissues	Daily 0-10
Isolation of bacteria	10
Stay as inpatient prolonged over 14 days	5

Total score	**Category of infection**
0-10	Satisfactory healing
11-20	Disturbance of healing
21-30	Minor wound infection
31-40	Moderate wound infection
> 40	Severe wound infection

Ans: (c) Induration

Ref: *Bailey and Love's Short Practice of Surgery, 27th Edition, Page 48*

20. Management of a renal cell cancer of size < 4 cm is:

(a) Radical nephrectomy
(b) Partial nephrectomy
(c) Chemotherapy
(d) Surgery followed by chemotherapy

Explanation:

- **Renal cell cancer (RCC)** arises from **epithelium of the proximal convoluted tubule** and coincidentally detected by radiology imaging.
- Has a **male preponderance.**
- Major subtypes are clear-cell, papillary and chromophobe RCC.
- **Surgery is the mainstay of treatment** for **tumors confined to the kidney.**
- Metastatic disease is treated with **tyrosine kinase inhibitors (TKIs) or mTOR inhibitors** (Targeted therapy).

AJCC TNM STAGING OF RCC

Primary Tumor (pT)

- **pTX:** Primary tumor cannot be assessed.
- **pT0:** No evidence of primary tumor.
- **pT1a:** ≤ 4 cm, limited to the kidney.
- **pT1b:** > 4 cm and ≤ 7 cm, limited to the kidney.
- **pT2a:** > 7 cm and ≤ 10 cm, limited to the kidney.
- **pT2b:** > 10 cm, limited to the kidney.
- **pT3a:** Invades renal vein / branches, perirenal fat, renal sinus fat or pelvicaliceal system.
- **pT3b:** Extends into vena cava below the diaphragm.
- **pT3c:** Extends into vena cava above the diaphragm or invades vena cava wall.
- **pT4:** Invades beyond Gerota fascia, including direct extension to adrenal gland.

Regional Lymph Nodes (pN)

- **pNX:** Cannot be assessed.
- **pN0:** No regional lymph node metastasis.
- **pN1:** Regional lymph node metastasis.

Distant Metastasis (pM)

- **pM1:** Distant metastasis, including non-contiguous adrenal involvement.

AJCC Prognostic Stage Groups

- **Stage group I:** T1a-1b N0 M0.
- **Stage group II:** T2a-2b N0 M0.
- **Stage group III:** T1a-3c N1 M0, T3a-3c NX-0 M0.
- **Stage group IV:** T4 any N M0, any T any N M1.

Staging of Renal Cell Carcinoma is Based on Size, Position and Lymph Node Involvement

- **Stage I:** Tumor <7 cm in the largest dimension, limited to the kidney.
- **Stage II**: Tumor >7 cm in the largest dimension, limited to the kidney.
- **Stage III**: Tumor in the major veins or adrenal gland with intact Gerota's fascia, or regional lymph nodes involved.
- **Stage IV:** Tumor beyond Gerota's fascia.

Partial Nephrectomy is Indicated for Patients with a T1 Tumor (Tumor < 7 cm Confined to Kidney/Stage 1)

- The goal of **partial nephrectomy** is to completely remove the primary tumor while preserving the largest possible amount of healthy renal parenchyma for a near normal kidney function.

Classic radical nephrectomy consists of removal of the entire kidney, perirenal fat, adrenal gland and regional lymph nodes.

- In patients with a tumor < 5 cm in size, located at the inferior pole, the adrenal gland can be preserved.
- Similarly, regional lymph node dissection can be reserved for patients with clinically positive nodes detected by CT.

Ans: (b) Partial nephrectomy

Ref: *Bailey and Love's Short Practice of Surgery, 27th Edition*

21. A male patient presents to the hospital with abdominal pain and is incidentally detected with an abdominal aortic aneurysm. What is the appropriate management of this patient?

(a) Immediate surgery

(b) Ultrasound surgery (USG) monitoring till size of the aneurysm reaches 70 mm

(c) USG monitoring till size reaches 40 mm

(d) USG monitoring till size reaches 55 mm

Explanation:

- Abdominal aortic aneurysm (AAA) is the **most common type of large vessel aneurysm** and is found in 2% of the population.
- **Mostly remains asymptomatic until rupture occurs.**
- These are **found incidentally** on physical examination, or during ultrasound investigation.
- Symptomatic aneurysms may cause minor symptoms, like back pain and abdominal discomfort.
- **Rupture of aneurysm produces severe back and abdominal pain along with hypotension**.
- The **annual incidence of rupture is 1%** or less in aneurysms that are < 55 mm in diameter.
- The **annual incidence of rupture is as high as 25%, in those that are 70 mm in diameter**.
- **Regular ultrasonographic assessment** is indicated **for asymptomatic aneurysms <55 mm** in diameter.
- **Repair of aneurysm** is considered **if diameter is > 55 mm in asymptomatic patients.**

Ans: (d) USG monitoring till size reaches 55 mm

Ref: *Bailey and Love's Short Practice of Surgery, 27th Edition, Page 961*

22. A 32-year-old man presents with cramping gluteal pain after walking 0.5 km. Which of the following vessel most likely involved?

(a) Arterial disease with aorto-iliac involvement

(b) Arterial disease with femoral artery involvement

(c) Femoral venous insufficiency

(d) Varicose vein

Explanation:

- **Cramping pain** after walking is referred to as **claudication pain** due to arterial insufficiency.
- The **muscle group affected by claudication** is classically **one anatomical level below the level of arterial disease.**
- If **claudication pain is felt in the calf,** the **superficial femoral artery** is the most commonly affected artery (70% of cases).
- **Gluteal claudication** is seen in **Aorto-iliac disease** (30% of cases) and if associated with sexual Impotence, it is called **Leriche's syndrome.**

RELATIONSHIP OF CLINICAL FINDINGS TO SITE OF DISEASE

Aorto Iliac Obstruction

- Also called **saddle thrombus.**
- **Bilateral claudication in buttocks, thighs and calves.**
- Femoral and distal pulses absent in both limbs.

- Bruit over aorto iliac region.
- Impotence (**Leriche Syndrome**).

Iliac Obstruction

- **Unilateral claudication in the thigh and calf and sometimes the buttock.**
- Bruit over the iliac region.
- Unilateral absence of femoral and distal pulses.

Femoropopliteal Obstruction

- **Unilateral claudication in the calf.**
- Femoral pulse palpable with absent unilateral distal pulses.

Distal Obstruction

- Femoral and popliteal pulses palpable.
- Ankle pulses absent.
- **Claudication in calf and foot.**

Ans: (a) Arterial disease with aorto-iliac involvement

Ref: *Bailey and Love's Short Practice of Surgery, 27th Edition, Page 944*

23. One of the following is a true statement about intermittent claudication:

(a) Felt at rest

(b) Most common site is calf

(c) Claudication distance cannot vary on day-to-day basis

(d) Relieved after getting out of bed and walking

Explanation:

- Intermittent claudication occurs as a result of **anaerobic muscle metabolism** and is **classically described as debilitating cramp-like pain** felt in the muscles and classically seen in **arterial insufficiency.**
- The distance that a patient is able to walk without stopping varies (**claudication distance**) only slightly from day-to-day. It is **decreased by increasing the work demand** and hence oxygen requirements of the muscles is affected.
- **Relieved by rest** both in the standing and sitting positions.
- **As disease progresses**, **claudication distance decreases** and perfusion to the leg may be so severely compromised that anaerobic respiration occurs even at rest, typically affecting the foot and/or calf. (**Rest Pain**).
- The muscle group affected by claudication is classically one anatomical level below the level of arterial disease and is usually felt in the calf because the **superficial femoral artery is the most commonly affected artery (70% of cases).**
- **Boyd's Clinical Classification of Claudication** indicated the severity and progression of the disease.

Boyd's Classification	
Grades	**Description**
I	The patient walks for a distance, gets the pain, continues to walk and the pain disappears
II	Patient walks for a distance, gets the pain and continues to walk with the pain (Limping)
III	Pain compels the patient to take rest
IV	Pain at rest (Due to involvement of Vasa Nervosum)
Claudication Distance: Distanc a patient is able to walk before the onset of pain.	

Ans: (b) Most common site is calf

Ref: *Bailey and Love's Short Practice of Surgery, 27th Edition, Page 943*

24. A patient presents with halitosis and swelling in the left side of neck. On pressing, it gives a gurgling sound. Barium image is shown below. What is the likely diagnosis?

(a) Zenker's diverticulum
(b) Laryngocele
(c) Dysphagia lusoria
(d) Schatzki ring

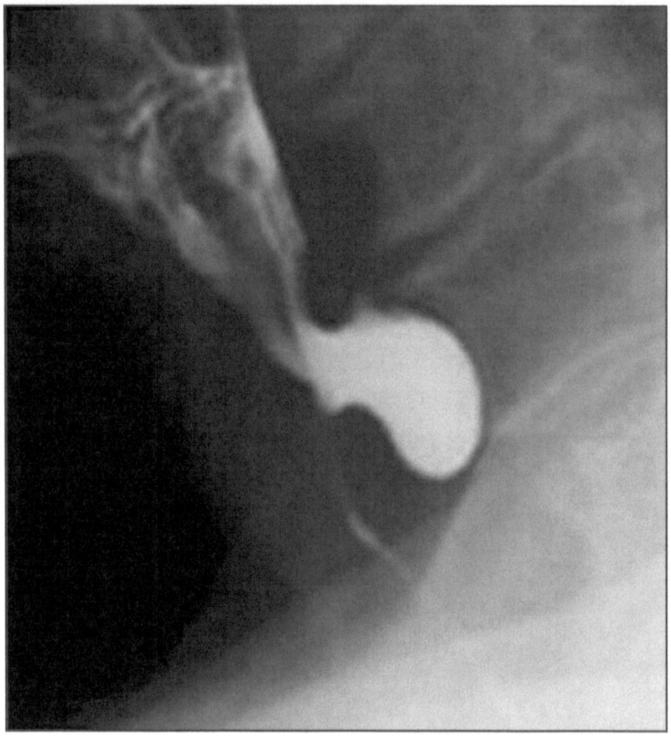

Explanation:

ZENKER'S DIVERTICULUM (PHARYNGEAL POUCH)

- **It** is the **protrusion of pharyngeal mucosa** through the natural weak point (**the dehiscence of Killian**) between **the oblique and horizontal (cricopharyngeus) fibres** of **the inferior pharyngeal constrictor.**
- When the diverticulum is small, **pharyngeal dysphagia** is common.
- As the pouch enlarges, it tends to fill with food on eating and produces **halitosis and esophageal dysphagia.**
- The **septum is formed by the cricopharyngeus muscle** and overlying mucosa and this septum forms the boundary between the posterior wall of the esophagus and the anterior wall of the pouch.

Treatment Options

- Endoscopic linear cutting stapler to divide the septum between the diverticulum and the upper oesophagus, producing a diverticulo-esophagostomy.
- Open surgery involving pouch excision.
- Pouch suspension (diverticulopexy) and/or myotomy of cricopharyngeus.
- All techniques have good results.

Recent Advances

Division of the 'bar' using **CO_2 laser**, as an alternative to stapling, is gaining popularity in some centres.

LARYNGOCELE

Laryngocele is a rare, benign **dilatation of the laryngeal saccule** that may extend internally into the airway or externally through the thyrohyoid membrane.

- Many laryngoceles are asymptomatic; sometimes, they may cause a **cough, hoarseness, stridor, sore throat** and may present as a **swelling on one or both sides of the neck.**
- Laryngocele may be **associated** with **supraglottic squamous cell carcinoma.**
- **Computed tomography scan** is the **most effective imaging** method for diagnosis.
- **Surgery** is the **treatment of choice.**

DYSPHAGIA LUSORIA

- **Congenital aberrant right subclavian artery (arteria lusoria)** causing compression of the esophagus resulting in dysphagia.
- **Dysphagia** usually presents **early in childhood**, although it can occur in the late teens.
- **Treatment** is usually by **division of the non-dominant component of vascular ring.**
- In adults, acquired causes include aneurysm of the aorta, diffuse cardiac enlargement and pressure from the left common carotid or vertebral arteries.
- It is rare that symptom severity justifies surgical intervention.

SCHATZKI'S RING

- It is a circular **ring in the distal esophagus** usually at the **squamo-columnar junction**.
- The cause is not clear, but there is a **strong association with gastroesophageal reflux disease.**
- The core of the ring consists of **variable amounts of fibrous tissue** and cellular infiltrate.
- Most rings are **incidentally found** while doing barium studies for other diseases.
- Some are associated with **dysphagia** and **respond to dilatation along with medical antireflux therapy.**

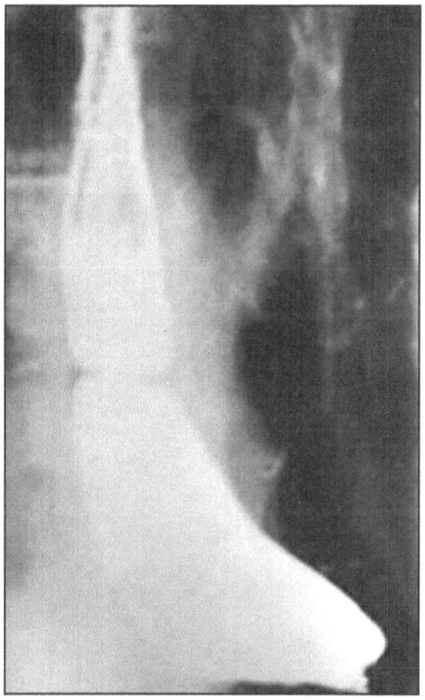

Barium swallow showing Schatzki's ring

Ans: (a) Zenker's diverticulum

Ref: *Bailey and Love's Short Practice of Surgery, 27th Edition, Page 1101*

25. Identify the Barium swallow image shown below:

(a) Achalasia cardia
(b) Carcinoma esophagus
(c) Eosinophilic esophagitis
(d) Post cricoid web

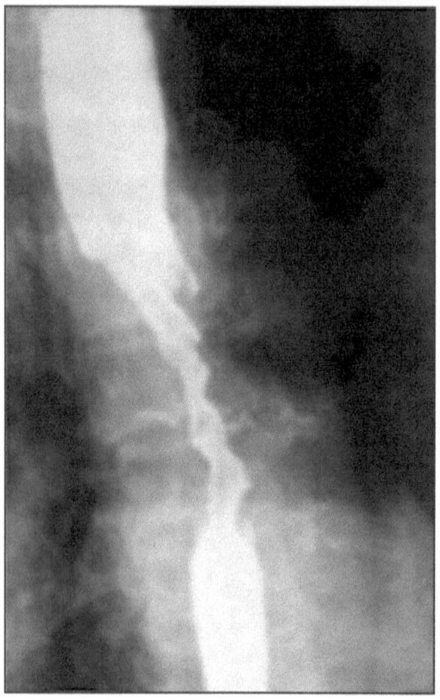

Explanation:

- Barium swallow showing **irregular filling defect**, narrowing with **shouldered margins.**
- **Squamous cell cancer and adenocarcinoma** are the **most common** types.
- **Squamous cell carcinoma** generally affects the **upper two-thirds** of the esophagus and **adenocarcinoma** the **lower third.**
- **Upper GI endoscopy and biopsy confirms the diagnosis.**
- Patients suitable for potentially curative therapies should proceed to staging investigations to rule out hematogenous spread (CT scan) and then to assess loco-regional stage (endoscopic ultrasonography / Endoscopic ultrasound +/- laparoscopy).

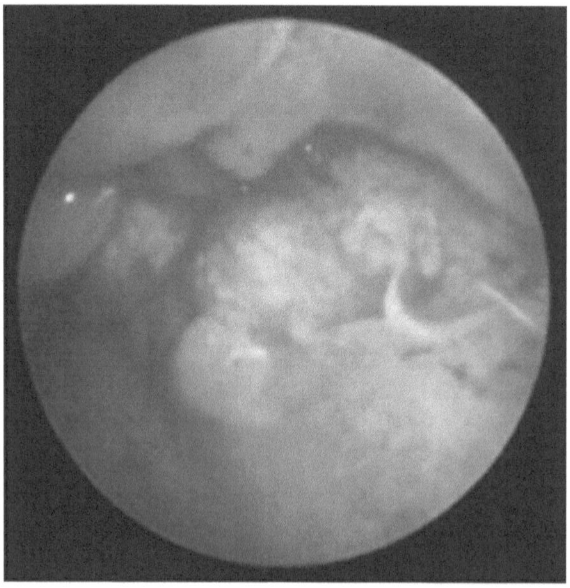

Endoscopic appearances of a mid-esophageal squamous cell carcinoma

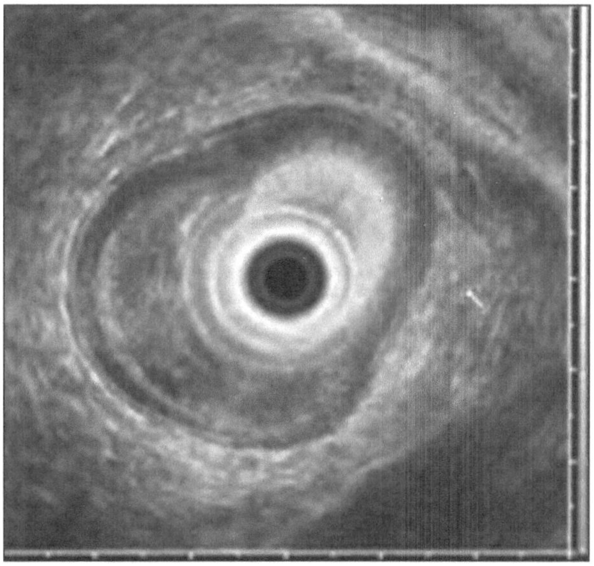

Endosonography demonstrating an 'early' tumor
Note the preservation of the outer dark wall layer that represents the muscle coat.

PLUMMER-VINSON SYNDROME

- This is also called the **Paterson-Kelly (or Paterson-Brown Kelly) syndrome or sideropenic dysphagia.**
- Dysphagia is said to occur because of the presence of **post cricoid web** that is associated with **iron deficiency anemia, glossitis and koilonychia.**
- Some patients may have **oropharyngeal leukoplakia** at risk of developing **hypopharyngeal cancer.**
- Webs occur in the **upper and middle esophagus**, usually without any kind of associated syndrome.
- They are nearly always thin diaphanous membranes detected coincidentally by contrast radiology.
- These require **endoscopic biopsy to rule out malignancy.**
- Few would require formal **endoscopic dilatation.**

Ans: (b) Carcinoma esophagus

Ref: *Bailey and Love's Short Practice of Surgery, 27th Edition, Page 1088*

26. Which of the following statements is true regarding retrosternal goitre?

(a) Operated only if patient is symptomatic
(b) Sternal incision is always required
(c) Majority of the goitres derive their blood supply from mediastinal vessels
(d) Majority of the retrosternal goitres can be removed by a neck incision

Explanation:

- Majority of patients with retrosternal goitre have minimal symptoms. Patient should be considered for surgery if there is significant airway compression, if symptoms are present or in young patients in whom symptoms are likely to develop.
- In **elderly patients** with **incidentally discovered retrosternal goitres, most surgeons would observe rather than treat.**
- Clearly a balance between risk and benefit must be made.
- If a decision is made to proceed to surgery, assessment of the extent of disease is critical. The **vast majority (>95%) of retrosternal goitres can be removed transcervically**.

- Those **at risk of requiring conversion to an open sternotomy approach** include malignant or revision cases, extension into the posterior mediastinum and those in which the diameter of the goitre exceeds that of the thoracic inlet.
- In such cases a joint case with thoracic surgery should be planned.

Ans: (d) Majority of the retrosternal goitres can be removed by a neck incision

Ref: *Bailey and Love's Short Practice of Surgery, 27th Edition, Page 811*

27. A middle-aged man complains of upper abdominal pain after a heavy meal. There is tenderness in the upper abdomen and on X-ray, widening of the mediastinum is seen with pneumo-mediastinum. What is the diagnosis?

(a) Spontaneous perforation of the esophagus
(b) Perforated peptic ulcer
(c) Foreign body in esophagus
(d) Rupture of emphysematous bulla

Explanation:

BAROTRAUMA (SPONTANEOUS PERFORATION OF ESOPHAGUS ALSO CALLED BOERHAAVE'S SYNDROME)

- This occurs classically **when a person vomits against a closed glottis.**
- The pressure in the esophagus increases rapidly, and the **esophagus bursts at its weakest point in the lower third**, sending a stream of **material into the mediastinum** and often the pleural cavity as well.
- The condition was first **identified by Boerhaave.**
- The clinical history is usually of severe pain in the chest or upper abdomen after a meal or a bout of drinking. Associated shortness of breath is common.
- **Boerhaave's syndrome is the most serious type of perforation** because of the large volume of material that is released under pressure. This causes rapid chemical irritation in the mediastinum and pleura followed by infection if untreated.
- Barotrauma has also been described in relation to other pressure events when the patient strains against a closed glottis (e.g., defecation, labour, weight-lifting).
- A **chest X-ray is often confirmatory** with air in the mediastinum, pleura or peritoneum.
- Pleural effusion occurs rapidly either as a result of free communication with the pleural space or as a reaction to adjacent inflammation in the mediastinum.
- A **contrast swallow or CT is nearly always required to guide management.**
- **General guidelines for non-surgical management** include:
  - Pain that is readily controlled with opiates.
  - Absence of crepitus, diffuse mediastinal gas, hydropneumothorax or pneumoperitoneum.
  - Mediastinal containment of the perforation with no evidence of widespread extravasation of contrast material.
  - No evidence of on-going luminal obstruction or a retained foreign body.
- **Surgical management** is required whenever patients:
  - Are unstable with sepsis or shock.
  - Have evidence of a heavily contaminated mediastinum, pleural space or peritoneum.
  - Have widespread intrapleural or intraperitoneal extravasation of contrast material.

Ans: (a) Spontaneous perforation of the esophagus

Ref: *Bailey and Love's Short Practice of Surgery, 27th Edition, Page 1072*

28. A middle-aged man presents with a swelling over scalp since childhood. On examination, the swelling has a bag of worm appearance. Bruit is heard over the swelling. What is your diagnosis?

(a) Plexiform neurofibroma
(b) Vasculitis
(c) Lymphangioma
(d) Cirsoid aneurysm

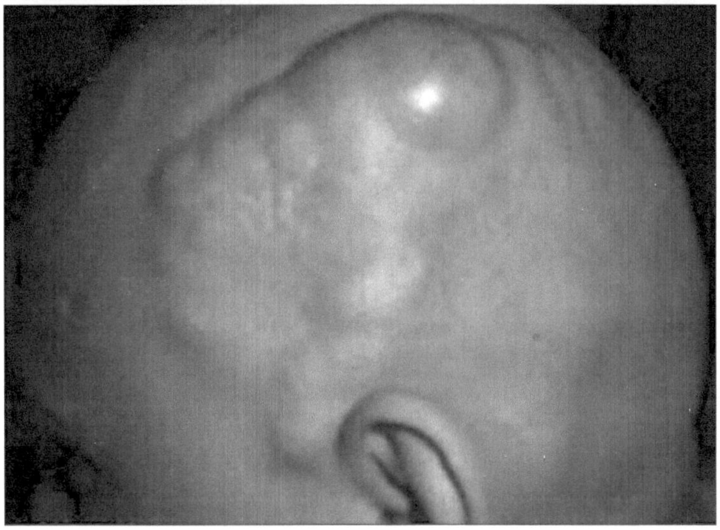

Explanation:

- **Anuerysms, AV malformations and AV fistula will have a bruit.**
- **Cirsoid aneurysms** are rare **arteriovenous fistulas** of the scalp. They are usually **congenital in etiology**. However, traumatic fistulas have also been described. In 90% of the patients, **the superficial temporal artery is the main supply** to the fistula in 71% of patients.
- **Surgical resection of the fistula is usually successful.**
- Endovascular and percutaneous occlusion of the fistulas have been described.
- **Angiography is the investigation of choice.**

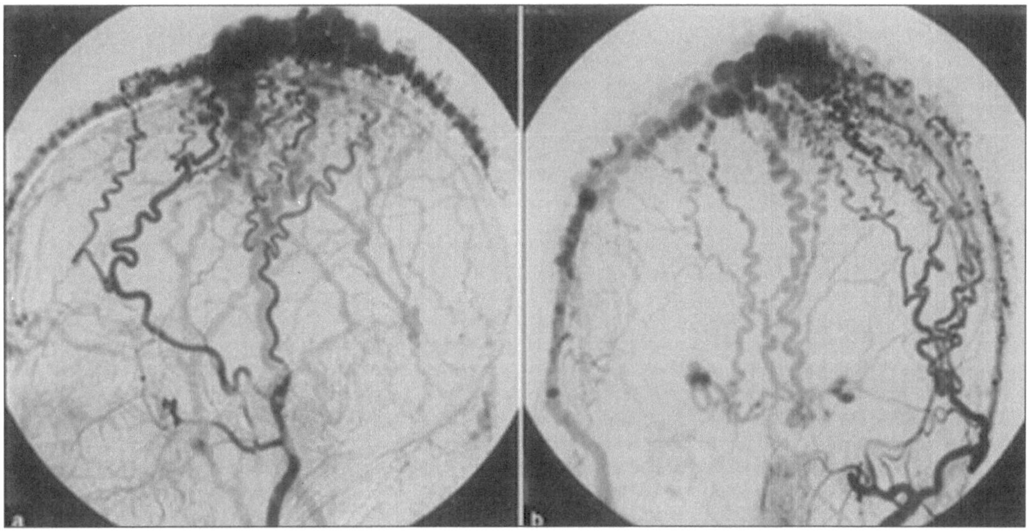

Cirsoid aneurysm of scalp. J Neurosci Rural Pract 2012;3(1)

Ans: (d) Cirsoid aneurysm

Ref: *Bailey and Love's Short Practice of Surgery, 27th Edition*

29. Which one of the following is not a component of Thoracoscore?

(a) Performance status

(b) Complication of surgery

(c) American Society of Anesthesiologists (ASA) grading

(d) Priority of surgery

Explanation:

Risk factors for in-hospital mortality in adult patients after thoracic surgery (based on Thoracoscore)	
Variable	**Risk factor**
Age	> 55 years
Gender	Male
ASA physical status	> 2
Performance Status Classification (WHO)	> 3
Dyspnea score (Medical Research Council)	> 3
Surgical priority	Urgent or emergency
Procedure class	Pneumonectomy
Diagnosis	Malignant
Comorbid diseases	> 3
Marc Giménez-Milà, Andrew A Klein, Guillermo Martinez. Design and implementation of an enhanced recovery program in thoracic surgery. Department of Anaesthesia and Intensive Care, Papworth Hospital, Cambridge, UK	

Ans: (b) Complication of surgery

Ref: *Bailey and Love's Short Practice of Surgery, 27th Edition, Page 915*

30. What is the T staging of a lung tumor than 2.5 cm in size as per American Joint Committee on Cancer (AJCC) classification?

(a) T1a

(b) T1b

(c) T1c

(d) T2

Explanation:

TNM 8th – Primary tumor characteristics	
T_x	Tumor in sputum/bronchial washings but not be assessed in imaging or bronchoscopy
T_0	No evidence of tumor
T_{is}	Carcinoma in situ
T_1	≤ 3 cm surrounded by lung/visceral pleura, not involving main bronchus
$T_{1a(mi)}$	Minimally invasive carcinoma
T_{1a}	≤ 1 cm

Contd.

Contd.

T_{1b}	> 1 to ≤ 2 cm
T_{1c}	> 2 to ≤ 3 cm
T_2	> 3 to ≤ 5 cm or involvement of main bronchus without carina, regardless of distance from carina or invasion visceral pleural or atelectasis or post obstructive pneumonitis extending to hilum
T_{2a}	> 3 to ≤ 4 cm
T_{2b}	> 4 to ≤ 5 cm
T_3	> 5 to ≤ 7 cm in greatest dimension or tumor of any size that involves chest wall, pericardium, phrenic nerve or satellite nodules in the same lobe
T_4	> 7 cm in greatest dimension or any tumor with invasion of mediastinum, diaphragm, heart, great vessels, recurrent laryngeal nerve, carina, trachea, esophagus, spine or separate tumor in different lobe of ipsilateral lung
N_1	Ipsilateral peribronchial and/or hilar nodes and intrapulmonary nodes
N_2	Ipsilateral mediastinal and/or subcarinal nodes
N_3	Contralateral mediastinal or hilar; ipsilateral/contralateral scalene/supraclavicular
M_1	Distant metastasis
M_{1a}	Tumor in contralateral lung or pleural/pericardial nodule/malignant effusion
M_{1b}	Single extrathoracic metastasis, including single non-regional lymph node
M_{1c}	Multiple extrathoracic metastases in one or more organs

Ans: (c) T1c

Ref: *Bailey and Love's Short Practice of Surgery, 27th Edition, Page 927*

31. Which is the most common pancreatic endocrine neoplasm?

(a) Insulinoma (b) VIPoma

(c) Glucagonoma (d) Gastrinoma

Explanation:

INSULINOMA

- **Most common pancreatic endocrine neoplasm –** Incidence is about 70–80%.
- Associated with weakness, sweating, tremor, tachycardia, anxiety, fatigue, dizziness, disorientation, seizures.
- Incidence of malignancy is < 10%.
- Criteria of Whipple's triad:

  (1) Hypoglycemia (plasma glucose < 50 mg/dl).

  (2) Neuroglycopenic symptoms; and

  (3) Prompt relief of symptoms following the administration of glucose.
- Following biological and biochemical confirmation of an insulinoma, preoperative localization is sought using computed tomography, magnetic resonance imaging, endoscopic ultrasonography (EUS), intra-arterial calcium stimulation test with hepatic venous sampling, and/or angiography and arterial stimulation venous sampling.

- **Surgical resection is the primary treatment modality for insulinomas.**

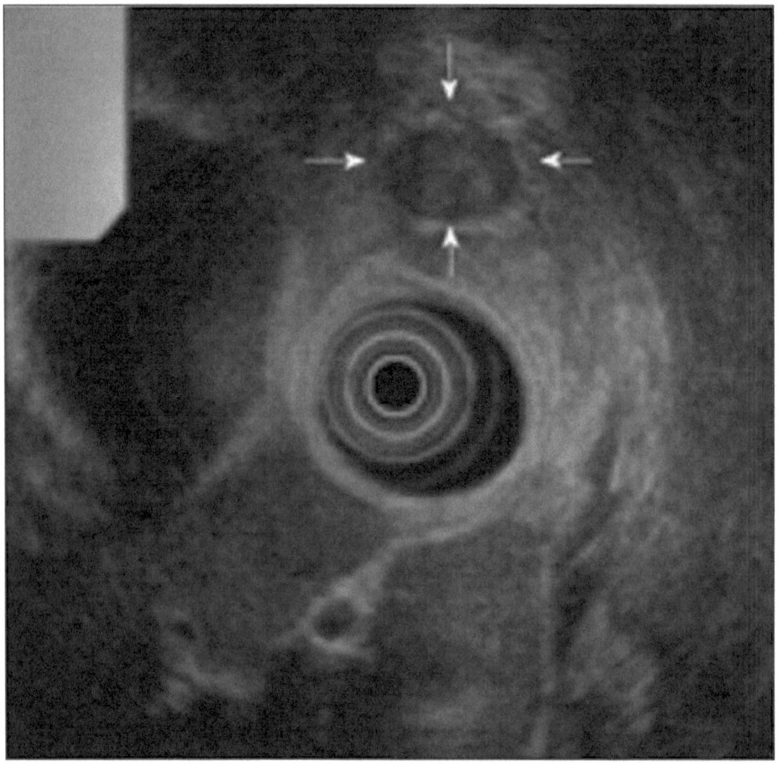

Endoscopic ultrasound features of insulinoma of the pancreas

Gastrinoma accounts for 20–25%. Associated with **intractable or recurrent peptic ulcer** disease that may result in gastrointestinal hemorrhage or intestinal perforation.

VIPoma accounts for 4%. Associated with profuse watery diarrhea, hypotension, abdominal pain.

Ans: (a) Insulinoma

Ref: *Bailey and Love's Short Practice of Surgery, 27th Edition*

32. What is the most common site of gastrinoma in MEN1 syndrome?

(a) Jejunum (b) Ileum

(c) Duodenum (d) Stomach

Explanation:

- **More than 70% of the gastrinomas in MEN 1 syndrome** are located in the **first and second part of the duodenum.**
- Therefore, **the anatomical area** comprising the **head of the pancreas, the superior and descending portion of the duodenum and the relevant lymph nodes** is referred to as the **'gastrinoma triangle'** because it harbours the **vast majority of these tumors.**
- All **patients with gastrinomas** should be **tested for MEN 1 syndrome.**
- **Surgical exploration** should be performed in all patients without diffuse metastases.

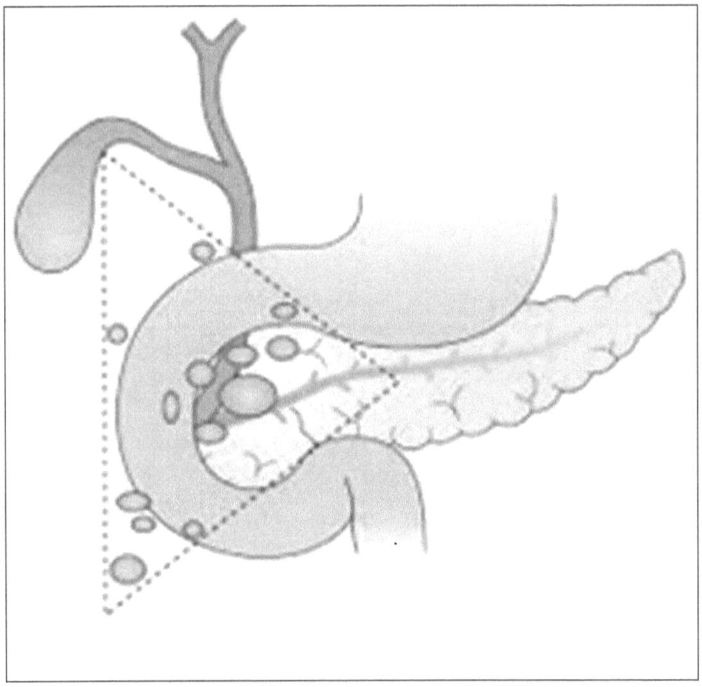

The gastrinoma triangle

Ans: (c) Duodenum

Ref: *Bailey and Love's Short Practice of Surgery, 27th Edition, Page 857*

33. A man was brought to the emergency after meeting with an accident and injured his perineum. He gets an urge to micturate but is unable to pass urine. On examination; blood was seen at the tip of urethra with swelling of penis and scrotum. This is because of:

(a) Penile urethra rupture
(b) Bulbar urethra rupture
(c) Membranous urethra rupture
(d) Urinary bladder rupture

Explanation:

- The signs of a ruptured bulbar urethra are **perineal bruising and hematoma.**
- There is usually **bleeding from the urethral meatus and retention of urine** is also typically present.

BULBAR URETHRAL INJURY

- **Suspect urethral injury** after **blunt perineal trauma** when the **man cannot void, when there is perineal bruising and when there is blood at the urethral meatus.**
- Confirmed by **urethrography** using **water-soluble contrast.**
- The safest initial management is to insert a **supra pubic catheter and drain the bladder.**
- Chances of **urinary extravasation** and **sepsis in the perineal hematoma is possible.**
- **Delayed urethroplasty** is **the preferred definitive management** of complete disruptions.

Ans: (b) Bulbar urethra rupture

Ref: *Bailey and Love's Short Practice of Surgery, 27th Edition*

OBSTETRICS AND GYNECOLOGY

1. Identify the image below:

(a) Diaphragm
(b) Male condom
(c) Female condom
(d) Chhaya

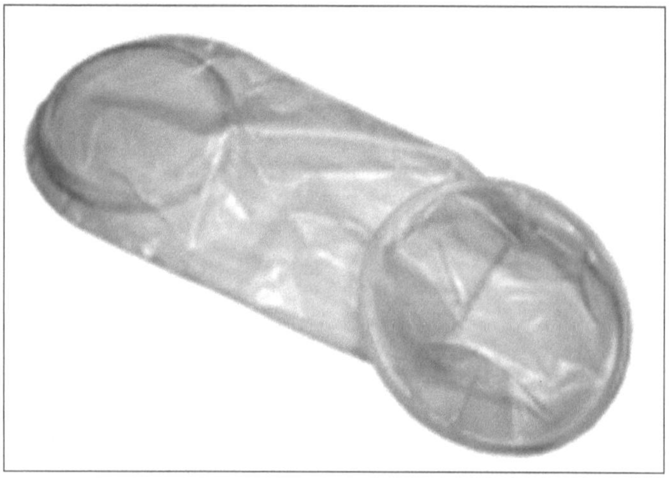

Explanation:

The given image is a **female condom,** a barrier contraceptive. Male condom and Diaphragm are other barrier contraceptives. **Chhaya is a nonhormonal contraceptive** containing **Ormeloxifene.**

Female Condom

- Female condom is a **barrier** contraceptive. It is made of transparent **polyurethane sheath** that is inserted into the vagina before sexual intercourse.
- It has two flexible rings, an inner ring and an outer ring. The **inner ring is at the closed** end, covers the cervix, and holds the condom in place.
- **The outer ring at the open end** is larger than the inner one. It stays outside the vagina and covers part of the perineum and labia during intercourse.
- In addition to contraception, it also has **non contraceptive benefits** like those of male condom–**prevention of transmission of STDs, HIV and hepatitis B infection.**
- However, because it is cumbersome to use, the female condom users are very less.
- **Failure rate** is higher than that of male condom: **5-20%.**

Male Condom

- Male condom is a **barrier method** of contraception.
- It is one of the **commonly used methods** of contraception.
- A male condom is a thin sheath made of latex or polyurethane. It is closed at one end with a teat and is open at the other end.
- The condom is put on an erect penis just before sexual intercourse.
- After sexual intercourse, the condom must be carefully taken off, so that the semen does not leak.
- Each condom is for **single usage.**

Advantages

- Not associated with any systemic side effects.
- Not expensive.
- Easily accessible (supplied free of cost by Government of India).
- **Non contraceptive benefits–**Condoms provide protection against **sexually transmitted diseases (STDs), HIV, hepatitis B, and human papillomavirus (HPV) infection**.

Side Effects

- Condoms can cause allergic reactions.
- May tear or leak during coitus.

Disadvantages

- **Failure rate** is high–**14 per HWY of use.**
- Concurrent use of spermicides reduces failure rate.

Diaphragm

- A diaphragm, a **barrier contraceptive** is a shallow rubber dome with a flexible rim that covers the cervix on insertion.
- It is often **used in combination with spermicidal jelly.**
- It is available in various sizes.
- It **can be inserted up to 6 hours before intercourse.** It should **remain in place for at least 6 hours** after intercourse. However, it must **not be left inside the vagina for more than 24 hours.**
- **Method of insertion:** The ring of the diaphragm is lubricated and then folded, so that the two sides of the ring are touching each other and then inserted into the vagina. Following insertion, the anterior rim of the diaphragm rests behind the pubic symphysis and the dome of the diaphragm covers the cervix.
- It **can be reused.** After usage, it is washed with soap and water, dried and stored in a case.

Side Effects

- It can cause irritation or allergic reaction.
- *Failure rate* is high.

Today/Vaginal Sponge (Contraceptive Sponge)

- The contraceptive sponge is marketed under the brand name **"Today Sponge",** which contains a **spermicidal agent (nonoxynol-9).**
- Spermicide in the sponge causes **immobilization of the sperms** and prevents sperms from entering the cervix.
- It is a **barrier contraceptive** which prevents entry of sperm into the cervical canal and contains a spermicidal agent.
- It contains 1 gm of nonoxynol-9 and is provided with a loop for easy removal.
- It should be placed high up in the vagina and **should be kept for 6 hours in vagina after intercourse.**
- It is for **single use.**

CHHAYA or CENTCHROMAN or SAHELI (Ormeloxifene)

- **Ormeloxifene is a nonhormonal contraceptive.** It is a **selective estrogen receptor modulator (SERM)** sold commercially in India as **Centchroman** or **Saheli.**
- It is a **once-a-week contraceptive** that acts by causing asynchrony between ovulation and endometrial changes, thereby preventing implantation. Initial dose is 30 mg twice a week for 3 months, followed by once a week thereafter.
- Ormeloxifene is **marketed only in India as a contraceptive.**

- The **failure rate** with typical use is **9%.**
- The **Ministry of Health and Family Welfare, India,** has launched two new contraceptives, an **injectable contraceptive medroxyprogesterone acetate (MPA) under the "Antara" program** and a **contraceptive pill, "Chhaya," containing centchroman** to expand the contraceptive choices offered to couples.
- It is a **safe and effective method** and can be given to **breastfeeding mothers.**
- During the first three months of taking Chhaya, women may notice lighter or irregular periods. This should be no cause of worry, as menstrual cycle gets normal after few months of usage.

Ans: (c) Female condom

Ref: *Clinical Obstetrics and Gynecology by Sharmila Arun Babu,1st Edition, Page 531*

2. All the following are estrogen dependent changes which occur during puberty *except:*

(a) Menarche (b) Thelarche

(c) Vaginal cornification (d) Axillary and pubic hair growth

Explanation:

Terminology used in physiology of puberty	
• Puberty	Time of sexual maturation
• Gonadarche	Activation of gonads by the pituitary hormones resulting in production of ovarian hormones
• Menarche	Onset of menstruation
• Thelarche	Onset of breast development
• Adrenarche	Activation of production of androgens by the adrenal cortex
• Pubarche	Appearance of pubic hair

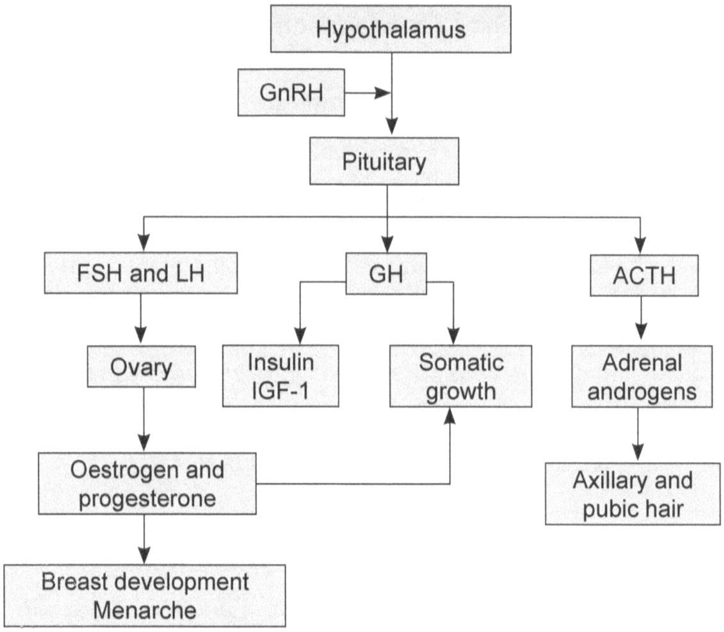

Endocrinal changes in puberty, ACTH, adrenocorticotropic hormone; FSH, follicle-stimulating hormone; GH, growth hormone; GnRH, gonadotropin-releasing hormone; IGF-1, insulin-like growth factor 1; LH luteinizing hormone

- **Estrogen dependent pubertal change:**
  - Breast (Thelarche).
  - Menstruation (Menarche).
  - Vaginal cornification.
  - Cervix mucosa → thin profuse , clear watery cervical mucous with spinnbarkeit effect (stretchability) and produces ferning pattern (microscopy) on drying up.
- **Androgen dependent pubertal change:**
  - Axillary hair.
  - Pubic hair.

Ans: (d) Axillary and pubic hair growth

Ref: *Lakshmi Seshadri, Essentials of Gynecology, 1st Edition, Page 248*

3. One of the following is not used as a post coital contraceptive:

(a) Copper T
(b) Danazol
(c) Ulipristal
(d) Mifepristone

Explanation:

Following agents are used for post coital contraception:

Various regimens used for emergency contraception		
Drug	**Dosage**	**Time period within which the drug has to be taken**
Levonorgestrel	0.75 mg given twice, 12 hours apart, or given as a single dose of 1.5	Up to 72 hours following unprotected intercourse
Yuzpe regimen	100 µg of ethinylestradiol + 500 µg levonorgestrel given twice, 12 hours apart	Up to 72 hours following unprotected intercourse
Mifepristone	10 mg single oral dose	Up to 72 hours following unprotected intercourse
Ulipristal	Single oral dosage of 30 mg	Up to 120 hours following unprotected intercourse
Copper intrauterine contraceptive device		Up to 5 days following unprotected sexual intercourse

Danazol is an **androgenic steroid.**

Mechanism of Action–By inhibiting the pituitary gonadotropins, danazol results in a hypoestrogenic state and causes endometrial atrophy.

Indications

- Endometriosis.
- DUB.
- Medical management of fibroid.
- Pre-operative thinning of the endometrium prior to endometrial ablation.
- Precocious puberty.

Ans: (b) Danazol

Ref: *Clinical Obstetrics and Gynecology, Sharmila Arun Babu, 1st Edition, Page 541*

4. Mention the usage of this instrument:

(a) Laparoscopic adhesiolysis
(b) Laparoscopic lymphadenectomy
(c) Laparoscopic sterilization
(d) Laparoscopic cystectomy

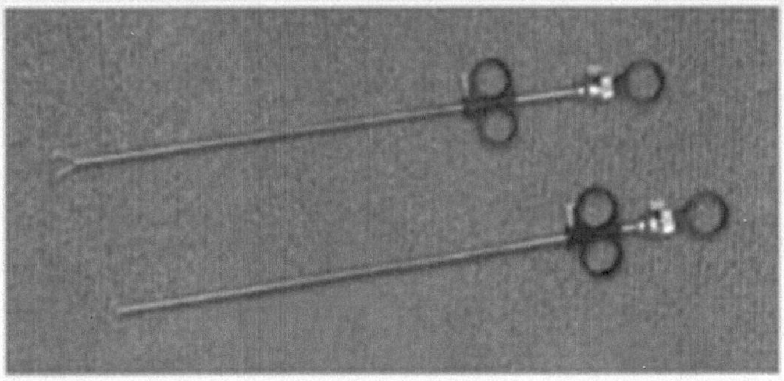

Explanation:

- It is the **laparoscopic ring applicator,** used to **apply Falope rings on fallopian tubes** during **laparoscopic sterilization.**

Laparoscopic Sterilization

- Done using laparoscope, usually performed for **interval sterilization.**
- It is **contraindicated during postpartum** period and **following 2nd trimester MTPs.**
- The patient is laid in lithotomy position and with a help of **Verres Needle** (introduced at an angle of 45°) pneumoperitoneum is created. Most **common gas used is CO_2.**
- The procedure is done on an outpatient basis.

Methods of Laparoscopic Sterilization

- **Electrocautery (unipolar or bipolar)**–Electrocoagulation is **not preferred due to high failure rate.** Bipolar is safer. Unipolar has lower failure rate but it is not done due to risk of intestinal burns.
- **Banding using Falope ring**–It is the **most common method for laparoscopic ligation in India.** The tube should be placed at the junction of **proximal and middle third of each tube** after drawing a sufficient "knuckle" of tube into Falope ring applicator. **Failure rate of 0.2-1.3%.**
- **Clip application using Hulka-Clemens clip and Filshie clip**–Clip placed around **isthmic portion of fallopian tube. Least damage to tube** but associated with **higher rates of failure.**

Advantages of Laparoscopic Sterilization

- A minimally invasive technique.
- Small incision.
- Reduced duration of hospital stay.
- Rapid recovery.
- Provides a chance to inspect the pelvis and upper abdominal organs.

Ans: (c) Laparoscopic sterilization

Ref: *Shaw's Textbook of Gynecology, 16th Edition, Page 283*

5. Which of the following test is used in modern era to monitor the Rh-isoimmunized pregnancy if the antibody titers exceed the critical level?

(a) Non stress test
(b) Amniotic fluid spectrophotometry analysis
(c) Percutaneous umbilical blood sampling
(d) Middle cerebral artery peak systolic velocity

Explanation:

Middle cerebral artery peak systolic velocity **(MCA PSV) Doppler** has **revolutionized the management of Rh-isoimmunized pregnancy** by minimizing the need for invasive tests by 70%.

Other Options:

- Amniotic fluid bilirubin assessment is performed through serial amniocentesis. It is now replaced with MCA PSV.
- Percutaneous umbilical blood sampling (PUBS) under ultrasound guidance is performed if MCA PSV or Amniotic fluid bilirubin assessment tests are abnormal.

Management of Rh-Isoimmunized Mother (ICT Positive)

The **main objective** of management of an Rh-negative pregnant woman who is already sensitized is **early detection and treatment of fetal anemia.**

Antenatal Management

- If ICT is positive, do **serial anti-Rh antibody titers (ICT in titers),** which can determine the risk of development of fetal anemia. As long as the **titer remains below the critical titer of 1:16,** the risk of fetal anemia or severe erythroblastosis or perinatal death is low.

Further Management is Based on ICT Titer Levels

- If the **antibody titer remains below the critical level,** repeat the titers every 4 weeks up to 28 weeks and then every 2–3 weeks thereafter.
  - The patient can be followed up with serial ultrasound till term. If no other indication for early termination exists, deliver the patient at term.
  - The pediatrician should be informed during delivery so that early evaluation and treatment of the newborn is started.
  - Keep the **umbilical cord long,** in case exchange transfusion is required.
  - The **cord blood** should be collected for **Rh typing, DCT, hemoglobin and serum bilirubin.**
- If at any point of time, **the antibody titers exceeds the critical level** or there is a significant rise in titers between two consecutive samples, **further evaluation is done by Doppler velocimetry of the middle cerebral artery peak systolic velocity (MCA PSV).**
- The **sensitivity of MCA PSV for prediction of moderate to severe fetal anemia is almost 100%. Further management is based on the interpretation of MCA PSV.**
  - If the **MCA PSV is <1.5 multiples of median (MoM),** repeat the study every 2 weeks and the patient may be delivered at 37–38 weeks.
  - If the **MCA PSV is ≥ 1.5 MoM,** further evaluation is required.
    - If the **MCA PSV is >1.5 MoM, and the patient is > 34 weeks,** the patient can be delivered and **exchange transfusion may be given postnatally** to the newborn.
    - If the **MCA PSV is >1.5 MoM, and the patient is < 34 weeks,** fetal blood sampling (FBS) is done by **cordocentesis** to estimate **cord blood hematocrit.**
    - If **cord blood hematocrit is > 30%,** FBS is to be repeated once a week. Delivery should be planned between 34 and 36 weeks.
    - If **cord blood hematocrit is < 30%, intrauterine transfusion (IUT)** is indicated.

Advantages of MCA PSV in the Detection of Affected Fetus

- Noninvasive technique to detect fetal anemia.
- Detects fetal anemia at an early stage.
- **Correlates directly with fetal anemia** while **spectrophotometric analysis of amniotic fluid correlates directly with fetal hyperbilirubinemia.**
- No worsening of fetomaternal hemorrhage.
- Fetal response to in utero transfusion can be monitored.

Evaluation and Management of Rh-Isoimmunization in Pregnancy

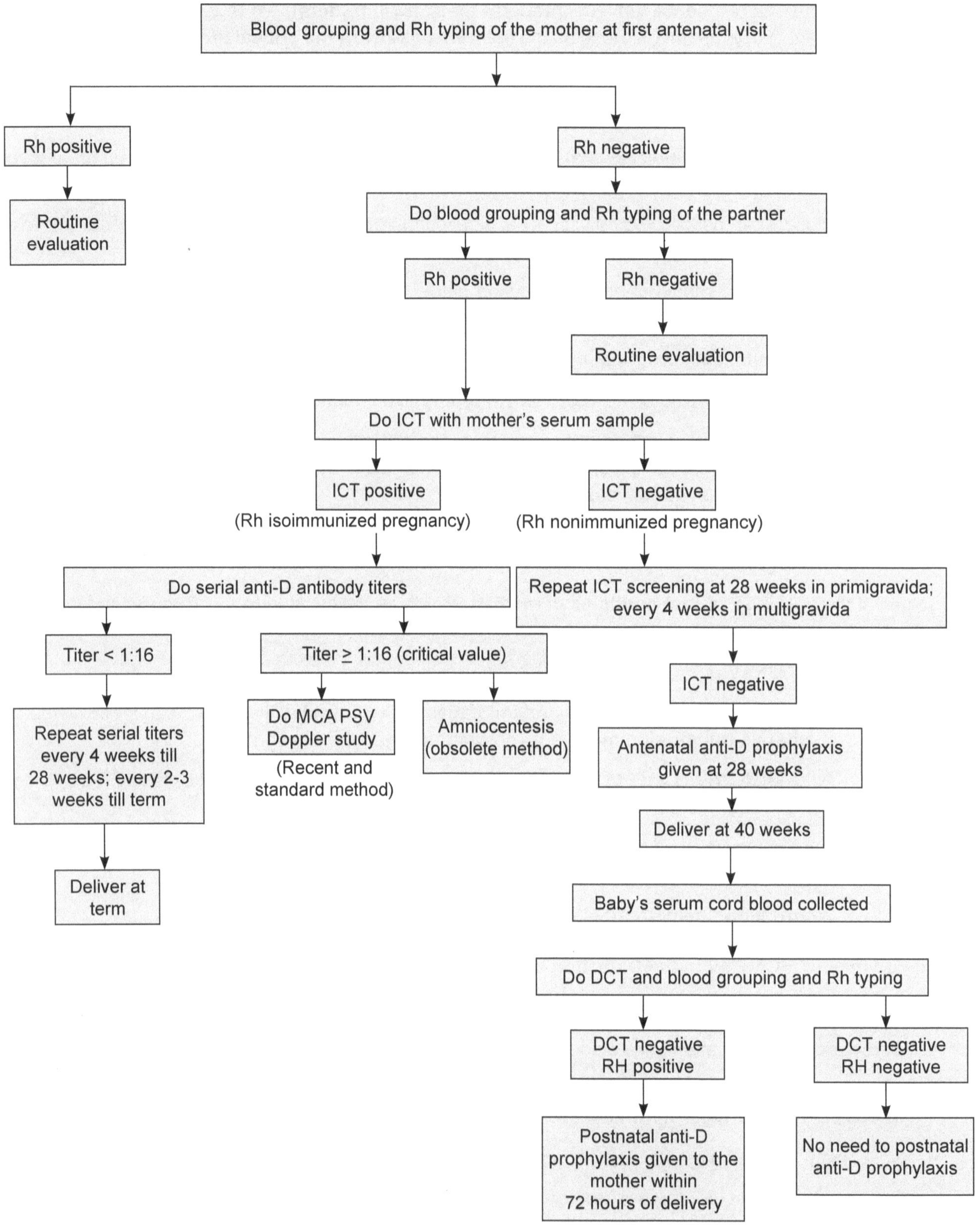

Flowchart: Management of Rh incompatible pregnancy; ICT, indirect Coombs test; MCA PSV, middle cerebral artery peak systolic velocity; DCT, direct Coombs test

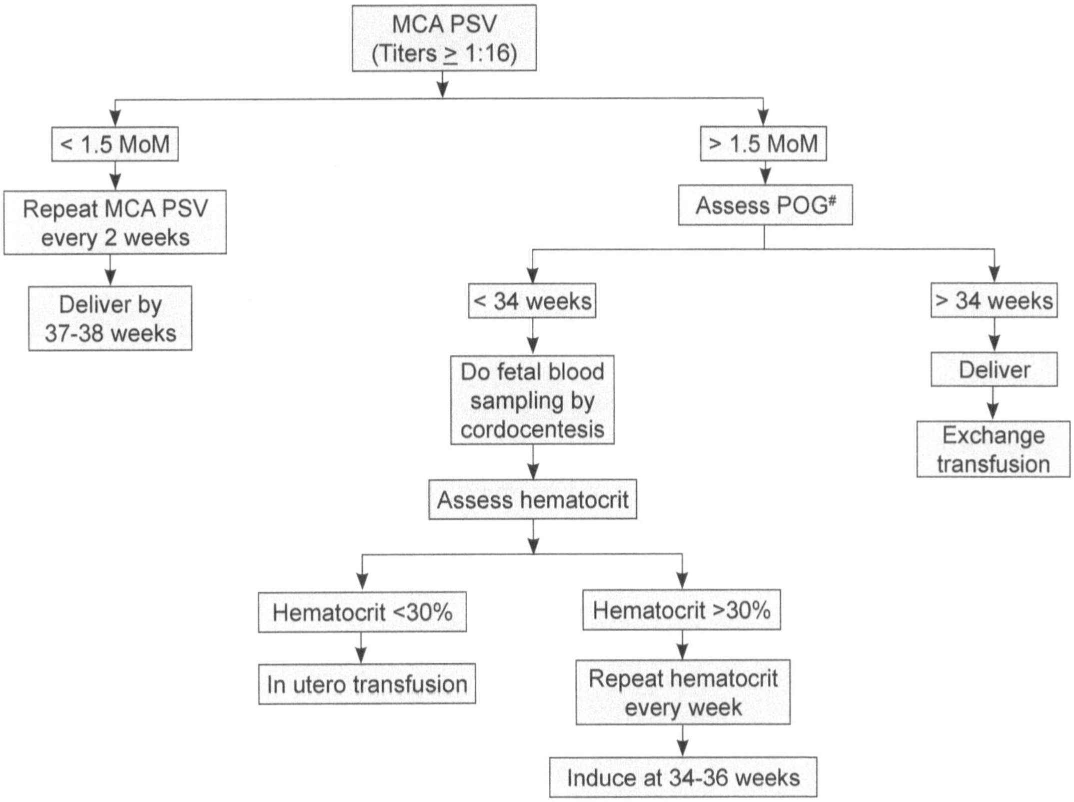

Flowchart: Management of Rh isoimmunized pregnancy based on MCA PSV. MCA PSV, middle cerebral artery peak systolic velocity; MoM, multiples of median; POG, period of gestation

Ans: (d) Middle cerebral artery peak systolic velocity

Ref: *Clinical Obstetrics and Gynecology, Sharmila Arun Babu, 1st Edition*

6. A 29-year-old woman married for 4 years was put on Clomiphene for infertility treatment. While on treatment, she developed dyspnea and abdominal pain. Her USG image is given below. What is the likely condition?

(a) PCOD
(b) Theca lutein cysts
(c) Ovarian hyperstimulation
(d) Malignant ovarian tumor

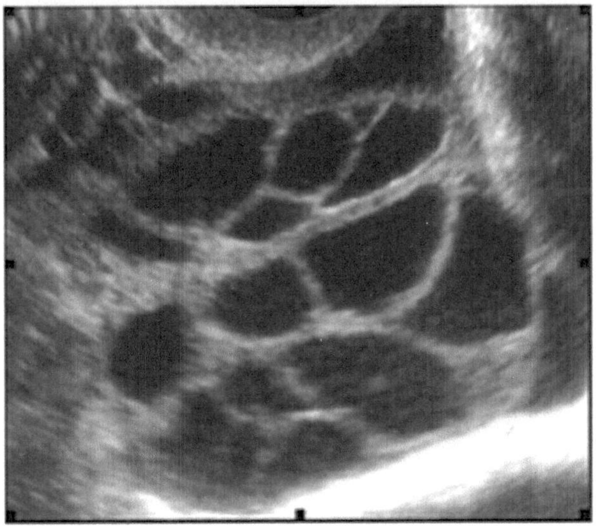

Explanation:

Complications of Ovulation Induction

- Ovarian hyperstimulation syndrome.
- Multifetal pregnancy.

Ovarian Hyperstimulation Syndrome

- This syndrome is characterized by ovarian enlargement with abdominal distension, ascites, hypotension, oliguria, hemoconcentration, gastrointestinal and respiratory problems.
- The condition **usually develops after treatment with ovulation induction** drugs and administration of hCG to trigger ovulation.
- **Classification:** According to **severity, OHSS is classified into grades 1–5.**
  - **Mild form:**
    - Grade 1 = Abdominal distension and discomfort.
    - Grade 2 = Grade 1 + Nausea, vomiting, diarrhea.
  - **Moderate OHSS:**
    - Grade 3 = Grade 2 + Sonographic evidence of ascites.
  - **Severe OHSS:**
    - Grade 4 = Grade 3 + Clinical ascites, hydrothorax, dyspnea.
    - Grade 5 = Grade 4 + hemo-concentration, renal insufficiency, oliguria, venous thromboembolism or RDS.
- Treatment is by **fluid replacement and supportive therapy.**
- **OHSS can be prevented** by close **monitoring of serum estradiol and follicular development,** and withholding hCG if there are too many follicles or if oestradiol levels are too high.

Ans: (c) Ovarian hyperstimulation

Ref: *Lakshmi Seshadri, Essentials of Gynecology, Page 322*

7. The following is an image of a fetal anomaly. What condition in the mother is associated with this fetal anomaly?

(a) Intake of ACE inhibitors
(b) Intake of phenytoin
(c) Maternal congenital heart disease
(d) Pregestational diabetes mellitus

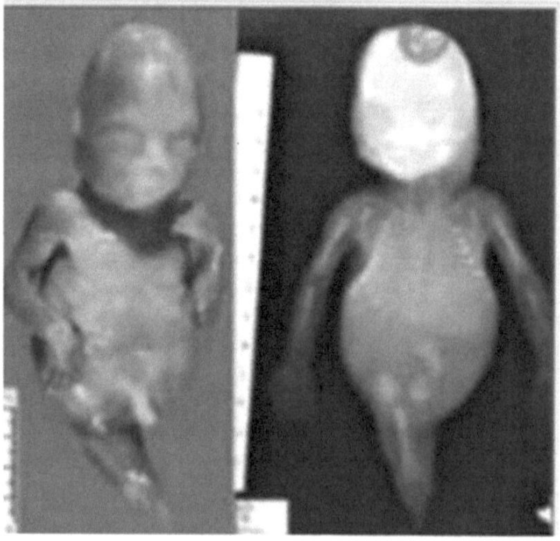

Explanation:

The image diagnosis is **caudal regression.**

Sacral agenesis/caudal regression: Abnormal development of lower fetal spine—**though rare, it is a specific anomaly to Pregestational diabetes.**

Fetal Complications Specific to Pregestational or overt DM

- Increased **risk of abortions and congenital anomalies** are specific to overt DM (in **true GDM,** hyperglycemia usually occurs in the second trimester and hence associated with late fetal complications such as **macrosomia and polyhydramnios).**
- Neonatal complications are similar in both true GDM and pregestational DM.

Congenital Malformations in DM

- These occur in overt DM when blood glucose levels are uncontrolled during organogenesis.
- *Incidence:* It is **6–10% in DM (in normal population–3%).**
- **HbA1c >10** is associated with **14% risk of congenital malformations.**

Common Congenital Anomalies in Fetuses of Diabetic Mothers

- **Cardiac anomalies (most common** anomalies)—Transposition of great vessels, ventricular septal defect, atrial septal defect, patent ductus arteriosus and coarctation of aorta.
- Neural tube defects—Anencephaly and microcephaly.
- Renal and gastrointestinal tract anomalies.

Ans: (d) Pregestational diabetes mellitus

Ref: *Clinical Obstetrics and Gynecology, Sharmila Arun Babu, 1st Edition, Page 66*

8. A 46-year-old female comes to gynecology OPD with history of heavy menstrual bleeding since 8 months, not controlled with tranexamic acid. Clinical examination reveal no abnormality and USG measured ET is 10 mm. Which of the following is the next step in management?

(a) Endometrial sampling (b) Hormonal therapy
(c) Endometrial ablation (d) Hysterectomy

Explanation:

Fractional curettage or endometrial sampling is indicated in perimenopausal women with AUB to rule out endometrial hyperplasia and endometrial carcinoma.

Other Options:

- **Hysterectomy** is generally the final resort in women with DUB not responding to any non surgical treatment.
- **Endometrial ablation** is an alternative to hysterectomy in women who do not desire future pregnancy.

Indications for Endometrial Sampling in AUB

- Women with AUB at > 45 years (perimenopausal AUB)—to exclude endometrial hyperplasia and carcinoma, as > 90% of endometrial cancers are seen in this age group.
- Women of reproductive age with persistent anovulatory AUB (> 6 months), associated with risk factors such as obesity, PCOD, or tamoxifen therapy, family history of colon/gynecologic cancer.
- Ultrasound showing increased ET (>12 mm) in perimenopausal women.
- Women not responding to medical therapy.

Methods for Endometrial Sampling

- **Fractional curettage (dilatation and curettage):** Requires cervical dilatation and is a blind procedure.
- **Endometrial aspiration biopsy:** Cervical dilatation not required and is a blind procedure. **ACOG recommends Pipelle office endometrial biopsy** for endometrial sampling in women older than 45 years with abnormal uterine bleeding (AUB).
- **Hysteroscopy-directed endometrial biopsy:** Gold standard method for evaluation of endometrial pathology as it allows direct visualization of the endometrium and targeted biopsies.

The Endometrial Histopathology in DUB Can Be of the Following Types

- **Normal endometrium 50% (most common histology).**
- Endometrial hyperplasia 30%.
- Irregular shedding 5–10%.
- Irregular ripening <5%.
- Atrophic endometrium <5%.
- Chronic endometritis 1–2%.

Ans: (a) Endometrial sampling

Ref: *Clinical Obstetrics and Gynecology, Sharmila Arun Babu, 1st Edition*

9. A 42-year-old woman presents to gynecology OPD with history of intermenstrual bleeding. USG shows a lesion within endometrial cavity with feeding vessel within endometrial cavity (image shown below). Which of the following is the probable diagnosis?

(a) Endometrial carcinoma
(b) Endometrial polyp
(c) Leiomyosarcoma
(d) Submucous fibroid

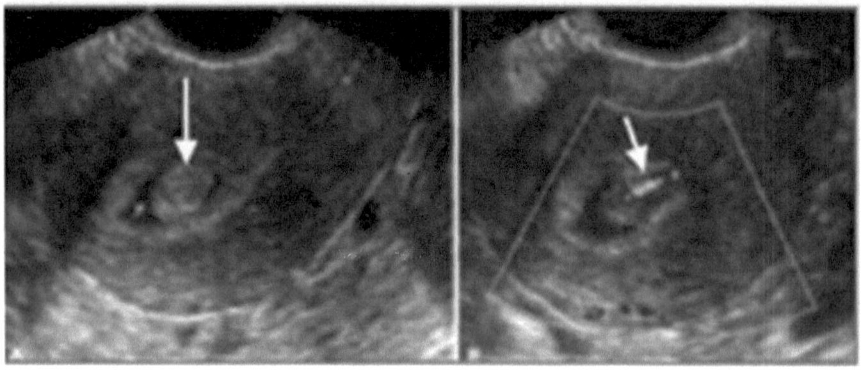

Explanation:

USG showing localized lesion with feeding vessel within the endometrial cavity is suggestive of endometrial polyp.

Endometrial Polyp

- Localized overgrowths of endometrial glands and stroma; usually arise at the uterine fundus.
- The **majority are asymptomatic,** but some present with irregular bleeding/postmenopausal bleeding.
- **Diagnosis:**
  - **Focal endometrial thickening** on ultrasound.
  - **Saline infusion sonography** allows **better visualization and demarcation of the endometrial polyp** within the endometrial cavity than transvaginal ultrasound. **Endometrial polyps** appear as **hyperechogenic pedunculated lesions** while **submucous fibroids have mixed echogenicity.**

- Directly visualization with **hysteroscopy.**
- Polyps are often difficult to identify with endometrial biopsy or curettage; because endometrial biopsy often misses polyps.

- **Treatment:**
  - **Polypectomy** is generally performed via curettage, blind avulsion, or hysteroscopic removal.

Ans: (b) Endometrial polyp

Ref: *Shaw's Textbook of Gynecology, 16th Edition*

10. A 28-year-old woman P1L1 who had a home delivery 2 weeks back, presents with fecal incontinence. Local examination reveals a complete perineal tear. What is the next line of management?

(a) Repair immediately
(b) Repair after 3 weeks
(c) Repair after 3 months
(d) Repair after 6 months

Explanation:

Classification of Perineal Laceration/Tears

Degree	Description
First degree	Involves skin and vaginal mucosa
Second degree	Involves skin, vaginal mucosa and perineal muscles (like an episiotomy)
Third degree	Involves the anal sphincter (complete perineal tear) 3a: Less than 50% thickness of external anal sphincter is involved. 3b: More than 50% thickness of external anal sphincter is involved. 3c: Internal anal sphincter is also involved
Fourth degree	Involves the rectal mucosa

Repair of 3rd and 4th Degree Tear:

- **Recent tear** should be **repaired immediately** following delivery of placenta.
- The complete perineal tear should be **repaired after 3 months if delayed beyond 24 hours.**
- Pregnancy should be avoided preferably for one year after 3rd or 4th degree perineal tear repair.

Principal Steps of Repair of Complete Perineal Tear

- Repair of rectal mucosa.
- Apposition and repair of the torn anal sphincters.
- Repair of perineal muscles.
- Repair of the vaginal mucosa and skin.

Ways to Prevent Perineal Tear During Delivery

- **Ritgen maneuver** (promoting flexion of fetal head with left hand and supporting perineum with right hand).
- **Episiotomy:** Not routinely recommended. Indicated only in selective cases.

Ans: (c) Repair after 3 months

Ref: *Clinical Obstetrics and Gynecology, Sharmila Arun Babu, 1st Edition, Page 613*

11. A 16-year-old girl is brought by parents to gynecology OPD with complaints of not having attained menarche. History of cyclical abdominal pain is present. Breast and secondary sexual characters are well developed. USG examination reveals hematocolpos and hematometra. Which of the following do you suspect?

(a) Imperforate hymen
(b) Longitudinal vaginal septum
(c) Vaginal agenesis
(d) Mullerian agenesis

Explanation:

- The girl presents with **primary amenorrhea and characteristic cyclical abdominal pain.** USG is suggestive of outflow tract obstruction, indicating cryptomenorrhea.
- Obstruction to the outflow of menstrual blood leads to collection of blood in the genital tract, a condition known as **cryptomenorrhea.**
- **Causes of cryptomenorrhea:**
  - Imperforate hymen (most common anatomic disorder of puberty).
  - Transverse vaginal septum.
  - Cervical atresia.
  - Vaginal agenesis.

Imperforate Hymen

- It is a **distal failure of vaginal vault canalization** during embryogenesis.
- It is the most **common single anatomic disorder of puberty.**
- Diagnosis is usually made at puberty when patients present with cyclic abdominal pain due to retained menstrual flow.
- The imperforate hymen can be seen as a **bluish bulging membrane at the introitus.**
- In girls with transverse vaginal septum and imperforate hymen, the **vagina distends with blood forming a hematocolpos** and pushes the uterus up into the abdomen. The collection of blood extends into the uterus and tubes forming **hematometra and hematosalpinx.**
- **Before menarche: Hydrocolpos or mucocolpos** may occur (build up of secretion behind hymen).
- **After menarche: Hematocolpos/hematometra** may occur (build up of blood behind hymen).
- Patient presents with primary **amenorrhea, pelvic pain, and difficulty with urination/defecation. Uterus is present and breasts are well developed.** Urinary retention can occur due to pressure on the urethra by the hematocolpos.
- Since development of kidneys and urinary tract is closely linked to development of Müllerian ducts, **anomalies of the kidneys and urinary tract are common in these girls.**
- Diagnosis is by **clinical examination** including per rectal examination and examination under anesthesia. Ultrasound can detect hematocolpos/hematometra, but **MRI has been found to be an excellent tool** for **diagnosing the exact site and nature of anomaly.** Serum FSH levels are in the normal range.

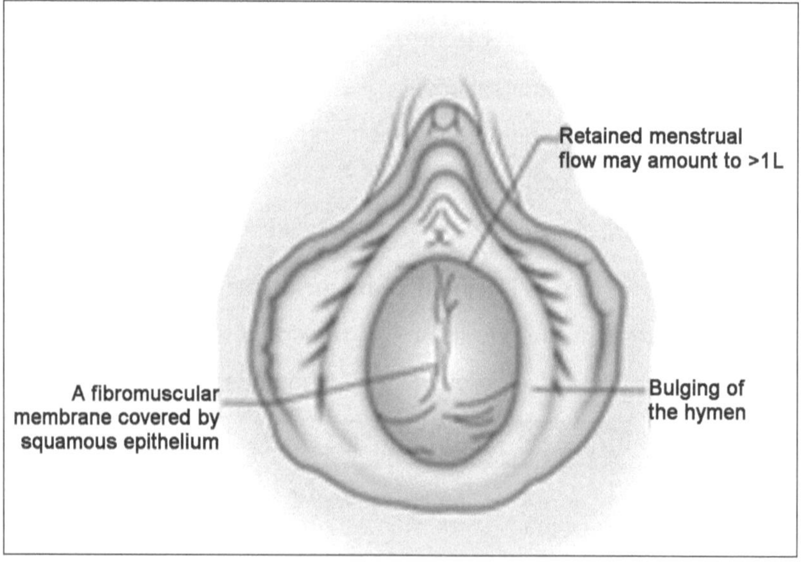

- **Complications:** Bilateral **ovarian endometriosis** can result due to prolonged retrograde menstruation.
- **Treatment:** Surgical hymenectomy.

Imperforate hymen

Transverse vaginal septum It is a more of a **proximal failure.** Sometimes it is difficult to distinguish an imperforate hymen from a transverse vaginal septum, and in such situations, examination under anesthesia (EUA) is required.

- **Longitudinal vaginal septum** usually does not cause cryptomenorrhea. It is usually noted incidentally during per speculum and pervaginal examination or during labour.
- **Mullerian agenesis (Mayer–Rokitansky–Küster–Hauser (MRKH) syndrome)** occurs when the **paramesonephric system fails to form in an otherwise normal 46,XX woman.** Characterized by **absence or hypoplasia of proximal vagina, cervix, uterus, fallopian tubes.**

Ans: (a) Imperforate hymen

Ref: *Lakshmi Seshadri, Essentials of Gynecology, Page 257*

12. A 29-year-old P1L1 presents to her OPD with c/o secondary amenorrhoea. She gives history of severe blood loss following delivery and failure of lactation in postpartum period. She is lethargic and has cold intolerance. What is the likely diagnosis?

(a) Androgen secreting ovarian tumor
(b) Asherman's syndrome
(c) Sheehan's syndrome
(d) Prolactinoma

Explanation:

- History of secondary **amenorrhea, failure of lactation, lethargy and cold in tolerance following severe blood loss during** delivery is suggestive of **Sheehan's syndrome.**

Sheehan's syndrome – A condition in which a woman following a delivery with severe postpartum hemorrhage, develops pan hypopituitarism because of **infarction and necrosis of the pituitary.**

- Clinical features occur due to **deficiency of all anterior pituitary hormones (GH, Prolactin, Gonadotropin (FSH, LH), TSH and adrenocorticotrophic hormones).**
- **Prolactin** is essential for lactation, and women with extensive pituitary necrosis (Sheehan syndrome) have failed lactation.
- **Gonadotropin deficiency** (LH and FSH) can lead to amenorrhea, genital atrophy, infertility, decreased libido, and loss of axillary and pubic hair.
- **Thyrotropin (TSH) deficiency** results in hypothyroidism with fatigue, weakness, hyperlipidemia, cold intolerance.
- **Adrenocorticotropin (ACTH) deficiency** occurs last and results in secondary adrenal insufficiency caused by pituitary disease.

Asherman's syndrome: It is a cause for secondary **amenorrhea.** It is most frequently associated with **scarring of uterine cavity** from **infection or dilation and curettage.**

Ans: (c) Sheehan's syndrome

Ref: *Shaw's Textbook of Gynecology, 16th Edition*

13. Identify the given image:

(a) Normal hysterosalpingogram
(b) Bilateral cornual block
(c) Bilateral hydrosalpinx
(d) Extravasation of dye

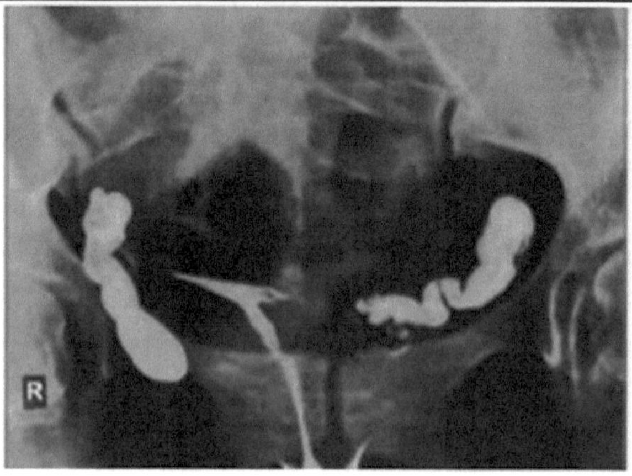

Explanation:

- The image shows an HSG film showing bilateral dilated fallopian tubes with no free spill into peritoneal cavity, suggestive of bilateral hydrosalpinx.
- **In Normal HSG:** Both the fallopian tubes are patent with **spill into the peritoneal cavity.**
- **In bilateral cornual block: No radiopaque shadow is visible in either fallopian tube.** Distal end will not be visualized. When HSG shows a cornual block, it may be due to tubal spasm. Bilateral cornual block with extravasation of the dye is highly suggestive of tubercular salpingitis.

HYSTEROSALPINGOGRAM

- **Hysterosalpingogram (HSG)** is a **contrast study to assess the uterine cavity and fallopian tubes.**

Procedure:

- HSG cannula **(Leech–Wilkinson's cannula) or No. 8 Foley's catheter** is inserted into the cervix, radiopaque dye is instilled slowly through the cervix and studied under fluoroscopic guidance.
- Two radiographic images are generally taken: The first one to show the filling of the uterine cavity. The second one after 10–15 minutes to show tubal filling and peritoneal spillage.
- Tubal patency is confirmed by peritoneal spillage of the dye.

Indications for HSG

- To assess tubal patency in infertility cases.
- To detect the side and site of block, if tubal block is present.
- To detect uterine malformations.
- For diagnosis of submucous fibroid or polyp.
- For diagnosis of uterine synechiae.

Time to Perform HSG: HSG is done between D4 and D10 of menstrual cycle.

Advantages of HSG

- Noninvasive test.
- Relatively simple to perform compared with laparoscopy, which is an invasive procedure.

Contraindications of HSG

- Pelvic infections.

- Pregnancy.
- Vaginal bleeding.

Complications of HSG

- Vasovagal attack.
- Pelvic pain.
- Flare-up of pelvic infection.
- Extravasation of dye into venous or lymphatic channel.

Advantages of Laparoscopy Over HSG

Besides testing for tubal patency, it helps in the following:

- Diagnosis of **peritubal adhesions and pelvic endometriosis.**
- Detection of **ovarian pathology.**
- Can perform **treatment procedures such as ovarian drilling for PCOD and lysis of peritubal adhesions** in the same sitting.

Disadvantages of Laparoscopy Over HSG

- Laparoscopy **cannot evaluate uterocervical factors** that can be diagnosed with HSG.
- It is an **invasive** procedure and needs **general anesthesia.**
- It is expensive compared with HSG and needs specialized training.

Hence, **HSG and laparoscopy are complementary to each other.**

Ans: (c) Bilateral hydrosalpinx

Ref: *Shaw's Textbook of Gynecology, 16th Edition, Page 251*

14. A 37-year-old primigravida who conceived after infertility treatment presents at 38 weeks POG with dichorionic diamniotic twin pregnancy with 1st twin in breech presentation. On examination, BP is 150/90 mm Hg with proteinuria +2. How do you manage this case?

(a) Wait and watch and perform LSCS at onset of labor

(b) Immediate LSCS

(c) Monitor BP and induce at 40 weeks

(d) Induction of labor

Explanation:

Twin I in non vertex presentation is an indication for LSCS.

Obstetric and Fetal Indications for Cesarean Section in Twin Pregnancy

Obstetric indications	Fetal indications
Twins with associated complications such as: • Previous lower-segment cesarean section • Severe preeclampsia • Placenta previa • Contracted pelvis • Bad obstetric history	• First twin in nonvertex presentation • Conjoint twins • Monoamniotic twins (as cord entanglement can occur) • Triplets or higher-order births • Discordant twins • Twin-to-twin transfusion syndrome • Fetal head collision–heads of both twins in vertex presentation trying to enter the pelvis leading to nonengagement of either head • Cord prolapse during labor

Indications for Performing Cesarean Section of the Second Twin Only

- Abruption following delivery of the first twin.
- Cord prolapse of 2nd twin

Ans: (b) Immediate LSCS

Ref: *Clinical Obstetrics and Gynecology by Sharmila Arun Babu, 1st Edition*

15. A 29-year-old pregnant woman, sure of her dates at 36 weeks POG, with previous history of twin delivery at term, attends the antenatal OPD for routine check-up. Which of the following is the obstetric score of the patient?

(a) G2 P1
(b) G2 P2
(c) G3 P1
(d) G3 P2

Explanation:

Obstetric history is suggestive of previous term delivery and present pregnancy at 36 weeks POG – G2 and P1.

Obstetric indices and their definitions	
Obstetric index	**Definition**
Gravida	Refers to the number of pregnancies including the present pregnancy the woman has had, irrespective of the period of gestation and pregnancy outcome
Para*,†	Refers to the number of pregnancies that have crossed the period of viability, excluding the present pregnancy
Live	Refers to the number of living children at present (while taking history)
Abortion#	Refers to the expulsion of products of conception before the period of viability (i.e., 28 weeks)

* Viability refers to the ability of the fetus to survive outside the uterus after birth. Period of viability varies in different countries:

- In developing countries such as India the period is 28 weeks.
- In developed countries such as the United States and the United Kingdom the period is 24 weeks.

† Previous history of multiple pregnancy: Parity is determined by the number of pervious viable pregnancies and not by the number of fetuses delivered. Hence, parity remains the same if previous twins or triplets were born.

\# Previous history of vesicular mole and ectopic pregnancy is included under abortion.

Various terminologies used in obstetrics	
Terminology	**Definition**
Primigravida	Woman who is pregnant for the first time
Multigravida	Woman who has had at least one previous pregnancy, irrespective of pregnancy outcome (she might have aborted/delivered a viable baby)
Nulliparous	Woman who has never carried a previous pregnancy up to the period of viability
Primiparous	Woman who has had one previous viable pregnancy
Multiparous	Woman who has had two or more previous viable pregnancies
Grandmultipara	Woman who has had five or more previous viable pregnancies
Nulligravida	Woman who has never been pregnant so far
Parturient	Woman who is in labor
Puerperal	Woman has just delivered a baby

Trimesters in pregnancy	
Trimester	**Time period during pregnancy**
First trimester	From the time of conception up to 12 completed weeks of gestation
Second trimester	From the 13th week up to 28 completed weeks of gestation
Third trimester	From the 29th week up to delivery

Ans: (a) G2 P1

Ref: *Clinical Obstetrics and Gynecology by Sharmila Arun Babu, 1st Edition, Page 4*

16. A 27-year-old female presents with profuse frothy foul-smelling vaginal discharge with intense itching. Per speculum examination reveals strawberry cervix. Which of the following is the most likely diagnosis?

(a) Bacterial vaginosis
(b) Candidiasis
(c) Trichomonas vaginalis
(d) Gonorrhea

Explanation:

Pruritus vulva and green frothy discharge in a young female with strawberry vagina on examination is suggestive of **Trichomoniasis** infection.

Distinguishing features of vaginitis			
	Bacterial vaginosis	**Trichomoniasis**	**Candidiasis**
Discharge	• White, thin, homogeneous • Foul odour	• Yellow, frothy • Foul odour	• Thick, curdy • No odour
Other symptoms		Pruritus, dysuria	Pruritus, dysuria
Signs	No erythema	Strawberry vagina	Erythema ++
pH	> 4.5	> 4.5	< 4.5
Diagnosis	• Wet mount • Clue cells • Amine odour with KOH	• Wet mount • Motile organisms	• KOH • Pseudohyphae or spores

Ans: (c) Trichomonas vaginalis

Ref: *Clinical Obstetrics and Gynecology by Sharmila Arun Babu, 1st Edition*

17. A 17-year-old adolescent girl comes to Gynecology OPD with history of low grade fever, generalized weakness, pain abdomen, weight loss and 6 months of secondary amenorrhea. On clinical examination, ascites is present and a pelvic mass is palpable on left side. Urine pregnancy test is negative. Which of the following is the probable diagnosis?

(a) Fibroid uterus
(b) Epithelial ovarian tumor
(c) Ectopic pregnancy
(d) TB pelvis with tubo-ovarian mass

Explanation:

Pelvic Tuberculosis

- **Most common causative organisms: M. tuberculosis** or M. bovis.
- **Most commonly seen in premenopausal women** in **developing countries.**
- Spreads via **hematogenous dissemination** from either the lung or GI tract.
- **Most common part affected: Fallopian tubes, endometrium and ovaries.**

- **Common symptoms** of pelvic tuberculosis: Infertility, abnormal uterine bleeding, pelvic pain and ascites.
- **Pelvic examination** is normal 50% cases; patients may have mild adnexal tenderness and/or bilateral adnexal masses.
- A **positive acid-fast stain and culture from menstrual blood or biopsy of the endometrium is diagnostic.**
- **Histopathology:** Classic giant cells, granulomas.
- **Treatment:** A multidrug regimen consisting of INH, rifampicin, pyrazinamide and ethambutol.
- **Complication:** Infertility and chronic endometritis.

Tuberculous peritonitis
• Wet – Straw-coloured ascitic fluid – Tubercles on the surface of viscera – Minimal adhesions – Can be mistaken for ovarian cancer – Histology typical of TB • Dry – No ascites – Dense adhesions – Pyosalpinx/tubo-ovarian mass – Mimics chronic PID
PID, pelvic inflammatory disease; *TB*, tuberculosis

Hysterosalpingography in genital tuberculosis
• Calcification in adnexa • Tubal block at the isthmus • Multiple constrictions (beaded appearance) • Rigid tube • Extravasation of contrast

Ans: (d) TB pelvis with tubo-ovarian mass

Ref: *Shaw's Textbook of Gynecology, 16th Edition*

18. Interpret the following partogram:

(a) Inadequate uterine contraction
(b) Uterine hyperstimulation
(c) Normal partogram
(d) Cephalopelvic disproportion

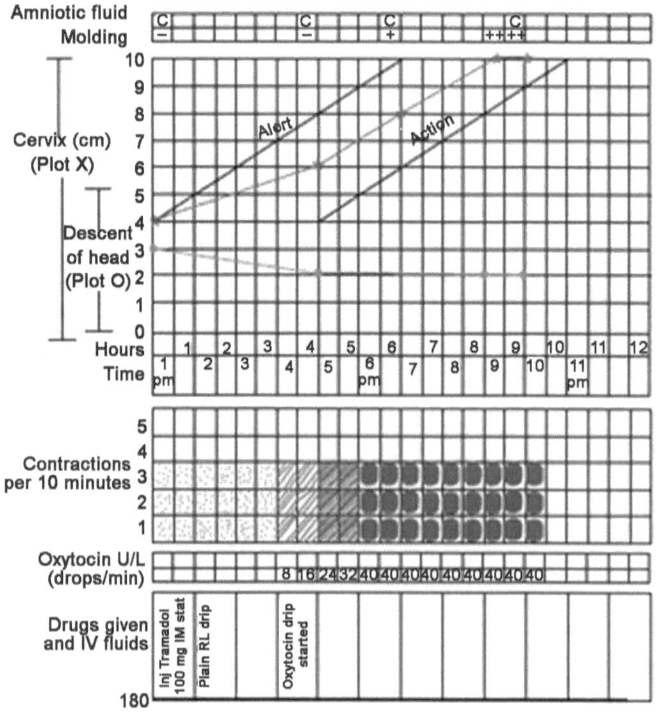

Explanation:

The Partogram is suggestive of cephalopelvic disproportion.

- The patient had no further descent of fetal head since the last observation at 5 pm. Fetal head moulding is observed. Partogram reveals full dilatation of cervix with arrest of descent despite adequate uterine contractions. This indicates that labor is obstructed probably due to CPD.

  In inadequate uterine contraction, the duration of uterine contractions will be <45 sec. **Inadequate uterine contractions** is the **most common cause for protraction disorders.**
- Minimum **cervical dilatation in nullipara = 1.2 cm/hour; Multipara= 1.5 cm/hours.**
- Minimum **descent in nullipara = 1cm /hour; Minimum descent in multipara = 2 cm/hour.**

Abnormal labor pattern			
Abnormal labor pattern	**Definition**	**Common causes**	**Management**
Disorders of the first stage of labor			
Prolonged latent phase	Prolonged latent phase is defined as that which lasts for > 20 hours in a primigravida and > 14 hours in a multigravida		Expectant management is recommended
Protracted disorders • Protracted dilatation • Protracted descent	• Protracted dilatation is when the rate of cervical dilatation is <1.2 cm/h in a primigravida and <1.5 cm/hour in a multigravida • Protracted descent is when the rate of descent of fetal heads is <1 cm/h in a primigravida and < 2 cm/hour in a multigravida	Hypotonic uterine dysfunction, malposition, big baby and CPD	• Abdominal and vaginal examinations are done to assess uterine contractions, to exclude malposition, big baby and CPD • In the absence of these factors, oxytocin augmentation with ARM achieves vaginal delivery in most of the cases
Arrest disorders • Arrest of dilatation • Arrest of descent (the cutoff limits for arrest disorders are the same for both primigravida and multigravida) • Prolonged deceleration phase	• Arrest of dilation is diagnosed when there is no dilation of the cervix for a period of > 2 hours in a woman in active phase of labor, despite adequate uterine contractions • Arrrest of descent is diagnosed when there is no descent of the presenting part for a period of >1 hour, despite adequate uterine contractions • Prolonged deceleration phase is that which lasts for > 3 hours in primigravida and > 1 hour in multigravida	Malposition, big baby, and CPD (in arrest disorders, hypotonic uterine dysfunction may be the result of obstruction; hence, augmentation should be done with caution)	• Abdominal and vaginal examinations are done to exclude malposition, big baby and CPD • Inadequate uterine contractions: Oxytocin augmentation is successful • Fetal malposition, CPD: Cesarean section is indicated
Disorders of the second stage			
• Protracted descent • Arrest of descent	• Descent of <1 cm/hour in a primigravida and < 2 cm/hour in multigravida • No progress in descent for > 2 hours in primigravida and >1 hour in multigravida	Big baby, malposition, CPD, and poor maternal expulsive forces (hypotonic uterine dysfunction may be the result of obstruction)	• Exclude CPD and malposition • IF CPD has been ruled out, judicious use of oxytocin and encouraging material expulsive efforts may achieve vaginal delivery • Instrumental delivery–if the head is below the level of ischial spines • Cesarean section–if there is CPD or malposition

ARM, artificial rupture of membranes; CPD, cephalopelvic disproportion

I stage of labor	*Slope of descent*
Latent phase	**Normal descent:** > 1 cm/h in primigravida; > 2 cm/h in multigravida
Normal duration: < 20 hours in primigravida; < 14 hours in multigravida	
	II stage of labor
Active phase *Slope of dilatation*	**Normal duration:** 2 hours if no regional anesthesia is used and 3 hours with regional anesthesia in a primigravida; 1 hour if no regional anesthesia is used and 2 hours with regional anesthesia in a multigraavida
Normal dilatation: 1.2 cm/h in primigravida; 1.5 cm/h in multigravida	A slope that is below these limits characterizes a labor with protracted dilatation or descent.

Principle Changes in the WHO Modified Partogram as Compared with WHO Composite Partogram

- Latent phase has been removed.
- Beginning of the active phase is considered at 4 cm dilatation of cervix instead of at 3 cm.
- There are two squares in 1 hour instead of one square in 1 hour, which means one square is equal to 0.5 hour in the modified partogram.

Ans: (d) Cephalopelvic disproportion

Ref: *Clinical Obstetrics and Gynecology by Sharmila Arun Babu, 1st Edition*

19. A 14-year-old child accompanied by her mother comes to gynecology OPD with complaints of failure to attend menarche. Local examination reveals clitoromegaly. Karyotype is 46XX. Which of the following enzyme is likely to be deficient in this case?

(a) 21-α hydroxylase
(b) 17-α hydroxylase
(c) 3-β hydroxyl steroid dehydrogenase
(d) 11-β hydroxylase

Explanation:

- **Clitorimegaly** is suggestive of excessive androgens (virilization); Testosterone levels should be checked.
- **The probable causes include:**
  - Congenital adrenal hyperplasia (CAH).
  - Androgen-producing ovarian or adrenal tumors.

Congenital adrenal hyperplasia is a life-threatening condition requiring mineralocorticoid supplementation to prevent salt wasting (hypovolemic-hyponatremia).

- The **most common (90%) form is 21-α hydroxylase deficiency;** 11-β hydroxylase defects can occur.
- **Accumulation of** androgenic precursors **(17 hydroprogesterone and DHEA)** occur due to deficiency of 21 hydroxylase.

Ans: (a) 21-α hydroxylase

Ref: *Berek and Novak's Gynecology, 16th Edition*

20. A primi at 20 weeks gestation presents to OPD for ANC check up. On abdominal examination, the uterine size is 16 weeks. USG is suggestive of severe oligohydramnios. Which of the following fetal anomaly is suspected?

(a) Tracheoesophageal fistula
(b) Spina bifida
(c) Anencephaly
(d) Renal agenesis

Explanation:

- The findings are suggestive of **oligohydramnios due to fetal renal agenesis**.
- Polyhydramnios (high amount of amniotic fluid: 2,000 ml in late pregnancy) is associated with inability of the fetus to swallow due to tracheoesophageal fistula, esophageal atresia, or anencephaly.

OLIGOHYDRAMNIOS

- **Definition:** Liquor volume is deficient in amount **(< 200 ml at term).**
- Ultrasonography definition of oligohydramnios: AFI **< 5 or Single deepest liquor pocket < 2 cm.**

Causes of oligohydramnios			
Maternal	**Fetal**	**Placental**	**Idiopathic**
• Preeclampsia, chronic hypertension • Post-term pregnancy • Placental insufficiency (IUGR) • Premature rupture of membranes • Drugs: ACE inhibitors (**Hint:** *Remember four "P"*)	• Chromosomal anomalies • Congential anomalies such as: – Renal agenesis – Obstruction of urinary tract	• Amnion nodosum	• Most common cause of mild oligohydramnios

ACE, angiotensin-converting enzyme; IUGR, intrauterine growth restriction.

Causes of polyhydramnios			
Maternal	**Fetal**	**Placental**	**Idiopathic**
• Maternal diabetes • RH incompatibility	• Congenital malformations–anencephaly (Figure 14.3), spina bifida, esophageal, or duodenal atresia • Fetal hydrops • Fetal aneuploidy • Parvovirus B_{19} infection • Multiple pregnancy	• Chorioangioma of placenta	• Accounts for 60% of cases (most common cause)

COMPLICATIONS IN OLIGOHYDRAMNIOS

Maternal Complications

- Increased operative interferences.
- Complications due to associated medical conditions such as preeclampsia.

Fetal Complications

- Fetal deformities due to intra-amniotic adhesions (clubfoot, amputation of limb, skull deformity).
- Pulmonary hypoplasia.
- IUGR.
- Fetal distress.
- Cord compression resulting in fetal hypoxia and asphyxia.
- Meconium aspiration syndrome.

Ans: (d) Renal agenesis

Ref: *Clinical Obstetrics and Gynecology by Sharmila Arun Babu, 1st Edition, Page 234*

21. A 62-year-old woman diagnosed with carcinoma cervix stage II B is advised for chemoradiation therapy. Which of the following is a true statement?

(a) Small bowel is radioresistant

(b) Small blood vessel is radioresistant

(c) Rapidly proliferating cells are radioresistant

(d) Dose/intensity of radiation is inversely proportional to the square of distance from source

Explanation:

Inverse Square Law

Dose or intensity of radiation is inversely proportion to the square of distance from the source.

- Small bowel, small blood vessels and rapidly proliferating cells are radiosensitive.

RADIOCURABILITY AND RADIOSENSITIVITY

- **Radiocurability: It is the elimination of tumor at the primary or metastatic site due to direct effect of radiation.**
- **Radiosensitivity: It refers to the response of tumor to irradiation.** Radiosensitivity is measured in terms of loss cellular proliferative capacity due to the DNA damage. Accumulation of sublethal injury following repeat radiation leads ultimately to DNA damage and cell death.

Radiosensitivity depends on the following factors:

Factors influencing radiosensitivity	
Factor	Effect
Tissue hypoxia	Hypoxic cells are more resistant to radiation compared to toxic cells; higher the hypoxic fraction of cells, the lesser is the radiation response
Proportion of mitotic (clonogenic) cells	Clonogenic cells are more radiosensitive
Cell cycle	**Mitotic cells (M phase) and G2 cells are more radiosensitive** compared to late S-phase cells
Tumor specificity	**Certain tumors (dysgerminomas) are more radiosensitive** than the others
Tumor volume	Smaller the tumor volume→esser the hypoxic cells→less the radiation dose→better the radiation response
Photon wavelength	**Lesser the photon wavelength** more is the penetrating power and energy of ionizing radiation

RADIATION DOSE

Inverse square law: Dose of radiation at a particular point varies inversely proportional to the square of the distance from the source of radiation.

According to the **"inverse square law"** there is reduction of radiation dose at a distance from the radiation source. This helps in **protection of normal tissues.**

MEASUREMENT OF RADIATION

- **Radiation absorption dose (Gray)** is the unit used to measure the amount of energy absorbed per unit mass of tissue.
- **One gray (Gy)** is equivalent to **1 Joule/kg which is equivalent to 100 rads.**
- **One centigray (cGy) is equivalent to one rad.**
- The amount of radiation the patient receives is calculated by **dosimetry.**

Ans: (d) Dose/intensity of radiation is inversely proportional to the square of distance from source

Ref: *Sharmila Arun Babu, Complete Review of Gynecological Oncology, 1st Edition 2020, Page 169*

22. A 28-year-old woman, married for 6 years presents with history of recurrent abortion. During evaluation, she is diagnosed to have Septate uterus. All the following are procedures done for septate uterus *except:*

(a) Strassmann's procedure

(b) Tompkin's procedure

(c) Transcervical hysteroscopic resection of septum

(d) Jones procedure

Explanation:

Septate uterus–Jones and Tompkins' septoplasty, hysteroscopic resection of septum.

Bicornuate uterus–Strassman's metroplasty.

Septate Uterus

- A septate uterus results from a problem in uterine development. The two müllerian ducts fused normally, but there is **failure in degeneration of the median septum.**
- **Complete septation:** A median septum persists in the entire uterus, separating the uterine cavity into two, that share one cervix.
- **Partial septation:** Resorption of the lower part of the median septum occurred, but the top of the septum has failed to dissolve. Thus, there is a single cervix and uterine cavity at the bottom, but at the top the cavity septum is present.
- **Hysteroscopic septal resection** (High live birth success rate–80-89%) has been shown to **improve pregnancy rates and outcomes.**
- At the time of hysteroscopy, **it may not be possible to differentiate a bicornuate from a septate uterus,** so **laparoscopy is usually performed** simultaneously to be able to look for **two separate uterine horns (bicornuate uterus)** as opposed to **normal fundus (septate uterus).**

Ans: (a) Strassmann's procedure

Ref: *Shaw's Textbook of Gynecology, 16th Edition*

23. Fertilization occurs in which part of the fallopian tube?

(a) Isthmus

(b) Ampulla

(c) Interstitial

(d) Infundibular

Explanation:

- Fertilization occurs in the **ampulla of the fallopian tube**.
- It includes Sperm penetration of corona radiata, Sperm binding and penetration of the zona pellucid and Fusion of sperm and oocyte cell membranes.
- Fertile period–**Begins 48 hours prior to ovulation** and Ends 24 hours after ovulation.

Clinical Implications

- Couples with infertility – Timed intercourse during fertile period is recommended.
- Couples desirous of contraception – Avoidance of intercourse during fertile period is recommended.

Ans: (b) Ampulla

Ref: *Essentials of Gynecology, Lakshmi Seshadri, Page 49*

24. All the following are distension media used in hysteroscopy *except:*

(a) 5% dextrose (b) Normal saline

(c) Mannitol (d) Glycine

Explanation:

- The popular liquid media used in hysteroscopy include **normal saline, 5% dextrose and Ringer lactate and Glycine**.
- The choice of medium depends on its availability, safety, effectiveness and cost as well as whether cautery or laser is used.
- Bipolar electrosurgical system works in normal saline, is cheap, has excellent hemostasis and causes instantaneous tissue vaporization.
- **Saline distension media** can lead to **electrolyte imbalance.**
- **Glycine is absorbed from the uterine cavity and peritoneum.** Excess glycine can lead to problems of **fluid overload and electrolyte disturbance.** So its input and output must be accurately documented and monitored.

ENDOMETRIAL ABLATION (MINIMAL INVASIVE SURGERY)

- Endometrial ablation involves destruction of the endometrium by resection or thermal energy.
- It is a safe and effective alternative to hysterectomy in women with DUB who do not respond to medical management.

Indications

- Failed medical therapy in DUB.
- Poor surgical candidates for hysterectomy.
- Patients who do not want surgery.
- Women with a desire to preserve the uterus.
- Endometrial ablation is especially beneficial in perimenopausal age group women who are not desirous of fertility or menstrual function.

Contraindications

- Premalignant or malignant lesion of the cervix and endometrium.
- Acute pelvic infection.
- Previous upper segment uterine scar (chance of perforation).
- Uterine size >12 weeks.
- Uterine malformations.
- Desire for future fertility.

Advantages

- Less morbid procedure.
- Short recovery time.

Preoperative Preparation

Prior therapy with GnRH analogues or danazol or Medroxy progesterone acetate for 4–6 weeks reduces endometrial thickness that facilitates the procedure.

Various Techniques

First-generation techniques: Resectoscopic endometrial ablation

- Transcervical resection of endometrium (TCRE).
- Rollerball endometrial ablation (REA).
- Laser endometrial ablation (LEA)–Nd: YAG laser commonly used.

Second-generation endometrial ablation: Non-resectoscopic endometrial ablation

- Thermal balloon ablation.
- Hydrothermal ablation.
- Microwave endometrial ablation.
- Radiofrequency–induced endometrial ablation.
- Cryotherapy.
- Photodynamic therapy.

Advantages of resectoscopic endometrial ablation methods

- Requirement of endometrial preparation is less as it is visually resected.
- Endometrial tissue is obtained for histopathology.
- Other uterine pathology such as polyps and submucous fibroid can be resected in the same sitting.

Disadvantages of resectoscopic endometrial ablation methods

- Require skilled personnel.
- Need general anesthesia.
- Distension media used, which has its own disadvantages (fluid overload).
- Complications such as uterine perforation, hemorrhage, and thermal injuries to adjacent structures.
- Expensive.

Advantages of nonresectoscopic endometrial ablation methods

- Can be done in OPD under local anesthesia.
- No distension media used (complications due to their usage are avoided).
- No bleeding during surgery.
- Duration of the procedure less compared with that in hysteroscopic methods.

Disadvantages of nonresectoscopic endometrial ablation methods

Endometrial tissue is not obtained for histopathology.

Outcome

- Improvement in symptoms occurs (reduced rate of dysmenorrhea, blood loss) in 90% of cases.
- Amenorrhea following the procedure occurs in 40–50% of cases.
- Success is not absolute and symptoms may recur or persist—20% of cases may require surgery later.

Complications of endometrial ablation

- Uterine perforation.
- Hemorrhage.
- Fluid overload (specific to resectoscopic endometrial ablation).
- Intrauterine scarring.
- Pelvic infection.
- Increased risk of complications if pregnancy occurs following the procedure.

Ans: (b) Normal saline

Ref: *Clinical Obstetrics and Gynecology by Sharmila Arun Babu, 1st Edition, Page 318*

ORTHOPEDICS

1. What is the most likely diagnosis of a 55-year-old female complaining of low backache?

(a) Hurler syndrome
(b) Paget's disease
(c) Renal osteodystrophy
(d) Osteoporosis

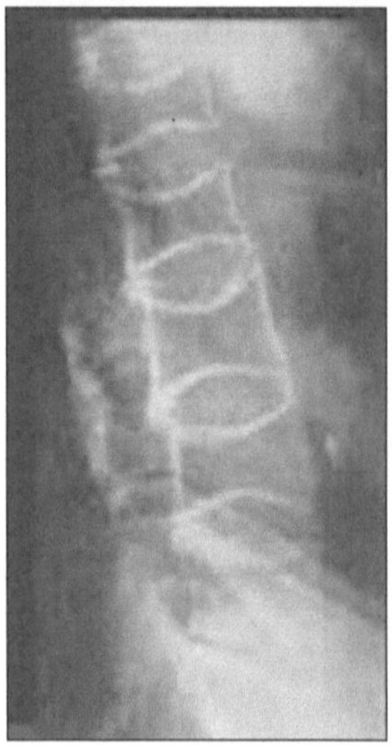

Explanation:

- The above image depicts ballooning of disc spaces leading to biconcave shape of vertebral body known as "**cod fish appearance**", classically seen in Osteoporosis.

DIAGNOSTIC TESTING OF OSTEOPOROSIS

Dual-Energy X-ray Absorptiometry (DEXA)

- This scan is the gold standard test for osteoporosis. It is very precise for measuring bone density.
- Most common site for measuring bone density: Femoral neck and lumbar spine.
- Indications for bone mineral density measurement:
  - All women aged 65 and older.
  - Postmenopausal women < 65 with one or more risk factors for fracture.
  - Men with risk factors for fracture.
- The results are reported as a T-score according to WHO's classification.
- The T-score is the bone density compared with what is normally expected in a healthy young adult of the same sex. The T-score is the number of units—standard deviations—that bone density is above or below the average.

BONE MINERAL DENSITY T-SCORE

Interpretation of T-Score

- T-score Greater than or equal to 1.0 – **Normal.**
- T-score Between -1.5 to -2.5 – **Osteopenia.**
- T-score ≥ –2.5 – **Osteoporosis.**

- T-score ≥ –2.5 and fragility fracture – **Severe osteoporosis.**
- T-scores are used in all postmenopausal and perimenopausal women, and in men over 50 years of age.
- In all other patients (including premenopausal women), z-scores are used.
- The Z-score is the number of standard deviations above or below what is normally expected for someone of the same age, sex, weight and ethnic or racial origin.
- Z-score ≤-2 may suggest that something other than aging is causing abnormal bone loss (consider drugs causing osteoporosis such as corticosteroids).

Ans: (d) Osteoporosis

Ref: *Apley's System of Orthopedics and Fractures, 10th Edition, Page132*

2. A 4-year-old child while playing suddenly spinned around his elbow from maid's hand and now continuously crying and not allowing anyone to touch the elbow. He is keeping the elbow in extended state. What is the most likely diagnosis?

(a) Radial head fracture
(b) Pulled elbow
(c) Supracondylar fracture
(d) Elbow dislocation

Explanation:

Pulled Elbow (or Nursemaid's Elbow)

- A pulled elbow is a result of the lower arm radius bone becoming partially dislocated (slipping out) of its normal position at the elbow joint. A pulled elbow is caused by a sudden pull on a child's lower arm or wrist, for example, when a child is lifted up by one arm.
- Refers to traumatic subluxation of the radial head produced by sudden traction on the hand, with the elbow extended and the forearm pronated.
- Pulled elbow is one of the most common musculoskeletal injuries in children younger than 4 years.
- Reduction is often unknowingly performed by the radiology technician, who passively forces the forearm into full supination in an attempt to obtain a true AP projection of the elbow.
- If the child escapes such treatment, the radial head is reduced by flexing the elbow to 90 degrees and rapidly and firmly rotating the forearm into full supination. As reduction is achieved, a palpable and sometimes audible click can be felt in the region of the radial head.

Ans: (b) Pulled elbow

Ref: *Tachdijian's Pediatric Orthopedics, 5th Edition, Page 1323*

3. Patient is presenting with deformity of the finger as shown. The PIP is involved but DIP is spared. What is the diagnosis?

(a) Osteoarthritis
(b) Rheumatoid arthritis
(c) Psoriatic arthritis
(d) Ankylosing spondylitis

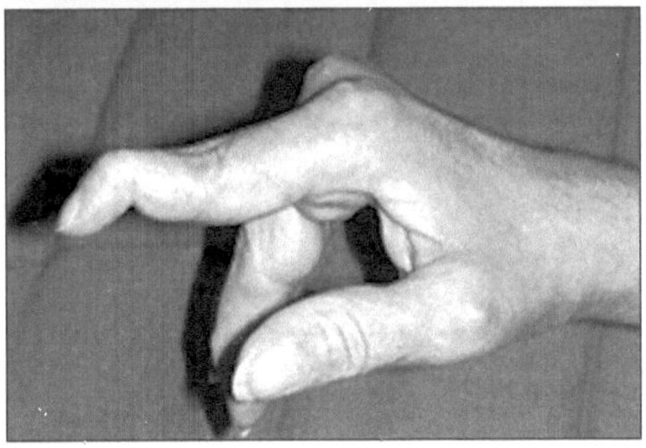

Explanation:

- The picture shows classic '**Swan neck deformity'** seen in **Rheumatoid arthritis.**

Rheumatoid Arthritis

- Autoimmune-inflammation induces formation of pannus (proliferative granulation tissue), which erodes articular cartilage and bone.
- Most commonly seen in women age > 50 years.
- Patients have complains of morning stiffness and joint pain seen in multiple joints of the hands lasting for more than 1 hour in the morning with the symptomatic episode going on for at least 6 weeks.
- RA is defined as having 4 or more of the following present for diagnosis:
  - Positive rheumatoid factor or anti-CCP.
  - Morning stiffness lasting more than 1 hour.
  - C-reactive protein (CRP) or ESR.
  - Inflammatory arthritis of 3 or more joints.
  - Duration of symptoms: More than 6 weeks.
- The more joints are involved, the more likely the diagnosis.
- Most common joints involves: Proximal interphalangeal (PIP) and metacarpophalangeal (MCP).

Joint Findings in Rheumatoid Arthritis

- Swelling and pain seen in metacarpophalangeal joint.
- Extension of the PIP with flexion of the DIP joint is known as **Swan neck deformity.**
- Outpocketing of synovium at the back of the knee is known as Baker cyst.
- Flexion of the proximal interphalangeal (PIP) with hyperextension of the distal interphalangeal (DIP) is known as Boutonniere deformity.

The Radiographic Hallmarks of Rheumatoid Arthritis are:

- **Erosions** are important early finding, in the "bare areas", frequently in the radial side of the metacarpophalangeal (MCP) joints.
- **Soft tissue swelling**
  - Fusiform and periarticular; it represents a combination of joint effusion, edema and tenosynovitis.
  - This can be an early/only radiographic finding.
- **Osteoporosis:** Initially juxta-articular, and later generalised; compounded by corticosteroid therapy and disuse.
- **Joint space narrowing:** Symmetrical or concentric.

Ans: (b) Rheumatoid arthritis

Ref: *Textbook of Orthopedics, 4th Edition, by John Ebnezar; Page 576*

4. History of arthritis with involvement of PIP and DIP and 1st MCP and spearing wrist as well as ankle are seen in:

(a) Osteoarthritis (b) Rheumatoid arthritis
(c) Psoriatic arthritis (d) Gout

Explanation:

Gout

- Acute inflammatory monoarthritis caused by precipitation of monosodium urate crystals in joints.
- Asymmetric joint distribution. Joint is swollen, red and painful. Classic manifestation is painful MTP joint of big toe (podagra).

Plain Radiographic Features of Gout

- Characteristic radiologic changes occur in the chronic stage, though not all patients progress to this. There is a predilection for the small joints of the hands and feet.
- Chondrocalcinosis is present in ~5%.
- **Joints:**
  - **Joint effusion (earliest sign).**
  - Preservation of joint space until late stages of the disease.
  - An absence of periarticular osteopenia.
  - Eccentric erosions.
  - The typical appearance is the presence of well-defined "punched-out" erosions with sclerotic margins in a marginal and juxta-articular distribution, with overhanging edges, also known as rat bite erosions.
- **Bone:**
  - Punched-out lytic bone lesions.
  - Overhanging sclerotic margins.
  - Osteonecrosis.
  - Mineralisation is normal.
- **Surrounding soft tissues:**
  - Tophi: Pathognomonic.
  - Olecranon and prepatellar bursitis.
  - Periarticular soft tissue swelling due to crystal deposition in tophi around the joints is common.
  - The soft tissue swelling may be hyperdense due to the crystals, and the tophi can calcify (uncommon in the absence of renal disease).

Ans: (a) Osteoarthritis

Ref: *Textbook of Orthopedics by John Ebnezar, 4th Edition, Page 576*

5. What is the most likely diagnosis for the image showing biceps tendon rupture?

(a) Rising sign (b) Griesinger sign
(c) Popeye's sign (d) Waddell sign

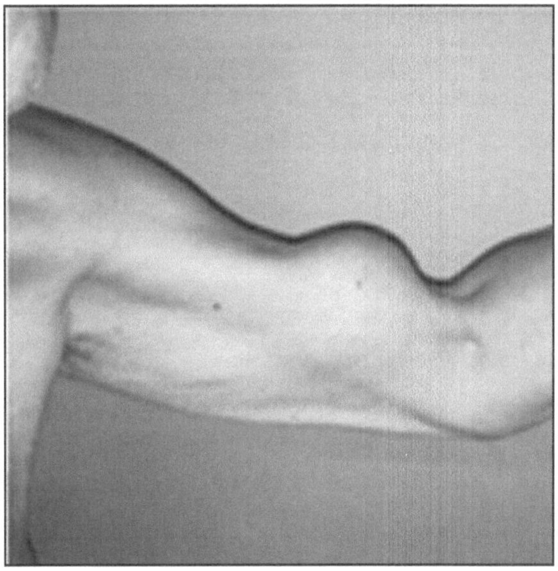

Explanation:

Popeye Deformity

- When a **tendon** in **biceps muscle tears**, the muscle can bunch up and form a large, painful ball in upper arm. This bulge is called a Popeye deformity or Popeye sign. It's named after the ball-shaped biceps of a popular cartoon character.
- Release or tear of the biceps tendon at its glenoid attachment causes severe "Popeye" deformity.
- The risk factors include older age, smoking and shoulder overuse or heavy overhead activities.
- Popeye deformity is due to the contracted belly of biceps brachii when it loses its attachment either at its origin or insertion.
- Biceps brachii flexes the elbow and is the chief supinator of the forearm in a semiflexed position of the elbow. It has two tendons (short head and long head) at the origin and a single tendon at the insertion.
- If there is a rupture of the single insertion tendon (i.e., bicipital tendon), neither of these actions will be possible with marked functional compromise. In contrast, if Popeye deformity is due to the rupture of one of the origin tendons [i.e., either long head of biceps (LHB) or short head of biceps (SHB)], these actions are possible but weak, causing less functional impairment because of the intact attachment of the other tendon at the origin that still allows some action of the muscle.
- In general, proximal biceps tendon rupture is managed non-surgically. Surgical intervention is indicated only if conservative therapy fails, or in a selected group of patients with concomitant shoulder pathology.

Ans: (c) Popeye's sign

Ref: *Campbell's Operative Orthopedics, 13th Edition, Page 2583*

6. A 30-year-old male came with complaints of swelling around the knee joint. Histopathological examination of the swelling demonstrated many giant cells interspersed with mononuclear cells. Your most probable diagnosis is:

(a) Osteosarcoma (b) Chondrosarcoma

(c) Ewing's sarcoma (d) Giant cell tumor

Explanation:

Giant Cell Tumor

- Most commonly seen in more than 20 years of age (80%) and the average age group is 35 years.
- It affects **epiphyseal** of long bones (Most common–**Distal femur**).
- **Sex:** Male : Female ratio = 1.5:1.
- **Egg shell crackling** on palpation.
- **Jaffe's criterion** is use for assessing the histological grading of the osteoclastoma.
- **Diagnosis:**
  - **Soap bubble** lesion on X-ray.
  - Cortex is expanded and thin seen in X-ray.
  - **X-ray shows:** Osteolytic area is seen near the epiphysis.
  - **X-ray reveals:** No periosteal new bone formation.
- Malignancy in GCT → Osteosarcoma/Malignant fibrous Histiocytoma/Fibrosarcoma.
- **Tumor with gaint cells:** Non-ossifying fibroma (Most common), Brown tumor, Aneurysmal bone cyst, Fibrosarcoma, MFH, Clear cell chondrosarcoma.

- **Treatment:**
  - Extended Curettage by PMMA or phenol or liquid nitrogen and bone grafting. It is procedure of choice for most lesions.
  - **Excision:** Lower end of ulna and Upper end of fibula.
  - **Excision and replacement by vascularized bone graft:** Lower end of radius where upper end of fibula is grafted.
  - Excision and arthrodesis or prosthetic replacement or Turn – O: Lower end femur and upper end tibia.
  - Treatment of recurrent lesions is the same as for primary lesions. After biopsy shows that the tumor is still benign, repeat curettage or resection should be performed.
  - **Amputation:** Malignant recurrent GCT of extremity.
  - **Radiotherapy:** Spine.

EXTRA EDGE

Image-Based Representation

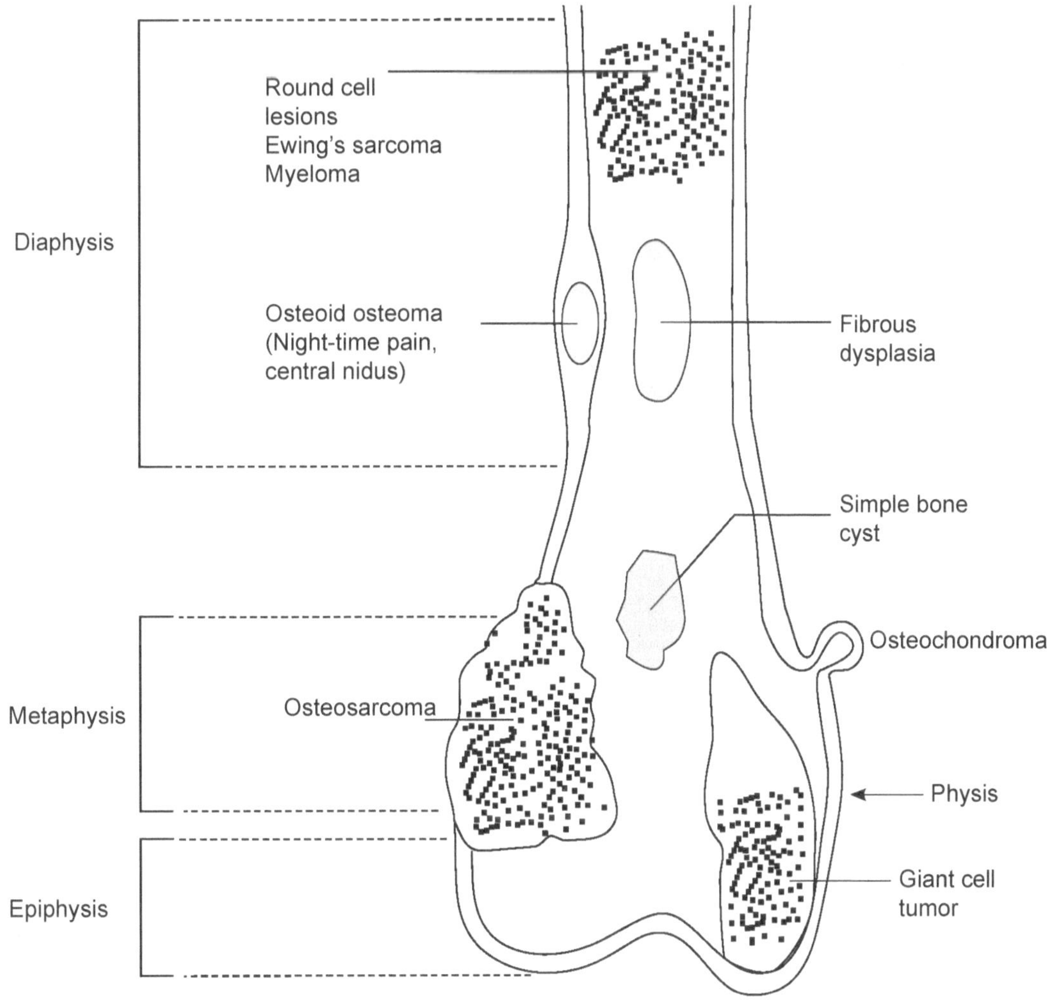

Ans: (d) Giant cell tumor

Ref: *Campbell's Operative Orthopedics, 13th Edition, Page 924*

7. Shown angle in the image is known as:

(a) Cobb's angle
(b) Baumann angle
(c) Ferguson angle
(d) Bohler angle

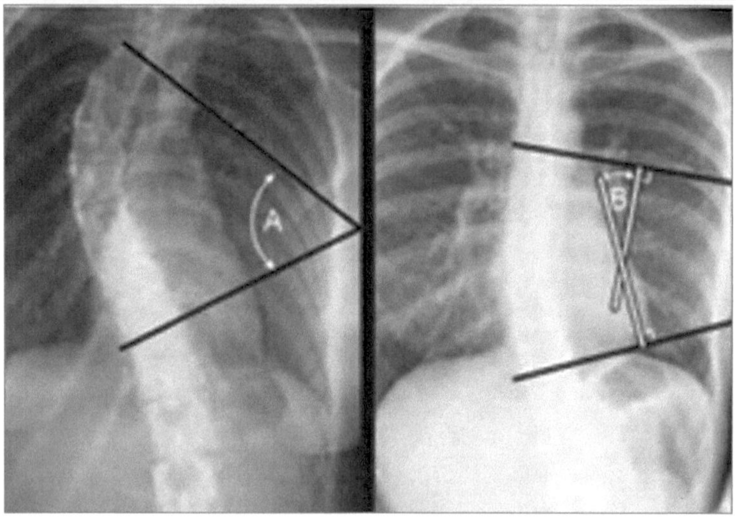

Explanation:

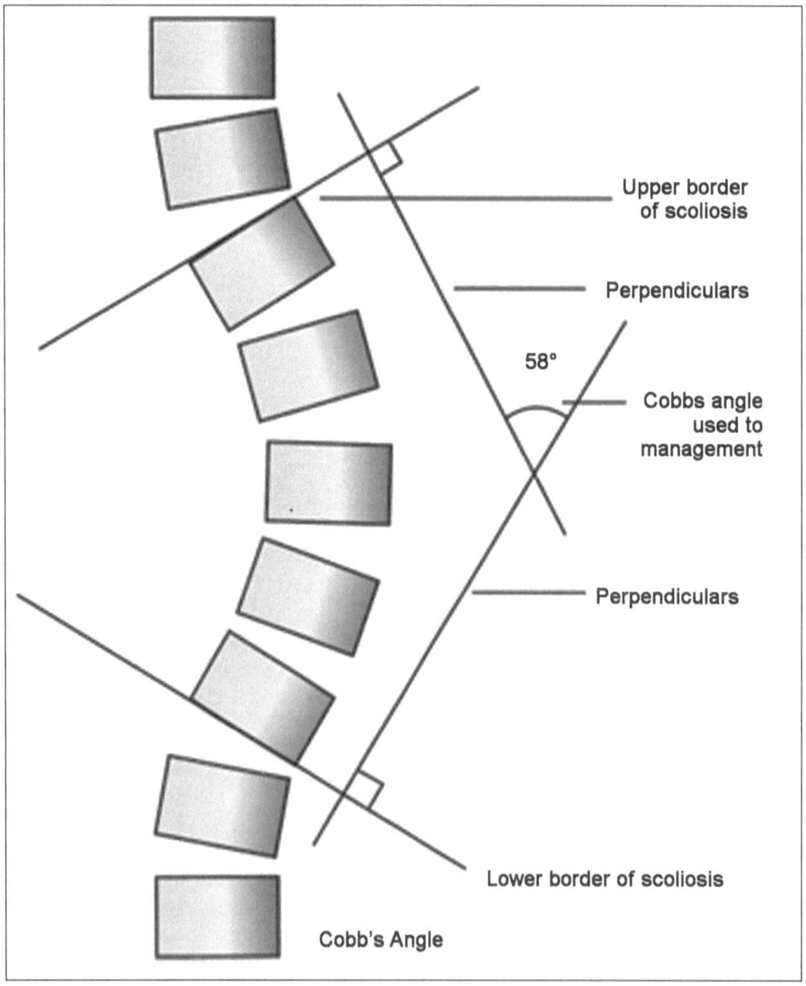

Cobb's angle

- **Cobb's angle:** Angle measured from the upper most vertebrae to lower most vertebrae. The angle between two gives Cobb's angle. It is a radiological assessment for scoliosis.
- **Ferguson angle:** Angle at lumbosacral area for the scoliosis.

Ans: (a) Cobb's angle

Ref: *Textbook of Orthopedics by John Ebnezar, 5th Edition, Page 421*

8. Patient present with pain in base of thumb. What is the tendon marked?

(a) APB and EPB
(b) APL and EPL
(c) APL and EPB
(d) APB and EPL

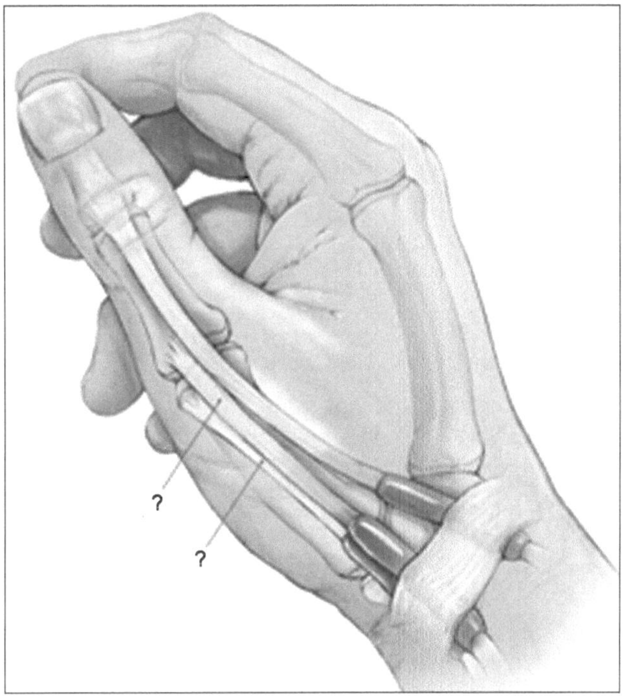

Explanation:

De Quervain Tenosynovitis

- De Quervain tenosynovitis is inflammation of the tendon sheaths located on the radial side of the wrist.
- This sheath surrounds two muscles of the thumb; the abductor pollicis longus and extensor pollicis brevis.
- De Quervain tenosynovitis is also called De Quervain tendinitis.

Etiology:

- De Quervain tenosynovitis is often related to a repetitive-motion injury.
- Some medical researchers assert that this condition is not related to repetitive motion but rather sustained weight bearing while the wrist is in a static position, such as young mothers who, as they carry their baby, force their hand into wrist flexion and thumb extension to hold the baby's head.
- Other cause includes direct injury to the wrist and inflammatory joint disease such as Rheumatoid arthritis (RA).

Sign and Symptoms:

- They complain of pain along the radial side of the wrist and the first dorsal compartment.

- On physical exam the pain can be reproduced by asking her to hold the thumb inside her closed fist, then forcing the wrist into ulnar deviation.

Treatment:

- Pain and inflammation are addressed by either anti-inflammatories or local injections of corticosteroids.
- The thumb and wrist are immobilized with a splint or brace for part of the day, and any motion that produces pain is eliminated while the area is healing.
- In severe cases, surgery is needed to release the tendons from the swollen sheath.

Ans: (c) APL and EPB

Ref: *Textbook of Orthopedics by John Ebnezar, 5th Edition, Page 401*

9. A patient presented 12 hours after fracture tibia is having PaO_2 of 60%. On rebreathing unit maintaining a saturation of 100%, but remains confused. Chest is clear. What is your diagnosis?

(a) Fat embolism syndrome
(b) Pulmonary contusion
(c) Atelectasis
(d) DVT

Explanation:

FAT EMBOLISM SYNDROME

- Fat embolism syndrome is synonym of Acute Respiratory Distress Syndrome.
- It's a post-traumatic stress disorder which occurs within 72 hours of skeletal trauma.
- After a long bone fracture the presence of fat globules which may be bone marrow fat or the platelet agglutination are sucked into the injured vessels and are transported to various sites as emboli giving rise to varied clinical manifestations.
- Most commonly occurs due to multiple fractures (10-45%).

MANAGEMENT

- **Nonspecific**
  - It includes: Keep airway to patient.
  - Don't mobilize the fracture (Keep immobilized by POP or external fixators).
  - Fluid resuscitation.
  - Careless handling of the injured (Avoid unnecessary transportation).
- **Specific**
  - Full-fledged ventilator support.
  - IV Steroids: It helps in gas exchange by decreasing inflammation in the lungs.
  - Low-molecular-weight heparin (LMWH).
  - Low molecular weight dextran.
  - Definitive fracture treatment.

Ans: (a) Fat embolism syndrome

Ref: *Textbook of Orthopedics by John Ebnezar, 4th Edition, Page 32*

PEDIATRICS

1. A term baby with birthweight of 2700 gms feeding exclusively on breast milk presented with jaundice on day 4 of life. Investigation showed total serum bilirubin of 14 mg/dl. What is the next line of management?

(a) Phototherapy
(b) Normal newborn care
(c) Exchange transfusion
(d) Stop breastfeeding

Explanation:

- Jaundice in breastfeeding term neonate weighing 2700 gm, on day 4 of life with a serum bilirubin of 14 mg/dl is **physiological**.
- This scenario doesn't need any intervention other than close monitoring for increasing severity.

Neonatal Jaundice:

- 60% of term and 80% of preterm neonates are clinically jaundiced in their neonatal period.
- While the physiological jaundice doesn't need intervention, pathological type needs immediate treatment.

Difference Between Physiological and Pathological Jaundice:

Physiological jaundice	Pathological jaundice
• Jaundice that first appears ***between 24-72 hours*** of age • Maximum intensity is seen on 4-5th day in term and 7th day in preterm neonates • Unconjugated Hyperbilirubinemia • Usually does ***not exceed 15 mg/dl*** • Clinically undetectable after 14 days • ***No treatment*** is required	• Clinical jaundice in ***first 24 hours of life*** • Total serum bilirubin (TSB) increasing by > 5 mg/dl/day or increasing at the rate of 0.5 mg/dl/hour • ***TSB >15 mg/dl*** • Conjugated serum bilirubin > 2 mg/dl • Clinical jaundice persisting for > 2 weeks in full term and > 3 weeks in preterm neonates

Causes of Jaundice

Jaundice appearing within 24 hours	Jaundice appearing after 24 hours
• Hemolytic disease of newborn: Rh, ABO and minor group incompatibility • Infections: Intrauterine viral, bacterial; malaria • G-6PD deficiency	• Extension of causes producing jaundice within 24 hours • Exaggerated physiological jaundice • Polycythemia • Concealed hemorrhages: Cephalhematoma • Sepsis • Neonatal hepatitis • Breast milk jaundice • Metabolic disorders

Clinical Assessment of Jaundice:

- **Jaundice is visible once the total serum bilirubin increase > 5 – 7 mg/dl.**
- ***Kramer's criteria*** – Used for clinical assessment of severity of jaundice in neonates not under phototherapy.

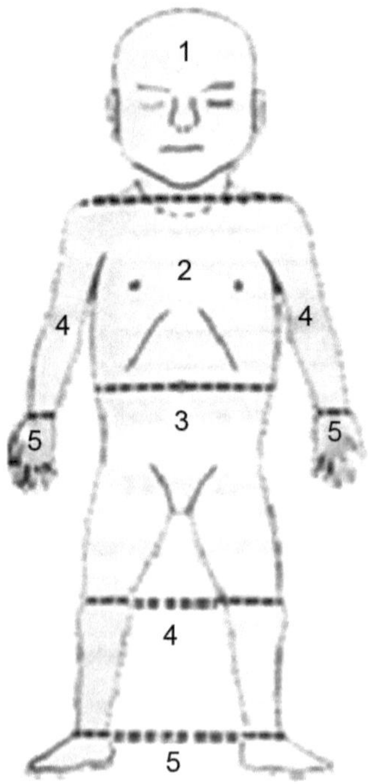

Grade	Extent of jaundice
0	None
1	Face and neck only
2	Chest and back
3	Abdomen below umbilicus to knees
4	Arms and legs below knees
5	Hands and feet

Management:

- **Goal** is to reduce the level of bilirubin so as to prevent its CNS toxicity by Phototherapy or Exchange transfusion.

Risk Factors for Severe Jaundice:

- Iso-immune hemolytic disease.
- G6PD deficiency asphyxia.
- Significant lethargy.
- Temperature instability.
- Sepsis.
- Acidosis.
- Serum albumin < 3.0 gm/dl.

Treatment Options:

Phototherapy	Exchange transfusion
Mechanism: • Light waves convert the bilirubin to water soluble nontoxic forms by ***photoisomerisation, structural isomerisation and photo oxidation***, which were excreted in stools. **Method:** • Exposure of the naked baby to blue, cool white or green light of wavelength 450-460 nm. • Eye / External genitalia should be covered. • Clinical assessment using ***Kramer's criteria is not possible*** as the babies skin will be bleached. Hence serum bilirubin must be used to monitor.	**Mechanism:** • Exchange transfusion ***removes partially hemolyzed and antibody-coated RBCs***, as well as unattached antibodies, and replaces them with donor RBCs, lacking the sensitizing antigen. **Indication:** • When phototherapy fails to prevent a rise in ***bilirubin to toxic levels*** (bilirubin level is rising > 1 mg/dl/hour despite phototherapy). • ***To stop hemolysis*** and bilirubin production by removing antibody and sensitized RBCs (bilirubin level is 20 mg/dl, or it appears that it will reach 20 mg/dl at the rate it is rising).

Contd.

Contd.

Complications: • Increased insensible water loss. • Loose stools. • Skin rashes. • ***Bronze baby syndrome***: In conjugated hyperbilirubinemia. • Hypo or hyperthermia: Monitor temperature frequently.	• ***To correct anemia*** and improve heart failure in hydropic infants with hemolytic disease (cord bilirubin level is >4.5 mg/dl and the cord hemoglobin level is under 11 g/dl). **Complications:** • Hypocalcemia / Hypomagnesemia / Hypoglycemia / Hyperkalemia / Sepsis.

EXTRA EDGE

Major Risk Factors for Developing Severe Jaundice in Neonates are:

- Jaundice observed in the 1st 24 hours of life.
- Blood group incompatibility with positive direct antiglobulin test.
- Elevated end-title CO concentration.
- Gestational age 35-36 weeks.
- Previous sibling received phototherapy.
- Cephalohematoma or significant bruising.
- Exclusive breastfeeding, particularly if nursing is not going well and weight loss is excessive.
- East Asian race.

Ans: (b) Normal newborn care

Ref: *Manual of Neonatal Care, John P Cloherty, 7th Edition, Page 304-31*

2. Two girls in the same class were diagnosed with meningococcal meningitis. Their 12-year-old close friend is in fear of contracting disease. What will you prescribe her?

(a) Two doses of polysaccharide meningococcal vaccines
(b) Single dose of polysaccharide meningococcal vaccines
(c) Chemoprophylaxis with chloramphenicol
(d) No vaccination is required as exposure has already occurred

Explanation:

Meningococcal Vaccine:

Vaccines against four specific antigens related to **sero types A, C, Y and W135** are currently available.

Vaccines against **sero type B** are still being evaluated.

- Two types of vaccines are in use:
  - Capsular polysaccharide vaccines; and
  - Conjugate vaccines.
- Only polysaccharides vaccines are licensed for use: (In our country)
  - Bivalent (A+C); and
  - Tetravalent forms (A+C+Y+W135).
- Vaccine contains 50 μg of each antigen.
- Dose of vaccine is **0.5 ml** given **subcutaneously** (deltoid region), in children > 2 years.
- Duration of immunity is 1-3 years.

Vaccination Recommended in High Risk Group:

Subjects with:

- Terminal complement component deficiency (C5-C9),
- Properdin deficiency; and
- Asplenemia/sickle cell disease.
- Vaccine for Haj Pilgrims.
- Certified vaccination status – not > 3 years and not < than 10 before arrival to Haj.
- Child > 2 years must be given one dose of quadrivalent vaccine (A+C+Y+W135).

Vaccine in Outbreak

- Polysaccharide vaccine:
  - (a) Single dose for children > 2 years.
  - (b) If children < 2 years need to be protected then 2 doses at 3 months interval is recommended during an outbreak.

Antimicrobial Chemoprophylaxis:

- Meningococcal prophylaxis should be implemented within 24 hours after contact.
- Secondary disease in contacts is highest immediately after the onset of disease in the index patient (as early as within 48 hours of diagnosis of index case).
- Close observation of this group of subjects is recommended for at least 10 days.
- Massive chemoprophylaxis is not recommended by any health authority during outbreaks.

Indication: **For close contacts**

Individuals who have had:

(a) Prolonged (>8 hours) contact while in close proximity (<3 feet) to the patient; or

(b) Directly exposed to the patient's oral secretions 7 days before the onset of the patient's symptoms.

(c) Until 24 hours after initiation of appropriate antibiotic therapy.

Close Contact:

- Household members living with a sick person.
- People who are in intimate contact with the patient.
- People sleeping in the same bedroom with the patient (students, soldiers, officers).
- People who have been in direct contact with secretions from the patient's respiratory tract during medical procedures, including mouth-to-mouth resuscitation, suctioning and endotracheal intubation, before or less than 24 hours after antimicrobial therapy was initiated.
- People travelling with the patient in the same plane, ship, bus or car for longer than 8 hours.

Invasive meningococcal disease with nasopharyngeal carriage, not treated with a 3rd generation cephalosporin should receive chemoprophylaxis for eradication of nasopharyngeal carriage prior to discharge from the hospital.

Drugs used:

Name	Dose	Route	Duration
Azithromycin	10 mg / kg	Oral	Single dose
Ceftriaxone	125 mg	Intra Muscular	Single dose
Rifampicin	10 mg / kg / dose, Q12H	Oral	2 days

EXTRA EDGE

- Mass chemoprophylaxis is **NOT** recommended routinely. Mass vaccination may be considered if the attack rate is > 10 cases per lakh population.

Ans: (b) Single dose of polysaccharide meningococcal vaccines

Ref: *Sachdeva A, Kukreja S, Jain V, Dutta AK, Meningococcal Disease–Outbreak in Delhi, Indian Pediatr 2005;42(6):547-556*

CD Alert – Monthly News of National Centre for Disease Control, DGHS, GOI – "Meningococcal Disease: Need to Remain Alert"

3. Maternal antibodies do not provide protective immunity to neonate from:

(a) Diphtheria (b) Pertussis

(c) Tetanus (d) Polio

Explanation:

*"Antibodies obtained in utero from mother protect against most childhood diseases, including **diphtheria, measles, tetanus** and **poliomyelitis**. In contrast, maternal antibodies against **whooping cough (pertussis)** are generally inadequate to protect the infant beyond 1 – 2 months." Medical Physiology, Boron WF, 2nd Edition*

Classically, pertussis is a prolonged disease, divided into catarrhal (1-2 weeks), paroxysmal (2-6 weeks), and convalescent stages (1-4 weeks).Clinical features of pertussis in infants <3 months of age do not display classical stages. Cough (expiratory grunt) may not be prominent. Whoop infrequently occurs in infants <3 months of age who at the end of a paroxysm lack stature or muscular strength to create sudden negative intrathoracic pressure. Cyanosis can follow a coughing paroxysm, or apnea can occur without a cough. Apnea may be the only symptom. The paroxysmal and convalescent stages in young infants are lengthy.

None of the other three options will present with recurrent apnea, bradycardia and cyanosis.

Pertussis (Whooping Cough)

- Caused by Bordetella pertussis.
- Has 3 clinical stages:
  - Catarrhal stages.
  - Paroxysmal stage.
  - Convalescent stage.
- The **catarrhal stage** (1-2 weeks) begins insidiously after an **incubation period ranging from 3-12 days** with nondistinctive symptoms of congestion and rhinorrhea variably accompanied by low-grade fever, sneezing, lacrimation and conjunctival suffusion.
- As initial symptoms wane, coughing marks the onset of the **paroxysmal stage** (2-6 weeks).
- The cough begins as a dry, intermittent, irritative hack and evolves into the inexorable paroxysms that are the hallmark of pertussis.
- ***Post-tussive emesis*** is common, and exhaustion is universal.
- The number and severity of paroxysms escalate over days to a week and remain at that plateau for days to weeks.
- At the peak of the paroxysmal stage, patients may have more than 1 episode hourly.
- As the paroxysmal stage fades into the **convalescent stage** (≥2 weeks), the number, severity and duration of episodes diminish.
- **Infants <3 months of age** do not display the classic stages.

- The catarrhal phase lasts only a few days or is unnoticed, and then, after the most insignificant startle from a draft, light, sound, sucking, or stretching, a well-appearing young infant begins to **choke, gasp, gag, and flail the extremities**, with face **reddened**.
- **Cough may not be prominent**, especially in the early phase.
- **Whoop** infrequently occurs in infants <3 months of age who at the end of a paroxysm lack stature or muscular strength to create sudden negative intrathoracic pressure.
- **Apnea** and **cyanosis** can follow a coughing paroxysm, or apnea can occur without a cough. Apnea may be the only symptom.
- **Apnea** and **cyanosis** both are more common with **pertussis** than with neonatal viral infections, including respiratory syncytial virus (**RSV**).
- The paroxysmal and convalescent stages in young infants are lengthy.
- Paradoxically, in infants, cough and whooping may become **louder** and **more classic** in **convalescence**.
- Convalescence includes intermittent paroxysmal coughing throughout the 1st year of life, including "exacerbations" with subsequent respiratory illnesses; these are not due to recurrent infection or reactivation of *B. pertussis*.
- **Adolescents** and previously immunized children have foreshortening of all stages of pertussis.
- Adults have **no distinct stages**.
- Classically, adolescents and adults describe a sudden feeling of **strangulation** followed by **uninterrupted coughs**, **feeling of suffocation**, bursting headache, diminished awareness, and then a gasping breath, usually without a whoop.
- **Post-tussive emesis** and intermittency of paroxysms separated by hours of well-being are specific clues to the diagnosis in adolescents and adults.
- At least 30% of older individuals with pertussis have nonspecific cough illness, distinguished only by duration, which is usually >21 days.
- Signs of lower respiratory tract disease are not expected unless complicating secondary bacterial pneumonia is present.
- **Conjunctival hemorrhages** and petechiae on the upper body are common.

DTwP VACCINE

- **Triple antigen** – **tetanus** and **diphtheria** toxoids as well as **killed whole cell pertussis bacilli** adsorbed on insoluble **aluminium salts** which act as adjuvants.
- Diphtheria toxoid varies from 20 to 30 Lf and that of tetanus toxoid varies from 5 to 25 Lf per dose.
- Stored at **2 to 8°C,** never be frozen, and if frozen accidentally, should be discarded 0.5 ml intramuscularly.
- **No/Minimal maternal antibody** for **protection** against **pertussis.**
- Three **primary doses** at **6, 10 and 14 weeks** and **two boosters** at **15-18 months** and **5 years**.
- Effectiveness against **diphtheria/tetanus** of **three doses** of the vaccine exceeds **95%.**
- Vaccine against **pertussis** is lower and as per data from international trials ranges from 70-90%.
- **Adverse effects (pertussis component):**
  - Fever more than 40.5°C.
  - Persistent crying.
  - Hypotonic hyporesponsive episodes.
  - Seizures.
  - Encephalopathy.
- No association with sudden infant death syndrome (SIDS), autism, chronic neurologic damage, infantile spasms, learning disorders and Reye's syndrome.

- **Absolute contraindications:**
  - History of **anaphylaxis;** or
  - Development of **encephalopathy within 7 days** following previous DTwP vaccination.
- **Relative contraindication:**
  - Progressive/evolving neurological illnesses.
- **Precautions but not contraindications:**
  - Persistent inconsolable crying of more than 3 hours duration.
  - Hyperpyrexia (fever > 40.50 C)/ HHE within 48 hours of DTwP administration; and
  - Seizures with or without fever within 72 hours of administration of DTwP.
- **Not recommended** in children **above 7 years.**

Ans: (b) Pertussis

Ref: *Nelson Textbook of Pediatrics, 21st Edition, Chapter 244*

4. A child presents with coarse facial features, hypercalcemia and cardiac findings/murmur, suggestive of Supravalvular aortic stenosis. Most likely diagnosis is:

(a) William's syndrome (b) DiGeorge syndrome
(c) Prader Willi syndrome (d) Angelman syndrome

Explanation:

- The abovementioned features are suggestive of **William's Syndrome.**
- The typical examples of **genomic imprinting** like **Prader-Willi syndrome** and **Angelman syndrome.**

Williams-Beuren Syndrome:

- Genetic defect; chromosome **7q11.23** (**elastin gene** deletion), sporadic.
- Associated congenital heart disease:
  - **Supravalvular aortic stenosis.**
  - **Peripheral pulmonic stenosis.**
- **Physical features:**
  - Microcephaly.
  - **Elfin facies** (full face, broad forehead, broad nasal bridge (anteverted nares), long upper lip and rounded cheeks).
  - Star-like (stellate) pattern in the iris.
  - Mental and growth retardation.
  - Hypoplastic nails.
  - Dental anomalies (partial anodontia, microdontia, enamel hypoplasia).
- **Other features:**
  - Idiopathic hypercalcemia.
  - Hypermobility of joint.
  - Excessive sensitivity to sound.
  - Precocious puberty.
  - Hypertension.

Diagnosis:

- Typical clinical features.
- Fluorescent in situ hybridization [FISH] – for deletion of one elastin gene on chromosome 7.

Treatment:

- No cure.
- Hypercalcemia – calcium and vitamin D restriction, steroids in severe hypercalcemia.
- **Surgical repair for cardiac defects.**
- **Endocrinology and developmental supportive care.**
- **Genetic counselling for the family.**

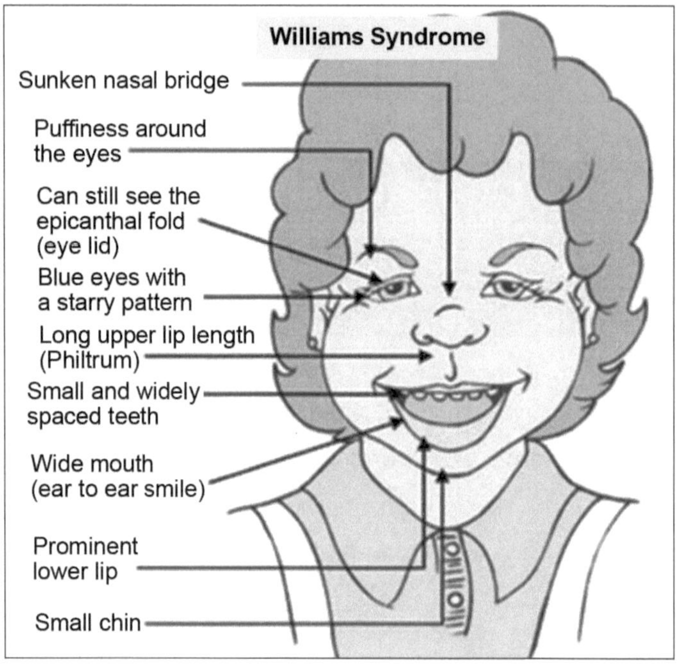

DiGeorge syndrome

- **Also known as 22q11.2 deletion syndrome and velocardiofacial syndrome.**
- Occurs in **both sexes.**
- **Microdeletions** from chromosome **22q11.2*.**
- Mutation of **T-box transcription family member**, ***TBX1,*** has been implicated as an etiology.
- Disorder of **T cell production***.
- **Basic pathology:**
  - **Dysmorphogenesis of 3rd and 4th pharyngeal pouches*.**
  - **Hypoplasia** of the **thymus** (**Recurrent infection**) and **parathyroid glands (Hypocalcemia**).
- **Associated anomalies:**
  - Right-sided aortic arch*.
  - **Esophageal atresia.**
  - **Bifid uvula***
  - Congenital heart disease (**conotruncal***, atrial and ventricular septal defects).
  - Cleft palate/a short philtrum of the upper lip.
  - Hypertelorism, antimongoloid slant, **mandibular hypoplasia,** and low-set, notched ears.

- **Complete DiGeorge syndrome:**
  - Aplasia of the thymus and parathyroid glands resemble **severe combined immunodeficiency (SCID*).**
  - **Associated with CHARGE syndrome** in 1/3rd patients (coloboma, heart defect, choanal atresia, growth or developmental retardation, genital hypoplasia, and ear anomalies including deafness).
- **Partial DiGeorge syndrome:**
  - Variable hypoplasia of the thymus and parathyroid glands.
- Concentrations of serum immunoglobulins are **normal***.
- **Absolute lymphocyte counts** are **low** for age. The CD3 T-cell counts are variably decreased in number.
- **Lymphocyte** responses to **mitogen** stimulation are **absent / reduced*.**
- **Treatment:**
  - Cultured unrelated thymic tissue transplants.

EXTRA EDGE

- **Maternal risk factors for cardiac anomalies in neonate:**
  - Family history of congenital heart disease.
  - Maternal metabolic disorders like (diabetes, phenyl ketonuira).
  - Maternal exposure to drugs (lithium, amphetamines, alcohol, anticonvulsant, isotretinoin).
  - SLE.
  - TORCH infections.

Ans: (a) William's syndrome

Ref: *Nelson Textbook of Pediatrics, 20th Edition, Page 2202*

5. Greenish-black thick stool in neonate was observed after delivery. Reason for this could be:

(a) Meconium
(b) Bile pigment like Biliverdin
(c) Bilirubin excretion
(d) Gut bacterial flora

Explanation:

- **Meconium** is **black-green** in colour, thick, viscous, sticky, odourless and acidic in nature **(pH 5.5 to 7.0).**
- The first passage of **meconium** occurs **within 48 hours** and first passage of **urine** occurs by **30 hours.**
- Green colour of meconium – due to **bile pigments** excreted by the biliary tract from the **12 weeks.**
- Primary bile acids are found more than secondary bile acids – due to absence of bacteria in meconium, this trend continue till 5th day of life.
- Meconium contains – water (72% - 80%), desquamated cells of the alimentary tract, bile, bile acids, pancreatic juices and swallowed materials such as lanugo hairs, vernix caseosa, amniotic fluid and blood.
- Protein content of meconium in less – 7% of dry weight (due to proteolytic activity of duodenal fluid).
- Protein content of the meconium is increased (upto 80%) in cystic fibrosis.
- Blood group substances are also present in meconium, 60 – 200 gm of meconium can be passed by a just born neonate.
- Among the minerals – sodium and zinc were found abundant in meconium.

Ans: (b) Bile pigment like Biliverdin

Ref: *Manual of Neonatal Care, John P Cloherty, 7th Edition, Page 106, 429, 811*

6. Meconium is passed:

(a) Soon after birth
(b) Within 12 hours of birth
(c) Within 24 hours of birth
(d) Within 48 hours of birth

Explanation:

- The first passage of **meconium** occurs **within 48 hours** and first passage of **urine** occurs by **30 hours.**

Causes of failure of passage of meconium:

- Imperforate anus.
- Microcolon.
- Mucous plug.
- Other causes of intestinal obstruction.

Causes of delayed passage of meconium:

- Hirshsprung's disease.
- Meconium ileus / Cystic fibrosis.
- Meconium plug syndrome.
- Hypothyroidism.
- Small left colon syndrome.

Causes of failure to develop transition stools after initial passage of meconium:

- Volvulus, other intestinal destruction.
- Malrotation.

EXTRA EDGE

- Dyselectrolemia causing failure to pass meconium – **Hypermagnesemia*.**
- 90% of infant with **meconium ileus** have – **cystic fibrosis*.**

Ans: (d) Within 48 hours of birth

Ref: *Manual of Neonatal Care, John P Cloherty, 7th Edition, Page 106*

7. A 5-year-old boy presents with complaints of prolonged fever for 7 days with palpable neck nodes. He also has bilateral watery eye discharge. Peelings of skin over palms are seen for the past 1 day along with macular rash over the trunk. What is the diagnosis?

(a) Dengue fever
(b) Rubella
(c) Scarlet fever
(d) Kawasaki disease

Explanation:

- Presence of fever for more than 5 days with features of **cervical lymphadenopathy, bilateral bulbar conjunctival injection, exanthema and peeling of skin** satisfies the criteria for the diagnosis of **Kawasaki's disease.**
- Though, the presence of **fever with rash and conjuctival suffusion** points towards **Dengue**, presence of lymphadenopathy and other features like peeling of skin are against dengue.
- The presence of skin peeling makes rubella less likely, even though fever, rash and lymphadenopathy can be seen.
- Scarlet fever, a common mimicker of Kawasaki Disease (KD), can usually be differentiated from KD by the swift clinical response to antibiotic in scarlet fever. Also, the appearance of ocular findings in scarlet fever is rare, while on KD it is common.

Difference Between Kawasaki's Disease and Scarlet Fever:

Features	Kawasaki's Disease	Scarlet Fever
Age group	Below 5 years	5 – 15 years
Etiology	Unknown	Streptococcus
Fever response to antipyretic	Donot respond	Responds
Lymphadenopathy	Painless	Tender
Rash onset	During the 1st week of illness	Within 24 – 48 hours
Rash type	Non-specific polymorphous	Blanching rash, fine papillae
Strawberry tongue	Present	Present
Treatment	Intravenous Immunoglobin, Aspirin	Antibiotics
Complications	Aneurysmal formation	Lead to Rheumatic fever or Glomerular nephritis

Kawasaki's Disease:

- Cause – unknown, may be related to infection (though not caused by).
- Now recently Kawasaki like illness associated with **COVID-19** – named as Multisystem Inflammatory Syndrome associated with COVID-19 (MIS-C).
- Common in winter season (male to female ratio 1.5:1).
- Occurs – young children < 5 years, with peak incidence of 1 – 2 years.

Pathology:

- Generalized **microvasculitis** occurs throughout the body, frequently **coronary arteries.**
- Less frequently involved arteries – iliac, femoral, axillary and renal arteries.
- **Coronary artery aneurysm** (proximal segment of the major coronary arteries) – may assume fusiform, saccular, cylindrical, or beads-on-a-string appearance.
- Aneurysm develops acute phase and persists for **1 to 3 weeks.**
- During the acute phase, there can be **pancarditis.**
  - Pericardium (pericardial effusion).
  - Myocardium (myocardial dysfunction, CHF); and
  - Endocardium (with aortic and mitral valve involvement).
- Late changes – Healing and fibrosis in the coronary arteries, with thrombus formation (elevated platelet adds to it) and stenosis leading to myocardial infarction (MI).

Clinical Features:

Acute Phase (first 10 days) – Fever persisting at least 5 days + presence 4 out of 5 the following:

No	Features	Description
1	Changes in extremities	**Acute**: Erythema of palms and soles; edema of hands and feet **Subacute:** Periungual peeling of fingers and toes in weeks 2 and 3
2	Exanthema	Polymorphous
3	Conjunctival injection	Bilateral bulbar without exudates
4	Changes in the lips and oral cavity	Erythema, lips cracking, strawberry tongue, diffuse injection of oral and pharyngeal mucosa
5	Cervical lymphadenopathy	(>1.5 cm in diameter), usually unilateral
Exclusion of other diseases with similar findings		
Measles, Scarlet fever, viral exanthems, drug reactions, juvenile rheumatoid arthritis and Rocky Mountain spotted fever		

Other Abnormalities:

- Signs of heart failure, LV dysfunction with cardiomegaly (myocarditis), Pericardial effusion and Mitral valve regurgitation murmur.

Other System Involvement:

- Arthritis or arthralgia.
- Sterile pyuria.
- Abdominal pain with diarrhea, liver dysfunction.
- Irritability, aseptic meningitis (25%) and sensory neuronal hearing loss.

Subacute Phase:

- Desquamation of the tips of the fingers and toes.
- Rash, fever and lymphadenopathy disappear.
- Cardiovascular changes – complicates (coronary aneurysm, pericardial effusion, Heart failure).
- Thrombocytosis – peaking at 2 weeks or more after the onset of the illness.

Convalescent Phase:

- Elevated ESR and platelet count return to normal.
- Beau's line appear in the finger and toe nails.

Laboratory Findings:

- Acute phase reactant (C-reactive protein [CRP] levels, erythrocyte sedimentation rate [ESR]) – elevated.
- Thrombocytosis (usually >450,000 /mm^3) occurs after day 7 of the illness.
- Pyuria (caused by urethritis).
- Liver enzymes are moderately elevated (more than two times the upper limit of normal).
- Elevated serum cardiac troponin I.

ECHO

During acute phase:

- Coronary arteritis – Perivascular brightness and ectasia (dilatation) (before aneurysm formation).
- Mild mitral valve regurgitation.
- Pericardial effusion.

After acute phase: (Aneurysm – left main coronary artery [LMCA], left anterior descending [LAD], left circumflex coronary artery [LCX] and right coronary artery [RCA]).

- Aneurysm and intraluminal or mural thrombi.
- Aneurysm > 8 mm – Giant aneurysm.

TREATMENT

Goal of Therapy:

- Reduction of inflammation within the coronary artery and myocardium – IV gamma globulin.
- Prevention of thrombosis by inhibition of platelet aggregation – aspirin.

Treatment of Choice:

High-dose (2 g/kg) as single infusion (given over 12-hour infusion) of IVIG.

with

Aspirin (80–100 mg/kg per day) given within 10 days.

Response:

- Fever abates within 24 - 48 hours.
- Repeat the dose if fever persists.

Precaution:

Defer live vaccine for 11 months after receiving high – dose IVIG.

Ans: (d) Kawasaki disease

Ref: *Nelson Textbook of Pediatrics, 20th Edition, Page 1209*

8. A 2-year-old boy presented with history of fever for 2 days. He developed oral lesion as shown in the image below. All of the following complications were anticipated in the acute phase of this disease, *except:*

(a) Pneumonia
(b) Acute otitis media
(c) Subacute sclerosing parencephalitis (SSPE)
(d) Diarrhea

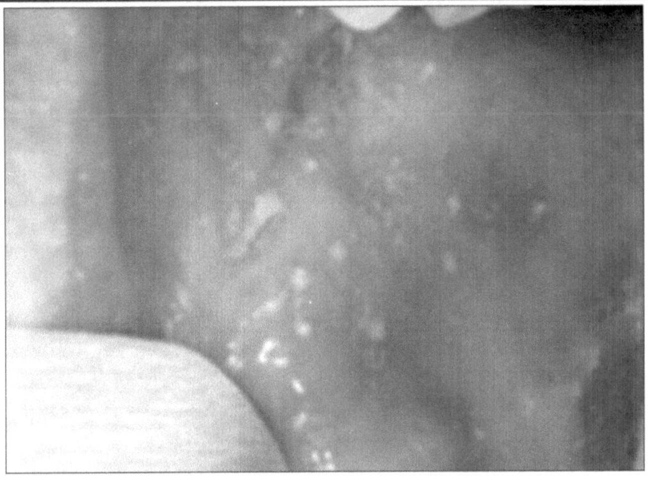

Explanation:

- The image shows tiny whitish grain like lesion with surrounding by red ring on the inner mucosa at the level of premolar suggests **koplik's spot.**
- These spots were pathognomonic of **measles**.
- All of the above mentioned complication (Pneumonia, Acute Otitis Media and Diarrhea) occurs during the measles infection except Subacute Sclerosing Parencephalitis (SSPE).

Measles (Rubeola)

- High fever, an enanthem, cough, coryza, conjunctivitis and a prominent exanthema.
- Caused by ***single-stranded lipid enveloped RNA virus*** of the genus Morbillivirus in the family Paramyxoviridae.
- ***Only one serotype*** is known.
- 6 major structural proteins – hemagglutinin (H) protein and the ***fusion (F) protein (important in inducing immunity***).
- Portal of entry – ***respiratory tract or conjunctivae*** in contact with virus suspended droplets.
- Virus is shed in nasopharyngeal secretions, blood and urine – ***3 days before the rash up to 4–6 days after its onset.***
- ***Face-to-face contact is not necessary*** – viable virus may be ***suspended in air up to 1 hour*** after a source case leaves a room.

- Virus remain viable for ***34 hours*** at room temperature.
- Mechanism of infection – attachment to ***the PVRL4 receptor (Nectin4)*** that is expressed on cells in the trachea, oral mucosa, nasopharynx and lungs.
- ***CD150 and PVRL4***, account for the lymphotropic and epitheliotropic nature of natural measles virus infection.

Pathology:

- Necrosis of the respiratory tract epithelium with lymphocytic infiltrate, small vessel vasculitis – skin and on the oral mucous membranes.
- Histology of the rash and exanthem – intracellular edema and dyskeratosis associated with formation of epidermal syncytial giant cells with up to 26 nuclei and lymphoid hyperplasia is prominent.
- Fusion of infected cells results in multinucleated giant cells, the ***Warthin-Finkeldey giant cells that are pathognomonic (up to 100 nuclei).***
- **Clinical Features:** Incubation period – 8 to 12 days.

Phase	Features
Incubation period	• Virus migrates to regional lymph nodes • Primary viremia – disseminates the virus to the reticuloendothelial system • Secondary viremia – spreads virus to body surfaces
Prodromal illness	• Begins with a mild fever followed by the onset of conjunctivitis with photophobia, coryza, a prominent cough and increasing fever • Features increase in intensity for 2–4 days until the 1st day of the rash
Exanthematous phase	• Enanthem, koplik spots (bluish white spots on the inner aspects of the cheeks at the level of the premolars) also in the lips, hard palate, gingiva, conjunctival folds and in the vaginal mucosa • Is the pathognomonic sign of measles and appears 1 to 4 days prior to the onset of the rash • Rash begins around the forehead (around the hairline), behind the ears, and on the upper neck as a red maculopapular eruption • Then spreads downward to the torso and extremities, reaching the palms and soles • Becomes confluent on the face and upper trunk • With the onset of the rash, symptoms begin to subside and the rash fades over about 7 days in the same progression as it evolved, often leaving a fine desquamation of skin in its wake • Virus shedding begins with onset of the rash
Recovery	• Cough lasts the longest, often up to 10 days • Generalized lymphadenopathy may be present, with cervical and occipital lymph nodes especially prominent

Inapparent Measles Infection:

- Rash may be indistinct, brief, or, rarely absent.
- Individuals with passively acquired antibody.
  - Infants, ***recipients of blood products, received vaccine.***
  - They ***do not shed measles virus and do not transmit infection to household contacts***.
- Recipient of formalin-inactivated measles vaccine - develop (**atypical measles** - severe form).
- Caused by the development of circulating immune complexes that formed due to an abnormal immune response to the vaccine.
- Onset of high fever, headache, maculopapular rash (petechial or purpuric) complicated by pneumonia and pleural effusions.

Hemorrhagic or "Black Measles":

- Hemorrhagic skin eruption and was often fatal.

- ***Keratitis and Thrombocytopenia*** are seen.

Diagnosis by Clinical and Epidemiologic Findings:

- Lab findings - ***Leukopenia***, Absolute neutropenia, normal erythrocyte sedimentation rate and C-reactive protein levels (in uncomplicated cases).
- Serologiccally - immunoglobulin M (IgM) antibody in serum. IgM (appears 1–2 days after the onset of the rash and remains detectable for about 1 month).
- By demonstration of a 4-fold rise in IgG antibodies in acute and convalescent specimens taken 2–4 weeks later.
- Viral isolation from blood, urine, or respiratory secretions can be accomplished by culture.

Complications:

- Due to pathogenic effects of the virus on the respiratory tract and immune system.
- Factors that make complications more likely.
  - Crowding – attributable to a larger inoculum dose following household exposure.
  - Severe malnutrition – suboptimal immune response.
  - Low serum retinol levels.
  - ***Common cause of death – Pneumonia.***
- **Respiratory Complication:**
  - ***Otitis media, pneumonia*** / Interstitial pneumonia – by the measles virus (***giant cell pneumonia***), superimposed bacterial infection **(S. pneumoniae, H. influenzae and S. aureus)**, ***laryngitis, tracheitis and bronchitis***.
  - May ***exacerbate underlying Mycobacterium tuberculosis*** infection.
  - Temporary ***loss of hypersensitivity reaction to tuberculin skin testing.***
- Gastrointestinal complications: ***Diarrhea***, vomiting and Appendicitis.
- Nervous system complication:
  - ***Febrile seizures.***
  - ***Encephalitis***: Greater numbers occurring in adolescents with unfavorable outcome.
  - ***Postinfectious*** immunologically mediated process rather than due to a direct effect by the virus.
  - Begins during the exanthem and presents with seizures, lethargy, coma and irritability.
  - In cerebrospinal fluid – lymphocytic pleocytosis and elevated protein concentration.
  - Majority suffer from long-term sequelae like mental retardation, motor disabilities and deafness.
- **Other Complications:** ***Myocarditis***, cellulitis and toxic shock syndrome, fetal wastage and stillbirths and congenital malformations.

Vitamin A in Measles:

- ***Hyporetinemia*** is present in more than 90% of cases of measles.
- There is an apparent inverse correlation between retinol concentration and measles severity.
- Treatment with oral vitamin A reduces morbidity and mortality in children with severe measles in the developing world.

Recommended regimen is a 2 doses, 24 hours apart:

1. ***100,000 IU orally for children 6 months to 1 year; and***
2. ***200,000 IU for children 1 year of age or older.***

EXTRA EDGE

Subacute Sclerosing Parencephalitis (SSPE)

- Fatal, delayed onset, neuro degenerative and chronic complication of measles (slow virus infection).
- Persistent infection with an altered measles virus that is harbored intracellularly in the CNS for several years.
- After 10 years the virus apparently regains virulence and attacks the cells in the CNS that offered the virus protection.

Clinical Features: After 10 years of primary infection.

- ***1st stage – Subtle changes*** (behavior or school performance, irritability, reduced attention span, or temper outbursts).
  - Fever, headache, or other signs of encephalitis are absent.
- ***2nd stage – Massive myoclonus*** (hallmark) begin in single muscle groups then massive spasms both axial and appendicular muscles.
  - ***Consciousness is maintained.***
- ***3rd stage*** – Involuntary movements are replaced by ***choreoathetosis***, immobility, dystonia and lead pipe rigidity.
  - Sensorium deteriorates into dementia, stupor, then coma.
- ***4th stage – Loss of critical centers*** that support breathing, heart rate and blood pressure.

Diagnosis:

- Documentation of a compatible clinical course and at least 1 of the following supporting findings:
  - ***Measles antibody detected in CSF (elevated IgG and IgM antibody titers*** in dilutions of >1:8).
  - Characteristic ***electroencephalographic findings (suppression-burst episodes)***; or
  - Typical histologic findings and/or isolation of virus or viral antigen in brain tissue obtained by biopsy or postmortem examination.

Management – Primarily supportive.

- ***Oral inosiplex and intraventricular interferon-α2b*** has been used with some benefit.
- Death usually occurs within 1–3 years of onset from infection or loss of autonomic control mechanisms.

Ans: (c) Subacute sclerosing parencephalitis (SSPE)

Ref: *Nelson Textbook of Pediatrics, 20th Edition, Page 1542*

9. Normal value of which of these parameter is specific in ruling out malnutrition:

(a) Total body water (b) Skin fold thickness

(c) Lean body mass (d) Body Mass Index

Explanation:

Body Mass Index (BMI) is used in diagnosis of malnutrition.

Malnutrition in Adults:

- Global consensus around core diagnostic criteria for malnutrition in adults in clinical settings:
- **5 ranked criteria includes:**
  - 3 phenotypic criteria:
    - Non-volitional weight loss.
    - Low body mass index.
    - Reduced muscle mass.

- 2 etiologic criteria:
  - Reduced food intake or assimilation.
  - Inflammation or disease burden.

Phenotypic Criteria			Etiologic Criteria	
Weight loss (%)	**Low body mass index (kg/m²)**	**Reduced muscle mass**	**Reduced food intake or assimilation**	**Inflammation**
>5% within past 6 months or >10% beyond 6 months	<20 if < 70 years or <22 if >70 years Asia: <18.5 if < 70 years or <20 if >70 years	Reduced by validated body composition measuring techniques	50% of ER > 1 week, or any reduction for >2 weeks, or any chronic GI condition that adversely impacts food assimilation or absorption	Acute disease/injury or chronic disease-related

ER – Energy Requirement, GI–Gastrointestinal.

To diagnose malnutrition at least one phenotypic criterion and one etiologic criterion should be present.

Ans: (d) Body Mass Index

Ref: *Cederholm T, Jensen GL, Correia MITD, Gonzalez MC, Fukushima R, Higashiguchi T, et al., GLIM Core Leadership Committee, GLIM Working Group. GLIM criteria for the diagnosis of malnutrition – A consensus report from the global clinical nutrition community, ClinNutr 2019;38:1e9*

10. All of the following were correct about fetal circulation, *except:*

(a) Ligamentum teres is the remnant of the umblical vein

(b) Functional closure of the ductus arteriosus occurs within 24 hours of life

(c) 3 shunts were present in the fetal circulation

(d) Lung expansion after the birth increases the Pulmonary Vascular Resistance (PVR)

Explanation:

- Lung expansion immediately after the birth decreases the Pulmonary Vascular Resistance (PVR) and thus closes the foramen ovale and ductus arteriosus.
- Ductus ateriosus, ductus venosus and foramen ovale are the 3 shunts present in the fetal circulation.

Fetal Circulation

- In fetal circulation, the right and left ventricles exist in a parallel circuit, whereas in children and adults, it is in series.
- Ductus venosus, foramen ovale, and ductus arteriosus are the important structures needed for maintaining this parallel circulation.
- Placenta provides gas and metabolites for exchange while the lungs do not provide gas exchange and vessels in the pulmonary circulation are constricted.

Fetal Circulatory Flow:

- Oxygenated blood from the placenta flows to the fetus through the umbilical vein (UV). Approximately 50% of UV blood enters the hepatic circulation while the rest bypasses liver and joins the inferior vena cava via the ductus venosus.
- This combined lower body plus umbilical venous blood flow enters the right atrium and is preferentially directed across the foramen ovale to the left atrium. The blood then flows into the left ventricle and is pumped into the ascending aorta.

- From fetal superior vena cava blood enters the right atrium and preferentially traverses the tricuspid valve, rather than the foramen ovale, and flows primarily to the right ventricle. From the right ventricle, the blood is ejected into the pulmonary artery.
- Since the pulmonary arterial circulation is vasoconstricted, only about 10% of right ventricular outflow enters the lungs. The major portion of this blood bypasses the lungs and flows through the ductus arteriosus into the descending aorta to perfuse the lower part of the fetal body, after which it returns to the placenta via the two umbilical arteries.

Oxygen Saturation (SPO_2) of Inferior Vena Cava	70%
Oxygen Saturation (SPO_2) of Superior Vena Cava	40%
Partial pressure of oxygen in Umbilical Vein	32 mm Hg (Highest)
Partial pressure of oxygen in Umbilical Artery	24 mm Hg
Partial pressure of oxygen Aorta	28 mm Hg
Partial pressure of oxygen Pulmonary artery	19 mm Hg

Circulatory Adjustments at Birth

- Removal of placenta
  - Increase in systemic vascular resistance (SVR) and closure of ductus venosus.
- Lung expansion results in:
  - Decrease in pulmonary vascular resistance (PVR).
  - Functional closure of foramen ovale.
  - Closure of Patent ductus arteriosus.

As a result of increase in SVR and decrease in PVR, there is reversal of shunt in ductus arteriosus from aorta to pulmonary artery, which was from pulmonary artery to aorta in fetal circulation.

PERINATAL CHANGES INFLUENCING LEFT TO RIGHT SHUNT

Before birth:

- Gas exchange in the fetus is primarily a placental function.
- Minimal pulmonary blood flow (PBF), higher pulmonary vascular resistance (PVR) and low systemic vascular resistance SVR (resistance in placental circuit is low) are characteristic.

After birth:

- Increase in **arterial PaO_2** decreases the PVR through arteriolar dilation but pulmonary artery pressure (PAP) remains elevated.
- Pulmoary smooth muscle regression and a postnatal increase in cross-sectional area of the pulmonary vascular bed allows progressive reduction in PVR over the initial 8–12 weeks and then till 4–5 years of age.
- Elimination of the low resistance placental circuit increases systemic vascular resistance (**SVR**) thereby promoting left-to-right shunting.
- Timing of changes in vascular resistances in the perinatal period dictates the onset of clinical symptoms. Hemodynamically significant left-to-right shunting starts at approximately 8–12 weeks.
- Size of defect is the primary determinant of the magnitude of shunting, larger defects allowing larger shunts leading on to earlier heart failure.

Structure	Functional closure	Structural closure	Remnant
Ductus venosus	Within minutes after birth	3 – 7 days	Ligamentum venosum
Ductus arteriosus	10 – 15 hours	Upto 3 weeks	Ligamentum arteriosum
Foramen ovale	3rd month of life	1 year of life	Fossa ovalis

EXTRA EDGE

FACTORS INFLUENCING THE CLOSURE OF DUCTUS

- **Oxygen and ductus arteriosus:**
  - Strongest stimulation for closure – Post natal increase in oxygen saturation in the ductus (from 25 to 500 mm of Hg due to lung expansion).
  - Responsiveness to oxygen induced closure is better in term than in preterm.
- **Prostaglandin E2 and closure:**
  - Decrease in PGE after birth result in ductal closure.
    - Removal of placental source of PGE.
    - Increased blood flow to the lung – effective removal of PGE in the lung.
  - Constriction effect of prostaglandin synthesis inhibitor (indomethacin, brufen, paracetamol) and dilator effect of PGE2 and PGI2 were greater in preterm than in term infant.

Ans: (d) Lung expansion after the birth increases the Pulmonary Vascular Resistance (PVR)

Ref: *Parks Cardiology for Practitioners, 5th Edition, Page 119 – 121*

11. Highest oxygen concentration in fetal circulation is in:

(a) Umbilical artery (b) Umbilical vein

(c) Pulmonary artery (d) Descending aorta

Explanation:

FOETAL CIRCULATION

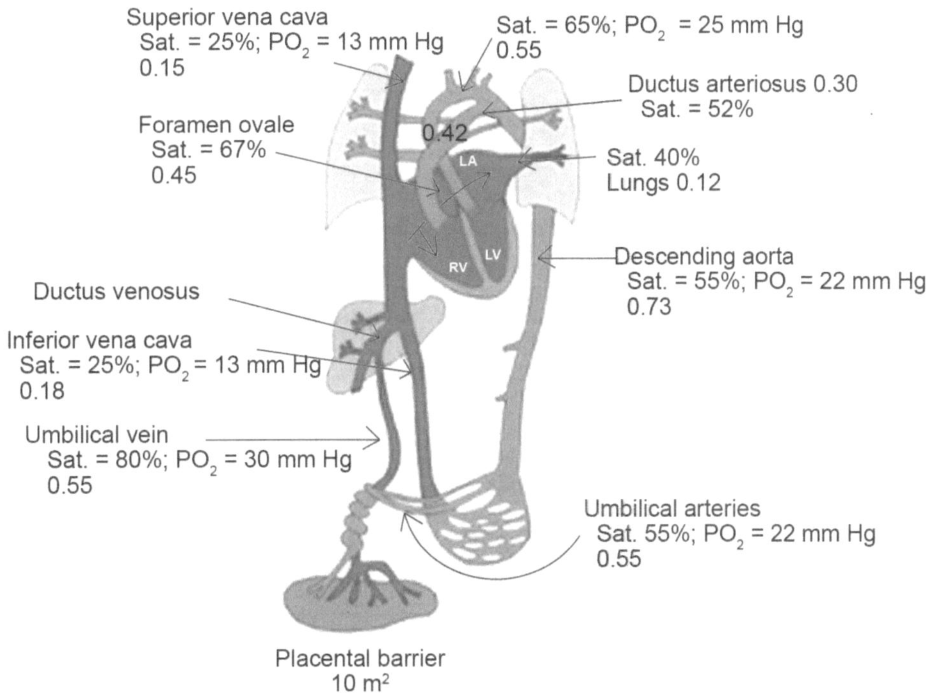

Ans: (b) Umbilical vein

Ref: *Parks Cardiology for Practitioners, 5th Edition, Page 119-121*

12. An 8-year-old boy presents with brown colored urine and oliguria for last 3 days. He has mild facial and pedal edema. His blood pressure is 126/90 mm of Hg. He has +3 proteinuria with 100 red cell and a few granular casts in urine examination. His creatinine is 0.9 mg/dl, urea is 56 mg/dl and C3 levels were reduced. He had skin infection before 2 weeks. What is the probable diagnosis?

(a) PSGN **(Post Streptococcal Glomerulonephritis)**

(b) Polyarteritis nodosa

(c) Good pasture syndrome

(d) Idiopathic rapidly progressive glomerular nephritis

Explanation:

The above clinical scenario is compatible with a diagnosis of **Post Streptococcal Glomerulonephritis (PSGN).** PSGN is quite likely in a child presenting with acute nephritic syndrome with a history of skin infection before 2 – 4 weeks.

In polyarteritis nodosa, Goodpasture syndrome and idiopathic rapidly progressive glomerular nephritis – serum ***complement levels will be normal***.

POST STREPTOCOCCAL GLOMERULONEPHRITIS (PSGN)

- **Second most common glomerular causes** of **gross hematuria** in children, **after IgA nephropathy***.
- It follows infection of the **throat (serotype 12**) or **skin (serotype 49**) by certain **"nephritogenic" strains of group A β-hemolytic streptococci.**
- Acute glomerulonephritis may also follow infection with **coagulase-positive and coagulase-negative staphylococci, Streptococcus pneumoniae and gram-negative bacteria*.**
- **Bacterial endocarditis** may produce a **hypocomplementemic glomerulonephritis** with **renal failure.**
- **Light microscopy findings:**
  - All glomeruli appear enlarged.
  - Relatively bloodless.
  - Diffuse mesangial cell proliferation.
  - Increase in mesangial matrix.
- **Immunofluorescence microscopy** reveals:
  - **'Lumpy-bumpy' deposits** of immunoglobulin and complement (GBM) and in the mesangium.
- **Electron microscopy:**
  - Electron-dense deposits, or "**humps**", seen on the **epithelial side** of GBM.

Clinical Features:

- Most common in children aged **5-12 years.**
- Presents with **acute nephritic syndrome (edema, hypertension and oliguria).**
- **1-2 weeks** after an antecedent **streptococcal pharyngitis** or **3-6 weeks** after a streptococcal **pyoderma.**
- Range from **asymptomatic microscopic hematuria** with normal renal function to **acute renal failure.**
- May develop **encephalopathy** and/or heart failure owing to hypertension or hypervolemia.
- The acute phase generally **resolves – 6-8 weeks.**
- Urinary protein excretion and hypertension usually **normalize – 4-6 weeks** after onset.
- Persistent microscopic hematuria may **persist – 1-2 years.**
- **Supportive Diagnosis.**
- Urinalysis shows **hematuria, RBC casts, proteinuria and polymorphonuclear leukocytes**.

- Normochromic anemia due to hemodilution and low-grade hemolysis.
- **Serum C3 level is reduced**.
- Confirmation of the diagnosis–clear evidence of invasive streptococcal infection (ALSO titer/Culture).
- The best single antibody titer to document **cutaneous streptococcal infection** is the deoxyribonuclease **(DNase) B antigen***.
- **The Streptozyme test** – detects antibodies to streptolysin O, DNase B, hyaluronidase, streptokinase and nicotinamide-adenine dinucleotidase using a slide agglutination test.

Complications:

- **Hypertension.**
- Heart failure.
- **Hyperkalemia*.**
- **Hyperphosphatemia*.**
- **Hypocalcemia*.**
- Acidosis.
- Seizures.
- Uremia.

Management:

- Treating the acute effects of renal insufficiency and hypertension (Sodium restriction, diuresis and pharmacotherapy with calcium channel antagonists, vasodilators, or angiotensin-converting enzyme inhibitors are standard therapies used to treat hypertension).
- Antibiotic therapy **does not affect** the natural history of glomerulonephritis.
- **Prognosis and Outcome:**
  - Complete recovery in >95% of children.
  - Glomerular hyalinization and chronic renal insufficiency.

EXTRA EDGE

Clinical features of acute glomerulonephritis	
Serum complement – low	**Serum complement – normal**
Renal diseases • Acute post-infectious GN (e.g., PSGN) • Membranoproliferative GN Type I	**Renal diseases** • IgA nephropathy • Idiopathic rapidly progressive (crescentic) GN • Postinfectious GN (non-streptococcal)
Systemic diseases • Lupus nephritis • Subacute bacterial endocarditis • Shunt nephritis • Essential mixed cryoglobulinemia	**Systemic diseases** • Polyarteritis nodosa • Hypersensitivity vasculitis • Henoch-Schönlein purpura • Goodpasture syndrome

Ans: (a) PSGN (Post Streptococcal Glomerulonephritis)

Ref: *Nelson Textbook of Paediatrics, 20th Edition, Page 2501*

13. A child presented with evisceration of bowel loops coming out of a defect in abdominal wall right to the umbilicus. The possible diagnosis is:

(a) Omphalocele (b) Umbilical hernia
(c) Gastroschisis (d) Patent urachus

Explanation:

Features	Omphalocele	Gastroschisis
Aetiology	Failure of the gut to return to abdomen	Vascular aetiology – ischemia in the right paraumbilical are leading to rupture of the abdominal wall
Gender	Frequent in females	Equal sex distribution
Family history	Present	Absent
Site of the defect	Central/umbilical	Paraumbilical/Right
Sac	Present (inner peritoneum and outer amnion)	Never
Herniated viscera	Bowel wall ± Liver / spleen / bladder	Bowel only
Umbilical cord	Inserted caudal to the hernia sac	No cord
Associated anomalies	Common (80%) – Cardiac / renal	Rare (10%)
Intestinal atresia	Less common	More frequent
Fluid resuscitation	Not needed	Needed
Surgical management	Not urgent	Urgent
Prognostic factor	Associated systemic anomalies	Condition of the bowel

- In umbilical hernia and patent urachus – evisceration of the bowel contents will be absent.

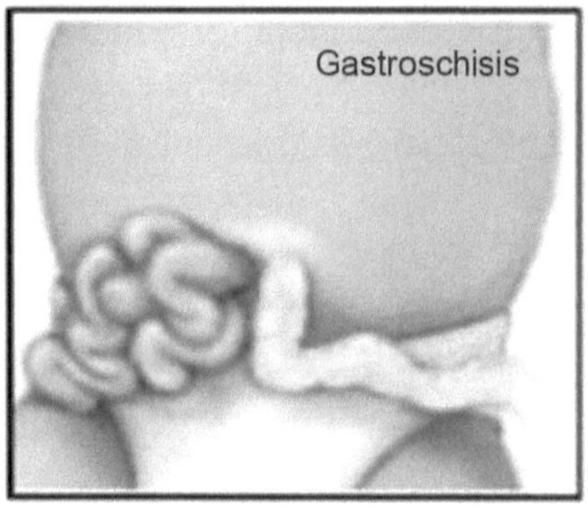

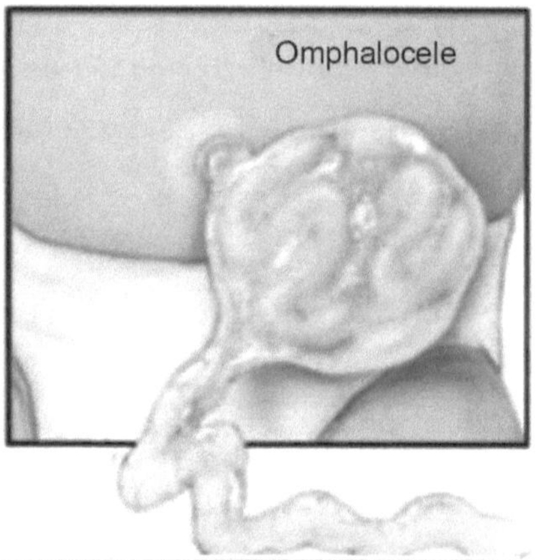

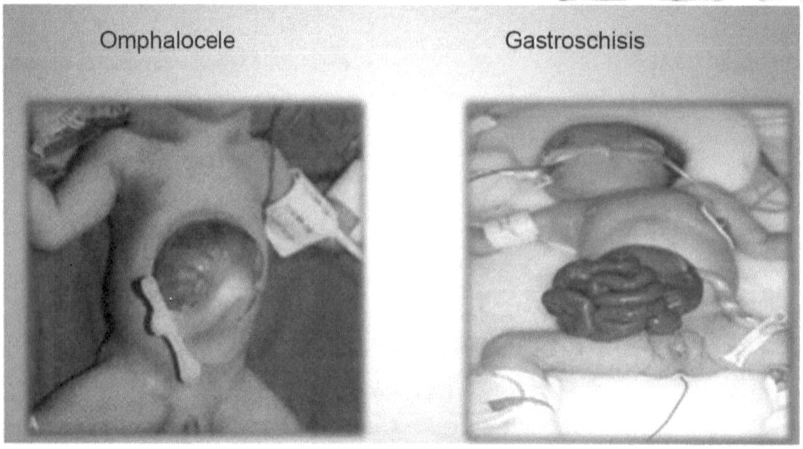

Ans: (c) Gastroschisis

Ref: *Manual of Neonatal Care, John P Cloherty, 7th Edition, Page 406-16*

14. Absence of dystrophin protein in muscle fiber causes:

(a) Duchenne muscular dystrophy
(b) Spinal muscular atrophy
(c) Myotonic dystrophy
(d) Tibialis myopathies

Explanation:

Duchenne Muscular Dystrophy (DMD):

- ***Most common hereditary neuromuscular disease*** / incidence 1 in 3,600 live born infant boys (***X-linked recessive trait***).
- Abnormal gene is at the ***Xp21.2 locus*** which encodes 427-kDa cytoskeletal protein (dystrophin).
- Common molecular defect is ***deletion***, followed by duplication and point mutation.
- Some female carrier, affected girls can have mild weakness (where the normal X chromosome becomes inactivated and the one with the gene deletion is active – ***Lyon Hypothesis***).
- ***Girls with Turner syndrome*** (single X chromosome have Xp21 gene deletion).
- Characteristic clinical features – progressive weakness, intellectual impairment, hypertrophy of the calves, and proliferation of connective tissue in muscle.
- ***Becker muscular dystrophy (BMD) similar to DMD, clinically milder.***

Clinical Features:

- ***Poor head control*** in infancy may be the first sign of weakness.
- Early gross motor skills – mildly delayed.
- At 1 year, walking is often accomplished.
- At 2 years, hip girdle weakness may be seen in subtle form.
- ***Toddlers assume alordotic posture*** when standing to compensate for gluteal weakness.
- At 3 years, early **Gowers' sign** is often evident and fully expressed by age 5 or 6 years.
- Classic features – enlargement of the calves (***pseudohypertrophy***) and wasting of thigh muscles.
- Pseudohypertrophy – enlargement is caused by hypertrophy of some muscle fibers, infiltration of muscle by fat, and proliferation of collagen.
- After the calves, ***tongue (no fasciculations)***, followed by muscles of the forearm.

Other Findings:

- ***Trendelenburg gait***, or hip waddle, frequent falling, toe walking, and trouble running or walking upstairs, developmental delay and ***malignant hyperthermia*** after anesthesia.
- Mostly confined to a wheelchair by 7 – 10 years of age.
- Ambulation – important for postponing the psychologic depression / scoliosis.
- ***Function of distal muscles / extraocular muscles – preserved.***
- ***Respiratory muscle involvement*** – weak and ineffective cough, frequent pulmonary infections and decreasing respiratory reserve.
- Smooth muscle dysfunction, particularly of the gastrointestinal tract, is a minor.
- Pharyngeal weakness – episodes of aspiration, nasal regurgitation of liquids, and an airy or nasal voice quality.
- ***Myalgias and muscle spasms do not occur***.
- Anal and urethral sphincter incontinence – very late event.
- Contractures – ankles (***ankle deep tendon reflexes preserved*** until terminal stages), knees, hips and elbows.

- Thoracic deformity further compromises – pulmonary capacity and compresses the heart.
- ***Intellectual impairment (in all patients) IQ <70***.
- Epilepsy, autism-like behavior – rare.

Cardiomyopathy

- Persistent tachycardia and myocardial failure.
- Severity of cardiac involvement / intellectually impairment, do not correlate with the degree of skeletal muscle weakness.

Death–18-20 years of age due to ***respiratory failure during sleep***, intractable heart failure, pneumonia, aspiration and airway obstruction.

In Becker Muscular Dystrophy:

- They remain ambulatory until late adolescence or early adult life.
- Calf pseudohypertrophy, cardiomyopathy, and elevated creatine kinase (CK) are similar to DMD.
- The ***onset of weakness is later in BMD than in DMD.***
- ***Death in BMD – late 20-40s.***

LAB FINDINGS

Serum Creatinine Kinase (CK) Level:

- ***Greatly elevated [15,000-35,000 IU/l*** (normal <160 IU/l)](presymptomatic stages and even at birth).
- Normal serum CK level – incompatible with the diagnosis of DMD (***except in terminal stages***).
- Some of the ***symptomatic carrier girls have elevated CK*** by 8 -12 years of age.
- ***Less specific elevation of aldolase and aspartate aminotransferase.***
- Cardiac assessment – echocardiography, electrocardiography (ECG) and radiography of the chest.
- Electromyography (EMG) – ***myopathic features*** without evidence of denervation.
- ***Nerve conduction velocities are normal.***

MRI (HEAD) – Cerebral atrophy appears late in the clinical course.

DIAGNOSIS

- ***Polymerase chain reaction (PCR) for the dystrophin gene mutation.***
- ***Immunohistochemical staining of frozen sections of muscle biopsy tissue.***
  - Common muscles sampled are the ***vastus lateralis (quadriceps femoris)*** and the gastrocnemius.
  - Changes include endomysial connective tissue proliferation, scattered degenerating and regenerating.
- Myofibers, foci of mononuclear inflammatory cell infiltrates and dense fibers.
- ***Dystrophin protein analysis on the muscle biopsy by western blot*** using fluorescent microscopy shows level of < 3% in DMD.
- ***Prenatal diagnosis at 12th week of gestation*** by sampling chorionic villi for DNA analysis by Southern blot or PCR.

TREATMENT

- No medical cure for this disease.
- Treatment to the complications and improving the quality of life of affected children.
- Cardiac decompensation – digoxin.
- Pulmonary infections prevented by immunizations for influenza virus and other bacterias.

- Good nutritional – adequate calcium / fluoride intake to minimise osteoporosis and prevention of obesity.
- Physiotherapy delays contractures.
- Avoid excessive exercise as this can accelerate the process of muscle fiber degeneration.
- External braces or corsets for scoliosis.

Another Recommended Treatment:

- Steroids like prednisone, **prednisolone, deflazacort.**
  - **Glucocorticoids** – decrease the rate of apoptosis and can decelerate the myofiber necrosis.
  - **Dexamethasone** or **triamcinolone** – avoided as they may induce **myopathy.**
- Injection of **antisense oligonucleotide drugs:**
  - Induce exon skipping during mRNA splicing in patients with susceptible mutations like **Drisapersen** and **eteplirsen.**

Ans: (a) Duchenne muscular dystrophy

Ref: *Nelson Textbook of Paediatrics, 20th Edition, Page 2967*

15. In a preterm baby with respiratory distress syndrome, which of the following lipid would be deficient?

(a) Sphingomyelin (b) Cardiolipin
(c) Dipalmitoylphosphatidyl choline (d) None of the above

Explanation:

- **Respiratory Distress Syndrome** in preterm are due to the deficiency of **surfactant**. The pulmonary surfactant is a complex mixture of **phospholipids** (mainly **dipalmitoylphosphatidylcholine**) and proteins (A, B, C and D) with neutral lipids and cholesterol.
- **Cardiolipin** (Culcutta antigen) is a component of the inner mitochondrial membrane and plays an important role in mitochondrial enzyme metabolism.
- **Sphingomyelin** are phosphosphingolipids present in increased concentration in nervous tissue, red blood cells and ocular lenses.

Respiratory Distress Syndrome (RDS) / Hyaline Membrane Disease (HMD)

Respiratory distress syndrome occurs primarily in premature infants.

- Risk for RDS increases
  - Maternal diabetes / previously affected infants.
  - Multiple births.
  - Cesarean delivery.
  - Precipitous delivery.
  - Asphyxia.
- Risk for RDS reduced
  - Pregnancy-associated hypertension.
  - Maternal heroin use.
  - Prolonged rupture of membranes.
  - Antenatal corticosteroid prophylaxis.

Etiology:

- Primary cause – **Surfactant deficiency.**

- Surfactant – Synthesized and stored in **Type II alveolar cells.**
- Constituents of surfactant – **dipalmitoyl phosphatidylcholine** (**lecithin**), **phosphatidyl glycerol**, **apoproteins** (surfactant proteins **SP-A, SP-B, SP-C and SP-D**) and **cholesterol**.
- Surfactant – reduces the surface tension and prevents collapse of small air spaces at end-expiration.
- Mature levels of pulmonary surfactant are present usually after **35 weeks** of gestation.
- Levels of surfactant present in immature preterm neonate were not sufficient to meet the postnatal demand.
- Alveolar atelectasis, hyaline membrane formation, and interstitial edema make the lungs less compliant in RDS.
- The chest wall of the preterm infant is more complaint and thus offers less resistance to collapse.

Pathology:

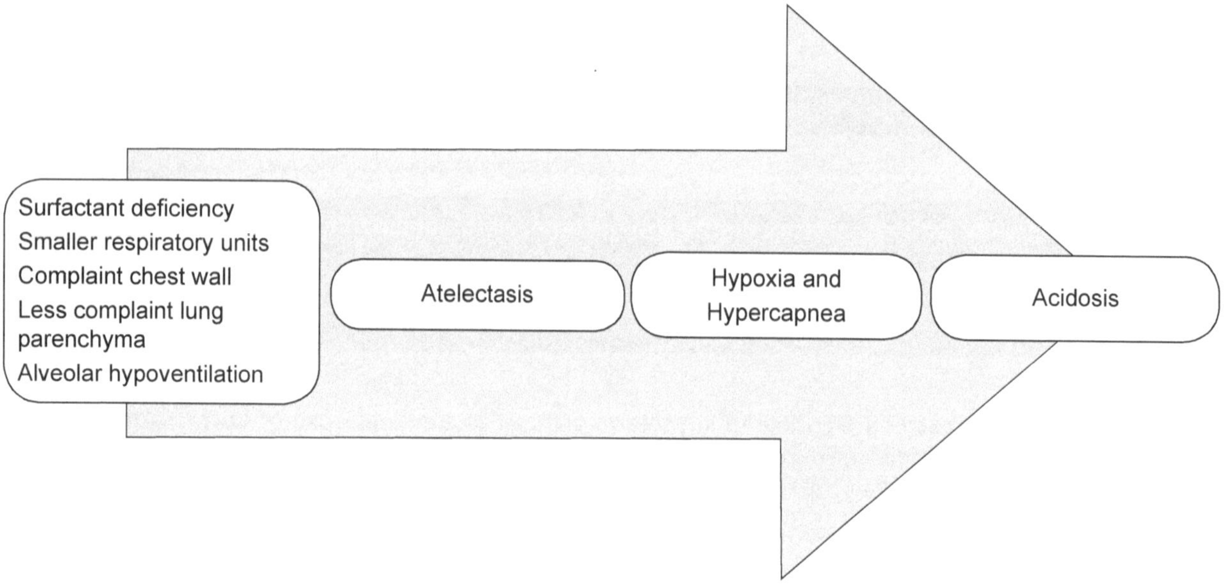

Clinical Features:

- Respiratory distress (characterized by tachypnea, prominent (often audible) grunting, intercostals and subcostal retractions, nasal flaring and cyanosis) usually develops within minutes after birth in preterm babies.
- If left untreated the dyspnea and cyanosis worsens and grunting decreases or disappears.
- These features reaches peak in 3 days (marked by spontaneous diuresis) then improves gradually.
- Death may be due to pulmonary hemorrhage, alveolar air leaks and severe respiratory acidosis.
- Some turn into chronic form of lung disease named **Bronchopulmonary Dysplasia (BPD).**

LABORATORY FINDINGS

Characteristic X-ray (Chest) Findings:

- **Fine reticular granularity** of the parenchyma and **air bronchogram.**
- **Small volume** and **white out lung** in severe disease.
- Other differential diagnosis based on X-ray findings – pneumonia, total anomalous pulmonary return, Meconium aspiration syndrome.

Arterial Blood Gas:

- Hypoxemia, hypercapnia, respiratory acidosis and variable metabolic acidosis.

PRENATAL PREDICTION: ASSESSMENT OF FETAL LUNG MATURITY

- **Lecithin / sphingomyelin (LIS) ratio – using chromatography**
  - If ratio is >2 – risk of RDS is very low.
- **TDx-FLM II** – Measures the surfactant to albumin ratio using fluorescent polarization technology.
  - Value of >55 mg surfactant/g albumin correlates with lung maturity.
- **Lamellar bodies count in amniotic fluid**
  - >50,000 lamellar body (pack of phospholipids produced by the Type II alveolar cells)/microliter predicts good lung maturity.
- **Phosphatidyl Glycerol Assay.**
- **Foam Stability Test:** Formation stable foam when the amniotic fluid is shaken with ethanol predicts lung maturity.

PREVENTIVE MEASURES

- **Indication:**
  - Pregnant mother of **24 – 34 weeks**, with intact membranes or preterm rupture of membranes without chorioaminitis, with at risk of preterm delivery in the next 7 days.
- **Contraindication:** Chorioamnionitis.
- **Action:** Induces production of surfactant and maturation of lung and other tissues.
- **Prevention:**
  - Respiratory Distress Syndrome.
  - Necrotising Enterocolitis.
  - Intraventricular Hemorrhage.
  - Perinatal mortality.
- **Drug and dose:**
  - **2 doses** of **betamethasone** (**12 mg IM**) separated by a **24-hour** interval.

    OR

  - **4 doses** of **dexamethasone** (**6 mg IM**) at **12-hour** intervals.

TREATMENT

- **Oxygen:**
  - To meet the target saturation of (88% to 92% for preterm < 30 weeks gestation and 88% to 95% for preterm > 30 weeks gestation).
- **Bubble – Continuous Positive Airway Pressure (CPAP) Therapy:**
  - Start at a pressure of 5 to 7 cm of H_2O, at flow rate of (5-10 l / minute), change pressure in increments of 1 to 2 cm of H_2O to a maximum of 8 cm of H_2O.
- **Surfactant Replacement Therapy:**
  - INSURE (Intubate, SURfactant replacement and Extubate) techniques.
  - Based on the timing of administration.
  - **Prophylactic** – within 15 minutes, before the appearance of respiratory distress (<32 weeks).
  - **Early rescue** – within 2 hours after the appearance of respiratory distress, within development of obvious RDS.
  - **Late Rescue** – after 2 hours of appearance if respiratory distress, after the development of obvious RDS.
  - The dose can be repeated after 6-8 hours for 2-4 times.

Complication: Bradycardia, apnea, single lung drug administration, pulmonary hemorrhage.

- **Mechanical Ventilation:**

  Indication:

  - Respiratory acidosis with a $PaCO_2$ >55 mm Hg or rapidly rising, a PaO_2 < 50 mm Hg; or
  - Oxygen saturation <90% with an FiO_2 above 0.50; or
  - Severe apnea.

  Complication:

  - Airleak syndrome.
  - Sepsis.
  - Intracranial hemorrhage.
  - Patent Ductus Arteriosus – non closure.

Ans: (c) Dipalmitoylphosphatidyl choline

Ref: *Manual of Neonatal Care, John P Cloherty, 7th Edition, Page 406-16 and Nelson Textbook of Pediatrics, 20th Edition, Page 850-58*

16. Which of the following cells are deficient in a premature infant with RDS?

(a) Alveolar capillary endothelial cells
(b) Type I alveolar cells
(c) Type II alveolar cells
(d) Alveolar macrophages

Explanation:

- **Alveolar capillary endothelial cells** – lines the surface of the vasculature and maintains hemostasis by preventing the coagulation of blood.
- **Type I alveolar cells** – is a component of air – blood barriers and are involved in the process of **gas exchange** between alveoli and blood.
- **Type II alveolar cells** – in the alveolar wall contain secretory organelles known as **lamellar bodies** that fuse with the cell membranes and secrete **pulmonary surfactant**.
- **Alveolar macrophages** – part of the innate immune system, clears the air space from the infectious, toxic and allergic particle and in addition they secrete interleukin 4 and 10 to check on uncontrolled inflammation.

Ans: (c) Type II alveolar cells

Ref: *Manual of Neonatal Care, John P Cloherty, 7th Edition, Page 406-16*

DERMATOLOGY

1. A 42-year-old female presents with a facial lesion as shown in the picture. Which of the following would be the ideal management for this condition?

(a) Topical retinoids
(b) Oral steroids
(c) Start on ATT
(d) Start on MDT for leprosy

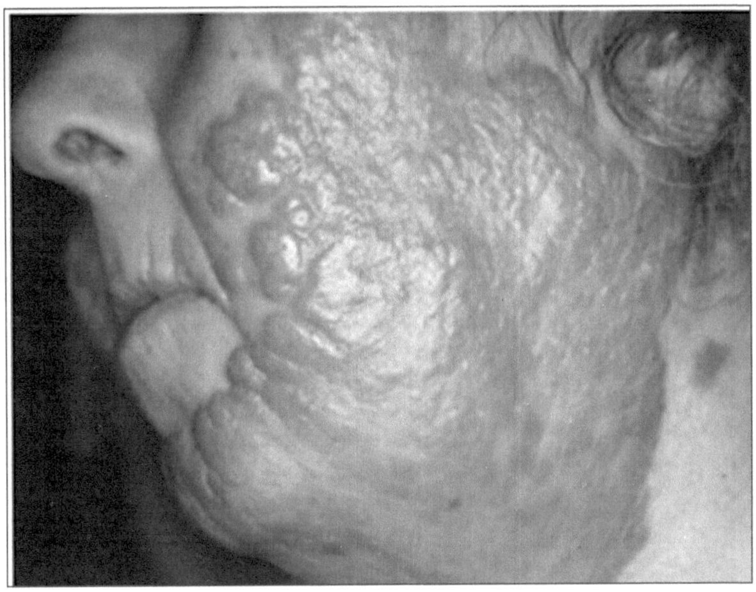

Explanation:

- The picture shows reddish brown plaque over face which is suggestive of **lupus vulgaris** (a form of **cutaneous TB**).

Types of Cutaneous TB:

- Lupus vulgaris.
- Scrofuloderma.
- Orificial tuberculosis.
- Acute military cutaneous tuberculosis.
- Tuberculous gumma (abscess).
- Tuberculosis verrucosa cutis.
- Tuberculids.
- Tuberculous chancre.

Lupus Vulgaris:

- It presents as **soft reddish brown papules** and **plaques**. The advancing edge shows infiltrated plaques resulting in **trailing central scarring**.
- **Most common site: Head and neck** in **Europe**; **buttocks** in **India.**
- **Types:** Plaque, Ulcerative, tumor-like, vegetating form and papulonodular forms.
- **Investigations:** Mantoux-usually positive, ***Diascopy–Apple jelly nodules*** in the periphery, Histopathology–Well defined epithelioid granuloma in dermis. Acid fast stain – Usually negative.
- **Treatment: ATT.**
- **Complications:** Scarring and contractures. Squamous cell carcinoma in long standing cases.

Scrofuloderma:

- It presents as **bluish or erythematous nodules** overlying **lymph nodes**, bones or joints which breaks to forms **skin ulcers** with undermining **edge.**

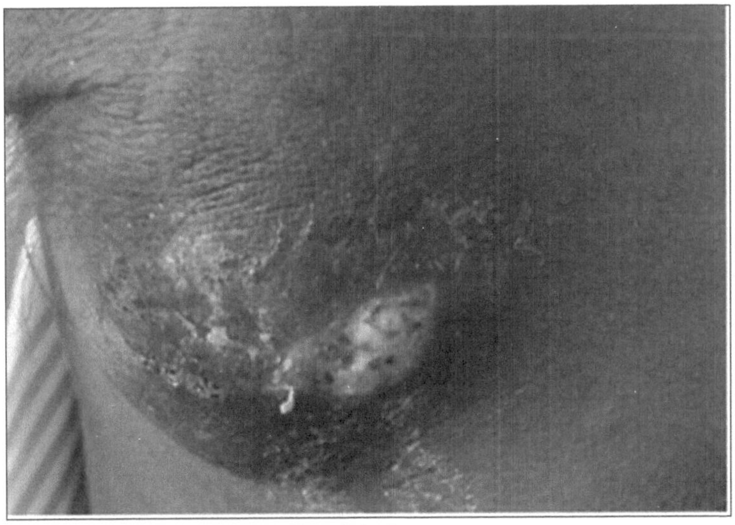

Scrofuloderma

Type 1 Lepra Reaction

- It presents as **erythema, edema** over **Hansen patches** associated with **tenderness** and **neuritis.**

Ans: (c) Start on ATT

Ref: *Rook's Textbook of Dermatology, 9th Edition, Page 27.6*

2. Examine the below picture carefully. Identify the condition shown in this image:

(a) SLE (b) DLE

(c) Rosacea (d) Vitiligo

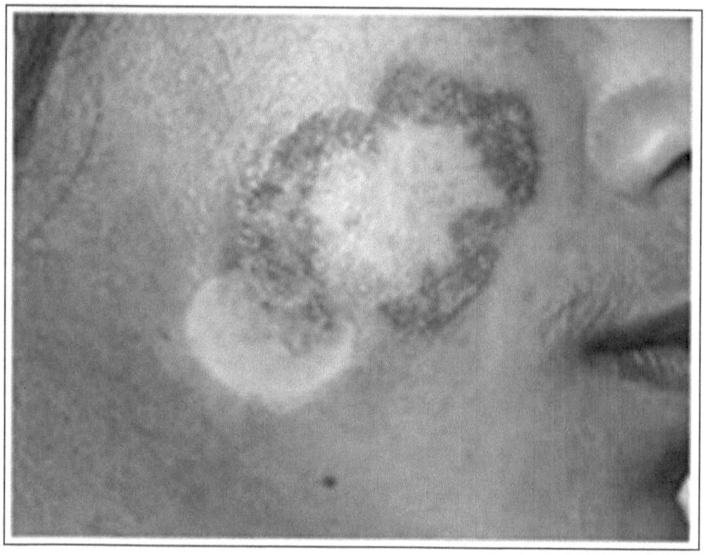

Explanation:

Classification of Cutaneous LE

- Acute.
- Subacute.
- Chronic cutaneous LE.

DLE (Discoid Lupus Erythematosus)

- It is a **chronic cutaneous LE lesion**.
- Most common form of cutaneous LE.
- It presents as erythematous to depigmented discoid plaque with adherent scaling usually occurring over face, scalp, 'V' area of chest.
- **Treatment:**
  - Photoprotection and sunscreens.
  - Topical steroid.
  - Topical tacrolimus.
  - Oral steroids.
  - Oral hydroxychloroquine.

Systemic Lupus International Collaborating Clinics Classification Criteria (SLICC) for Systemic Lupus Erythematosus (SLE), 2012

Clinical Criteria

- Malar rash.
- Discoid rash – depigmented plaque with adherent scaling [***cat tongue or tin tack or carpet tack sign*** – when scaling is removed from a DLE lesion the under surface shows horny plugs similar to carpet tack].
- Oral ulcers or nasal ulcers.
- **Non-scarring alopecia.**
- Synovitis.
- **Serositis:** Pleurisy or pericarditis.
- **Renal disorder:** Persistent proteinuria (> 500 mg/day) or cellular casts.
- Neurological disorder, seizures, psychosis.
- Hemolytic anemia
- Leukopenia (< 4000/mm^3 at least once) or lymphopenia (<1000/mm^3).
- Thrombocytopenia (<100000/mm^3 at least once).

Immunological Criteria

- ANA above reference laboratory range.
- Anti-dsDNA antibody above reference laboratory range.
- Anti-Sm: Presence of antibody to Sm nuclear antigen.
- Antiphospholipid antibody positivity.
- Low complement.
- Direct Coombs' test in the absence of hemolytic anemia.

*A patient is classified as **SLE** if **four** of **clinical** and **immunological** criteria, including **at least** one **clinical** criteria.*

Rosacea:

- Usually presents as episodic flushing, papules and pustules over face.
- **Types:**
  - Papulopustular.
  - Erythematotelangiectatic.
  - Phymatous.
  - Ocular.
- **Treatment:**
  - Photoprotection and sunscreens.
  - Metronidazole gel, oral doxycycline for papulopustular lesions.
  - Topical brimonidine and vascular lasers (PDL) for telangiectatic lesions.
  - Electrosurgery, ablative CO_2 laser for rhinophyma.

Vitiligo

- Presents as hypopigmented to depigmented milky white macules.
- **Types:** Segmental and non-segmental.
- Non-segmental: Vitiligo vulgaris, Acrofacial vitiligo, Lip tip vitiligo, Universal vitiligo.
- ***Trichrome sign:***

  Between normal skin and depigmented macules there is tan color intermediate zone.
- Quadrichrome: Presence of dark brown perifollicular repigmentation in addition.
- Pentachrome: Presence of depigmentation, tan color, brown, blue-grey hyperpigmented and normal skin.
- ***Koebner's phenomenon.***
- **Treatment:** Topical steroids, Topical calcineurin inhibitors, NBUVB phototherapy, PUVA therapy.

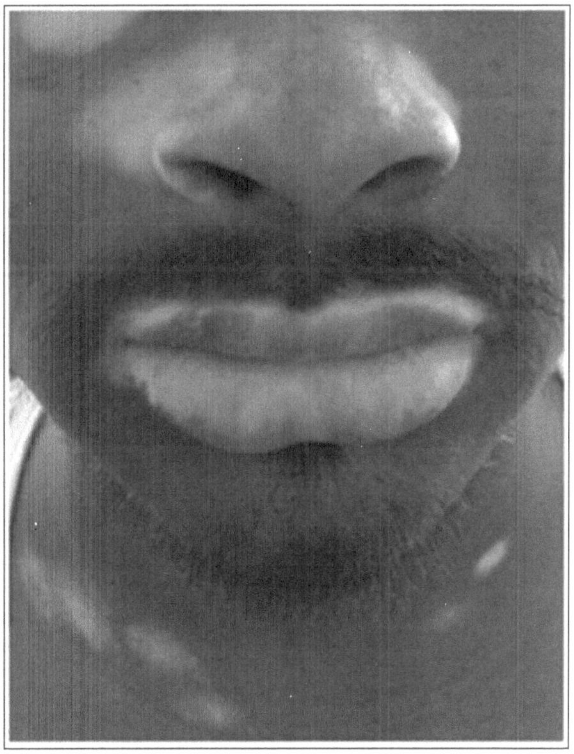

Vitiligo

Ans: (b) DLE

Ref: *Fitzpatrick's Dermatology in General Medicine, Page 1910; Rook's Textbook of Dermatology, 9th Edition, Page 88, 39*

3. A 32-year-old woman presented with these lesions shown in picture. Identify this phenomenon:

(a) Isomorphic phenomenon (b) Reverse isomorphic

(c) Gottron's papule (d) Nikolsky sign

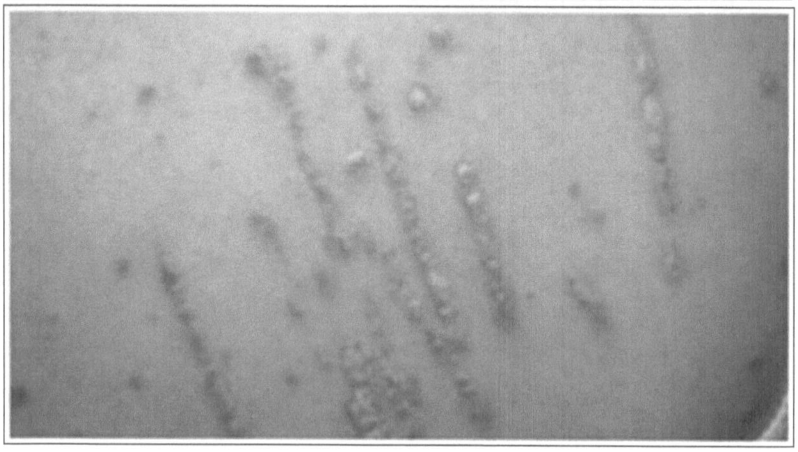

Explanation:

Isomorphic Phenomenon or Koebner Phenomenon:

- The development of morphologically similar lesions following trauma to uninvolved skin.
- Seen in ***psoriasis, lichen planus, vitiligo***.

Reverse Isomorphic or Koebner Phenomenon:

- The clearance of skin lesions following trauma to lesional skin.
- Seen in ***psoriasis, granuloma annulare.***

Gottron's Papule:

- They are pathognomic skin lesion in ***dermatomyositis.***
- Presents as flat topped violaceous papules over interphalangeal region, knuckles, elbows, knees.
- **Gottron's sign:** Confluent violaceous macules over elbows and knees.

Nikolsky Sign:

- Seen in **pemphigus vulgaris, pemphigus foliaceous.**
- Peeling of skin followed by application of tangential pressure over normal appearing skin near blisters.

Ans: (a) Isomorphic phenomenon

Ref: *DM Thappa's Essentials in Dermatology, 2nd Edition, Page 26*

4. Identify the lesion associated with scaling and itching:

(a) Granuloma annulare (b) Pyoderma gangrenosum

(c) Ichthyosis vulgaris (d) Tinea corporis

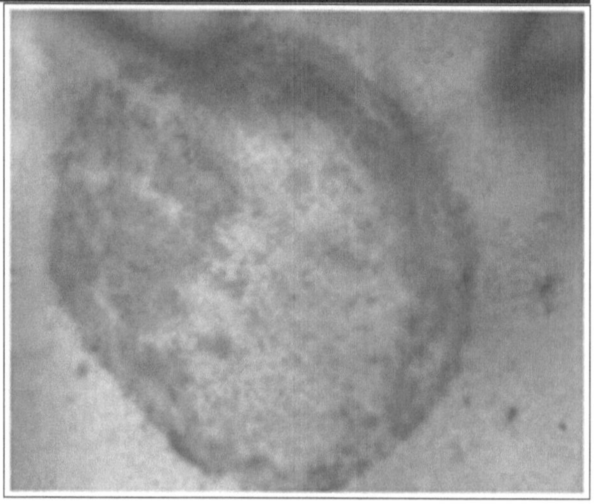

Explanation:

TINEA

Etiology:

- **Microsporum** – affects **Hair, Skin.**
- **Trichophyton** – affects **Hair, Skin, Nails.**
- **Epidermophyton** – affects **Skin, Nails.**

Tinea Corporis:

- It presents as itchy well defined annular plaques with peripheral papulopustules, scaling and central clearing.

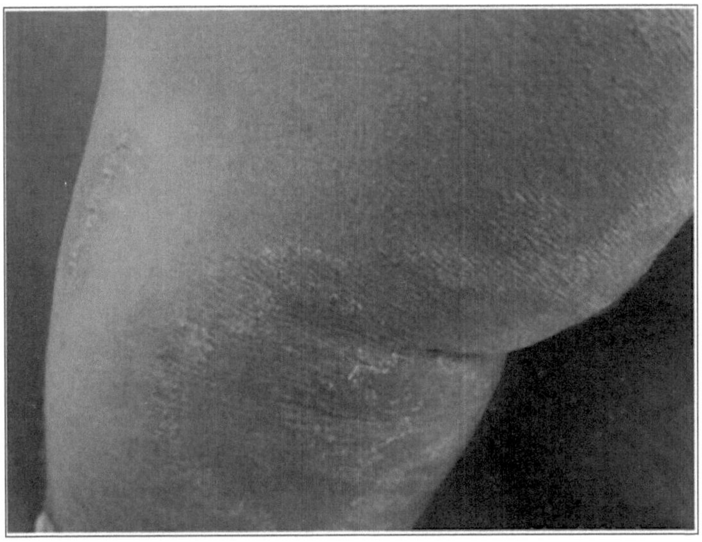

- Caused by dermatophytes (***T. rubrum*** is the most common organism).
- **Variants**:
  - ***Tinea imbricata*** – Caused by ***Trichophyton concentricum*** presenting as large concentric ring lesion.
  - **Majocchis granuloma** – Perifollicular granulomatous nodules.
- KOH smear–*branched septate hyphae.*
- **Treatment:** Oral terbinafine, itraconazole and griseofulvin.
- **Topicals:** Clotrimazole, terbinafine, eberconazole, luliconazole, sertaonazole.

  Depending on sites:
  - Tinea cruris (Dhobi's /Jock's itch) – groin.
  - Tinea facei – face.
  - Tinea barbae – beard.
  - Tinea pedis–Athlete's feet.
  - Tinea mannum–hands.
  - Tinea capitis – scalp.

Tinea Capitis:

- ***T. violaceum:*** Most common organism in India.
- Patchy hair loss, scaling, easy pluckability of hair, ***Exclamation mark hair*** are typical findings.
- **Types:** Black dot, grey patch and seborrheic dermatitis like presentation.
- **Endothrix:** Arthroconida within hair shaft (most commonly seen).

  Ectothrix: Arthroconidia outside hair shaft.
- **Kerion:** Presents as inflammatory pustules and *boggy swelling.*

  Caused by ***T. verrucosum and mentagrophyte.***
- **Favus:** Presents as scutulae (sulphur yellow crust) over scalp caused by ***T. schonlenii*** seen usually in Kashmir.

Granuloma Annulare:

- It usually presents as asymptomatic annular reddish papules and plaques with central clearing with dorsa of hands, feet and fingers being the more common sites.

Pyoderma Gangrenosum:

- It presents as painful ulcers with bluish edge.
- Can be associated with inflammatory bowel disease, arthritis, hematological dyscrasias.
- Treatment: Oral steroids, cyclosporine.

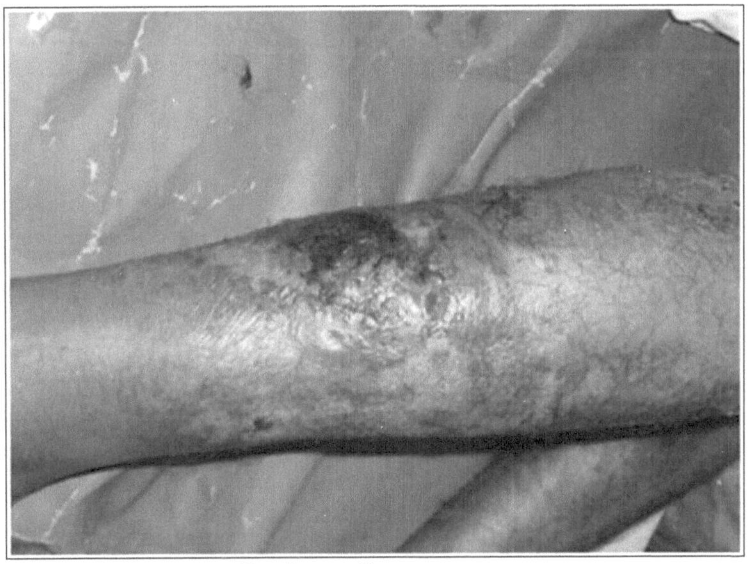

Pyoderma Gangrenosum

- The following picture shows ulcer in leg with violaceous margin.

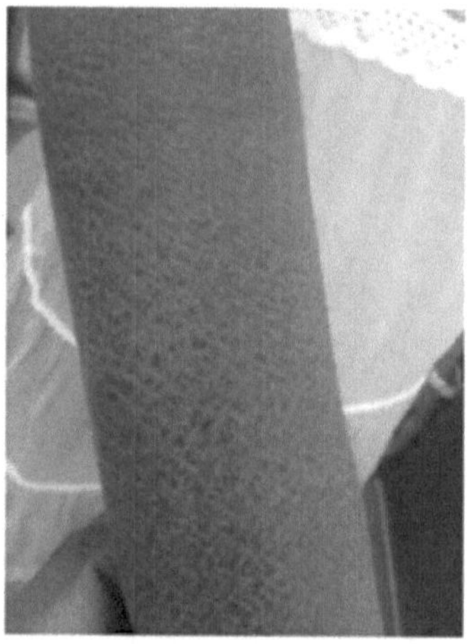

Ichthyosis Vulgaris

- Inherited disorder.
- Fish like scales predominantly seen over extensor aspect of extremities especially legs.
- Associated with hyperlinear palms.

Ans: (d) Tinea corporis

Ref: *DM Thappa's Essentials in Dermatology, 2nd Edition, Page 57; Rook's Textbook of Dermatology, 9th Edition, Page 97.3*

5. A 23-year-old woman presented with peri-oral lesions as shown in the picture. What is the diagnosis?

(a) Impetigo contagiosa
(b) Herpes labialis
(c) Pemphigus vulgaris
(d) Varicella zoster

Herpes Simplex:

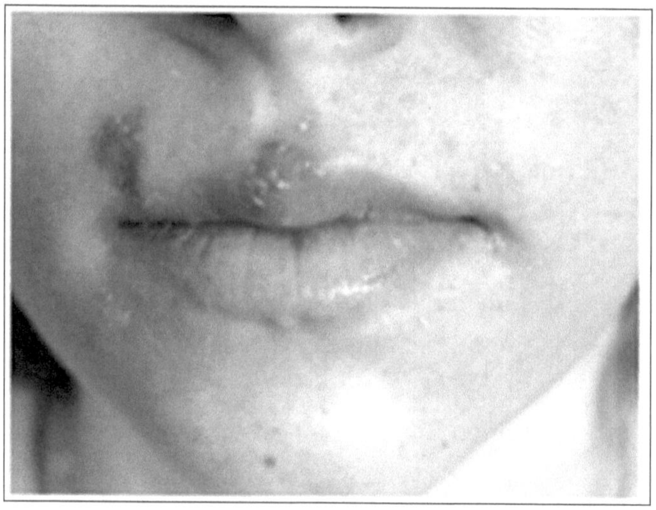

- It usually presents as *painful grouped vesicles.*
- Causative agent: HHV 1 and 2.
- Herpes labialis is caused by HHV 1. It presents as painful grouped vesicles around mouth.
- Herpes genitalis is caused by HHV 2.
- **Eczema herpeticum or Kaposi's varicelliform eruption:** Widespread herpes infections in certain dermatologicsl disorders like atopic dermatitis, pemphigus vulgaris.
- Multinucleated giant cells in tzanck smear.
- Acyclovir, valaciclovir, famciclovir are used in treatment.

Pemphigus Vulgaris:

- Autoimmune intraepidermal blistering disorder.
- **Pathogenesis**
  - Ig G directed against desmoglein 3 leading to acantholysis and suprabasal cleft.
- **Clinical features**
  - Painful oral erosions.
  - Flaccid bullae rupturing to leave painful erosions.
  - ***Nikolsky sign – positive.***
- **Investigations**
  - Tzanck smear: *Acantholytic cells.* They are large, rounded epidermal cells with a large nucleus, perinuclear halo and peripheral condensation of cytoplasm.
  - **Histopathology**
    - Suprabasal cleft with acantholytc cells.

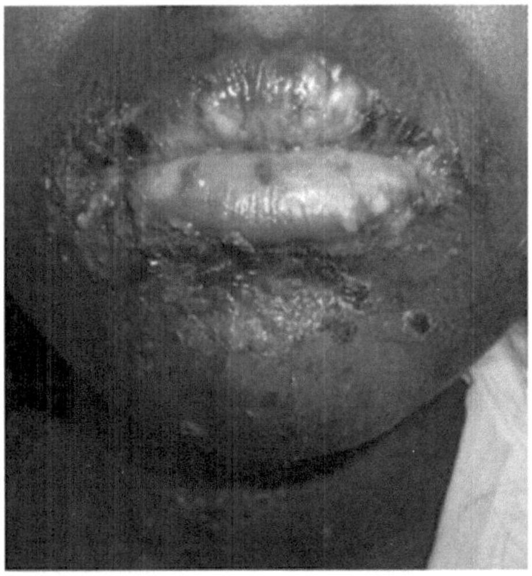

   - ***'Row of tomb stone'*** appearance of basal keratinocyte.
   - ***Fish neat pattern*** is seen in direct immunofluorescence.
- **Treatment**
  - Oral/I.V. steroids.
  - Immunosuppressants like azathioprine, cyclophosphamide, mycophenolate mofetil, rituximab.
  - The following picture shows crusting and oral erosion in a case pemphigus vulgaris.
- The following picture shows **flaccid bullae** and **erosions** in **pemphigus vulgaris.**

Herpes Zoster

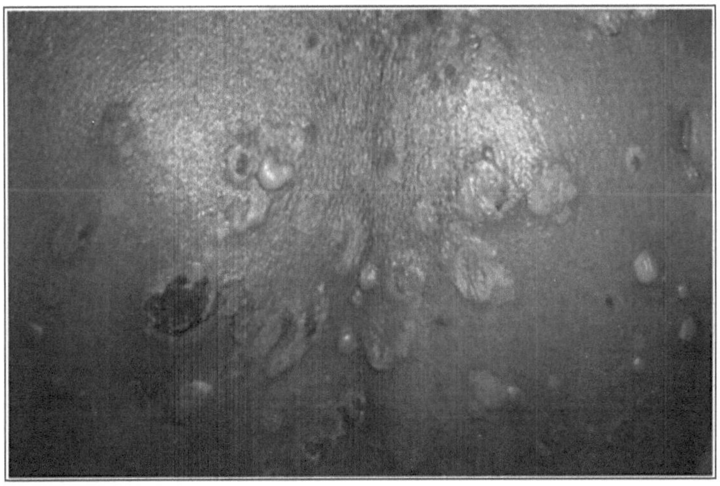

- **Causative agent:** Varicella zoster virus (HHV-3)
  - Caused by reactivaton of latent virus from dorsal root ganglion.
- **Features**
  - It presents as grouped painful vesicular eruption in dermatomal distribution. It can be unidermatomal, multidermatomal or disseminated.
  - The decreasing order of frequency of dermatomal involvement is thoracic (53%), cervical (20%), ophthalmic (15%) and lumbosacral (11%).
  - **Hutchinson's sign:** When patients develop ophthalmic herpes zoster, if tip of nose is involved then there is increased possibility for the patient developing ocular complications.
- **Ramsay Hunt syndrome:** Herpes zoster oticus with facial palsy.
- **Tzanck smear:** Multinucleated giant cells and intra-nuclear inclusion bodies.
- **Treatment:** Oral acyclovir, Valacyclovir.
- **Complications:** Motor weakness, post herpetic neuralgia, secondary bacterial infection.

Impetigo

Impetigo – 2 types	Causative organism	Features	Treatment
Bullous	***Staphylococcus aureus**** **Grams:** Gram positive cocci arranged in clusters	1. Newborn and infants commonly affected 2. Blisters and erosions in flexures are typically seen	**Localised –** Topical fusidic acid cream or mupirocin
Non Bullous (Impetigo contagiosa)	*Streptococcus pyogenes* (more common in warm climatic regions) Staphylococcus **Grams:** Gram positive cocci arranged in chains	1. Preschool and young school age children affected commonly 2. Honey colored crusted lesions are typically seen over face	**Extensive disease** – Oral cloxacillin, cephalexin, co-amoxiclav

Ans: (b) Herpes labialis

Ref: *DM Thappa's Essentials in Dermatology, 2nd Edition, Page 45, 49, 116*

6. A patient presented to the dermatology OPD with complaints of papular lesions in fingers. On examination the lesions were soft and non-tender. Image of the lesion is shown below. What is the probable diagnosis of this case?

(a) Condylomata lata
(b) Molluscum contagiosum
(c) Condylomata acuminata
(d) Common warts

Explanation:

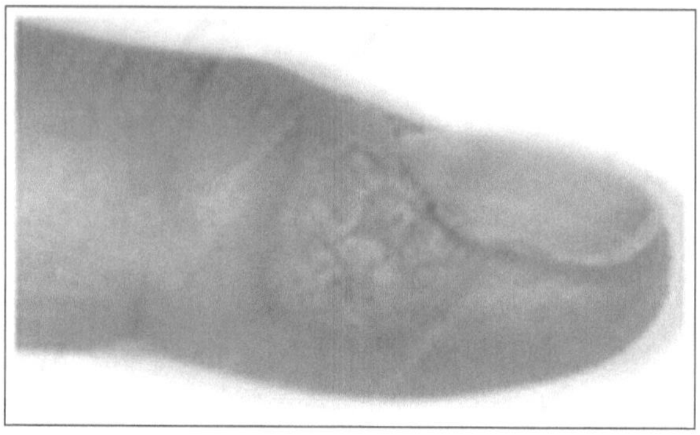

- Common warts (***verruca vulgaris)*** are caused by human papilloma virus (HPV). It presents as verrucous papules and plaques.

WART

Etiology

- Human papillomaviruses

Types of Warts (HPV types):

- Common warts (2, 4).
- Filiform wart.
- Anogenital warts (6,11).
- Flat warts (3,10).
- Palmoplantar warts (1).
- Butcher's warts (7).
- Epidermodysplasia verruciformis (5).

Plantar Warts

- Several contiguous warts may fuse to form a large plaque called ***mosaic wart.***

Epidermodysplasia Verruciformis (*EVER1, EVER2* genes):

- HPV types 5 and 8.
- Autosomal recessive, but an X-linked recessive form also has been postulated.
- Presents as ***plane warts, pityriasis versicolor like lesions and reddish plaques.***
- Progress to **squamous cell carcinoma** in 10% of patients.

Anogenital Warts

- HPV types 6 and 11.

Condyloma Acuminata

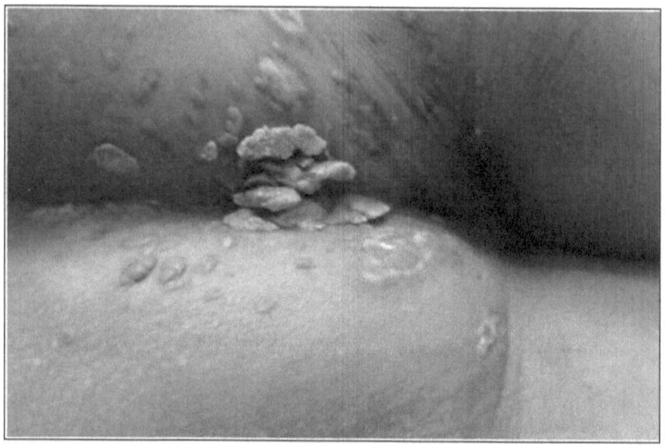

- **Presents as finger like projections in mucosal surfaces in** perianal mucosa, labia, vaginal introitus, glans penis.
- Laryngeal papillomas (same HPV types as in anogenital papillomas).
- Transmission from mothers with a genital HPV infection to neonates who aspirate infectious virus during birth.
- **Buschke Lowenstein tumor or giant condyloma:** It is locally invasive.
- **Histology:**
  - Koilocytes seen in stratum spinosum and granulosum.

- Basophilic intranuclear inclusions.
- ***Pseudo-koebnerization or autoinoculation is seen.***

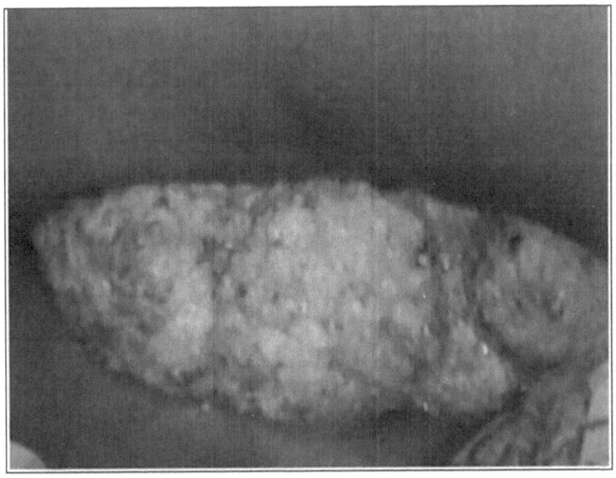

- **Treatment**
  - More than 65% of warts disappear spontaneously within 2 years.
  - Electrosurgery, Radiofrequency ablation, CO_2 laser, Cryotherapy with liquid nitrogen.
  - 40% salicylic acid plasters.
  - ***Condyloma acuminata*** – podophyllin, Imiquimod cream.
  - Immunotherapy with intralesional candida/MMR vaccine/BCG when lesions are numerous or resistant to other therapies.

Molluscum Contagiosum

- The following picture shows umbilicated papules over chest.

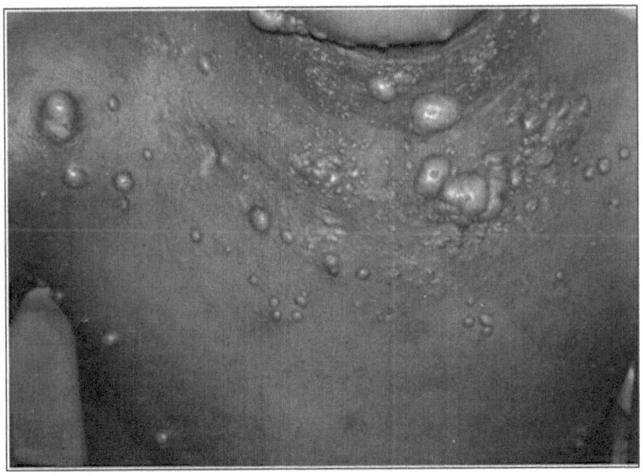

Molluscum Contagiosum

- **Etiology:**
  - Double-stranded DNA poxvirus.
  - Replicates in the cytoplasm of host epithelial cells.
  - Type 1 virus causes most infections.
  - Direct contact with an infected person or from fomites.
- **Clinical Manifestations:**
  - Pearly, skin-colored, dome-shaped, papules.
  - Central umbilication with cheesy white material.
- **Investigations:**
  - Intracytoplasmic ***Handerson Paterson*** inclusion bodies.
- **Differential Diagnosis:**
  - Cryptococcosis, Histoplasmosis, *Penicillium marneffei.*
- **Treatment:**
  - Self-limited.
  - KOH, TCA application, curettage are used in the treatment.

Disseminated lesions are seen in atopic dermatitis or immunodeficiency.

Condylomata Lata

- It is secondary syphilis presenting as moist greyish plaques in intertriginous regions.
- **Other presentations of secondary syphilis** are asymptomatic symmetrical hyperpigmented macules with scaling over palms and soles, papular syphilide (demonstrate ***Ollendorff sign),*** mucous patches, split papules in labial commissures, 'moth-eaten" alopecia, generalised lymphadenopathy including epitrochlear nodes.

Ans: (d) Common warts

Ref: *DM Thappa's Essentials in Dermatology, 2nd Edition, Page 43*

ANESTHESIOLOGY

1. A person was given a muscle relaxant that competitively blocks nicotinic receptors. Which of the following drug is used for reversal of muscle relaxation after surgery?

(a) Neostigmine
(b) Carbachol
(c) Succinylcholine
(d) Physostigmine

Explanation:

- Normal neuromuscular transmission critically depends on acetylcholine binding to nicotinic cholinergic receptors on the motor end plate.
- **Nondepolarizing muscle relaxants** act by **competing** with **acetylcholine** for these binding sites, thereby blocking neuromuscular transmission.
- Reversal of blockade depends on gradual diffusion, redistribution, metabolism, and excretion from the body of the nondepolarizing relaxant (***spontaneous reversal***) or on the administration of specific reversal agents (***pharmacological reversal***).
- **Cholinesterase inhibitors indirectly** increase the amount of acetylcholine available to compete with the nondepolarizing agent, thereby reestablishing normal neuromuscular transmission.
- Commonly used cholinesterase inhibitors are **Neostigmine** and **Edrophonium.**
- Cholinesterase inhibitors **inactivate acetylcholinesterase** by reversibly binding to the enzyme.
- The stability of the bond influences the duration of action:
  - The electrostatic attraction and hydrogen bonding of Edrophonium are short-lived.
  - The covalent bonds of Neostigmine are longer lasting.
- The lipid solubility and CNS penetration of Physostigmine limit its usefulness as a reversal agent for nondepolarizing blockade, but make it effective in the treatment of central anticholinergic toxicity caused by overdoses of atropine or scopolamine.

Ans: (a) Neostigmine

Ref: *Clinical Anesthesiology, 4th Edition, Chapter 10*

2. A patient of biliary colic presented to emergency room. The pain worsened after an injection was given by doctor. Which is the most likely injection given?

(a) Diclofenac
(b) Nefopam
(c) Morphine
(d) Etoricoxib

Explanation:

- Opioids act through specific opioid receptors on neuronal tissues such as peripheral nerves and neurons in the spinal cord and brain.
- Examples of opioids: Morphine, Fentanyl, Sufentanyl, Alfentanyl, Remifentanyl etc.
- The most important receptors include the:
  - μ opioid receptor.
  - δ opioid receptor.
  - κ opioid receptor.
- For anesthesia and pain relief, the μ is most important.

- Opioids also act through non-neuronal pathways, such as those affecting the immune system, which may be of relevance in the treatment of inflammatory pain.
- Administration of opioids can potentially lead to life-threatening respiratory depression. The incidence of serious perioperative respiratory events is approximately 0.5% (1 in every 200 patients).
- Apart from respiratory depression, opioids cause a large number of side effects that require attention:
  - **Nausea** with or without **vomiting**, **smooth muscle spasms**, **skeletal muscle rigidity** (fentanyl and congeners).
  - **Histamine release** (morphine, codeine, meperidine).
  - **Itching** (especially after spinal administration).
  - **Miosis**, sedation and dizziness.
  - The **cardiovascular side effects** of opioids include bradycardia and hypotension (especially when combined with anesthetics, even at usual clinical doses, or in severely ill patients), opioids may produce hemodynamic instability.
  - **Delayed gastric emptying**, constipation, bowel distension and paralytic ileus.
  - Due to spasms of the sphincter of Oddi and common bile duct, opioids may cause **acute upper abdominal pain** and colic-like complain.

Ans: (c) Morphine

Ref: *Barach's Clinical Anestheisa, 7th Edition, Chapter 19*

3. A 55-year-old female patient on Angiotensin-Converting Enzyme (ACE) inhibitors for hypertension. She had Coronary Artery Bypass Graft (CABG) 4 years back. Now the patient is scheduled for hernia surgery. She has good tolerance. What is the proper investigation to be ordered?

(a) Routine preop, clinical evaluation and V/Q scan

(b) Routine preop, clinical evaluation and angiography to look for patency

(c) Routine preop, clinical evaluation and stress testing

(d) Routine preop, clinical evaluation

Explanation:

(See Flowchart on the next page)

ASA PS class 1	Normal healthy patient. No organic, physiologic, biochemical, or psychiatric disturbance
ASA PS class 2	Mild-to-moderate systemic disease that is well controlled and causes no organ dysfunction or functional limitation (e.g., treated hypertension)
ASA PS class 3	Severe systemic disease of at least one organ system that does cause functional limitation (e.g., stable angina)
ASA PS class 4	Severe systemic end-stage disease of at least one organ system that is life threatening with or without surgery (e.g., congestive heart failure or renal failure)
ASA PS class 5	Moribund patient who has little chance of survival but is submitted to surgery as a last resort (resuscitative effort; e.g., ruptured aortic aneurysm)
ASA PS class 6	A declared brain-dead patient whose organs are being removed for donor purposes
Emergency operation (E)	Any patient in whom an emergency operation is required
Modified from American Society of Anesthesiologists: New classification of physical status. Anesthesiology 1963;24:111	

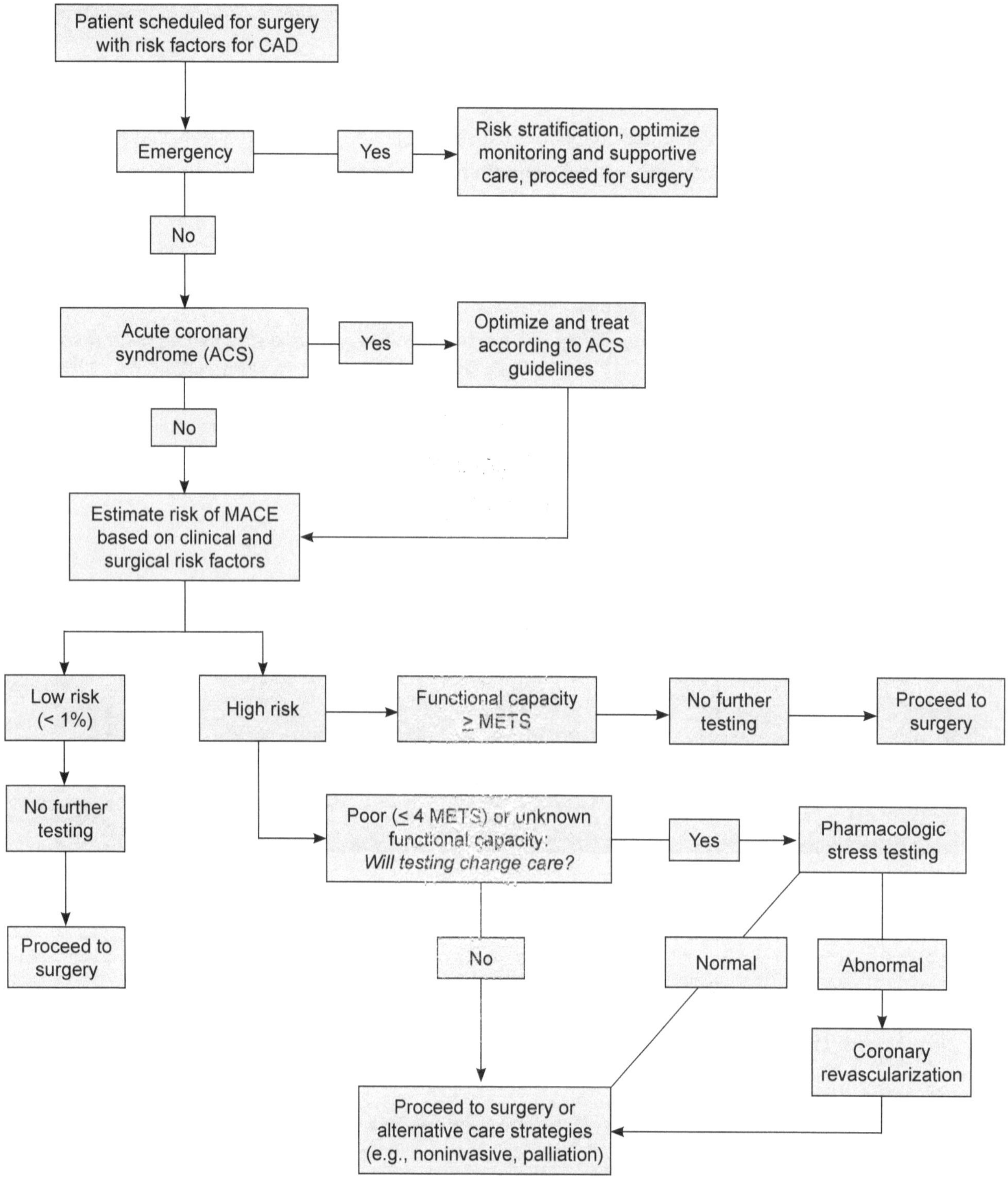

Key: MACE, major adverse cardiac event; MET, metabolic equivalent

This Flowchart is showing the preoperative assessment of the cardiac patient for non cardiac surgery.

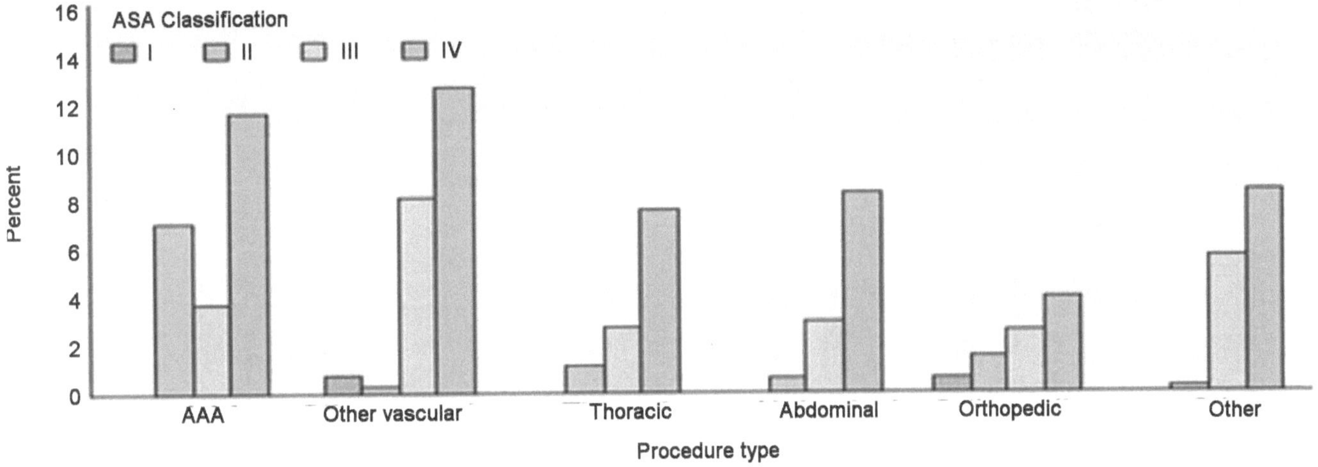

According to these Flowchart

Ans: (d) Routine preop, clinical evaluation

Ref: *2014 ACC/AHA Guideline on Perioperative Cardiovascular Evaluation and Management of Patients Undergoing Noncardiac Surgery*

4. What does the following ETCO$_2$ depict?

(a) Esophageal intubation
(b) Spontaneous efforts
(c) Bronchospasm
(d) Cardiac arrest

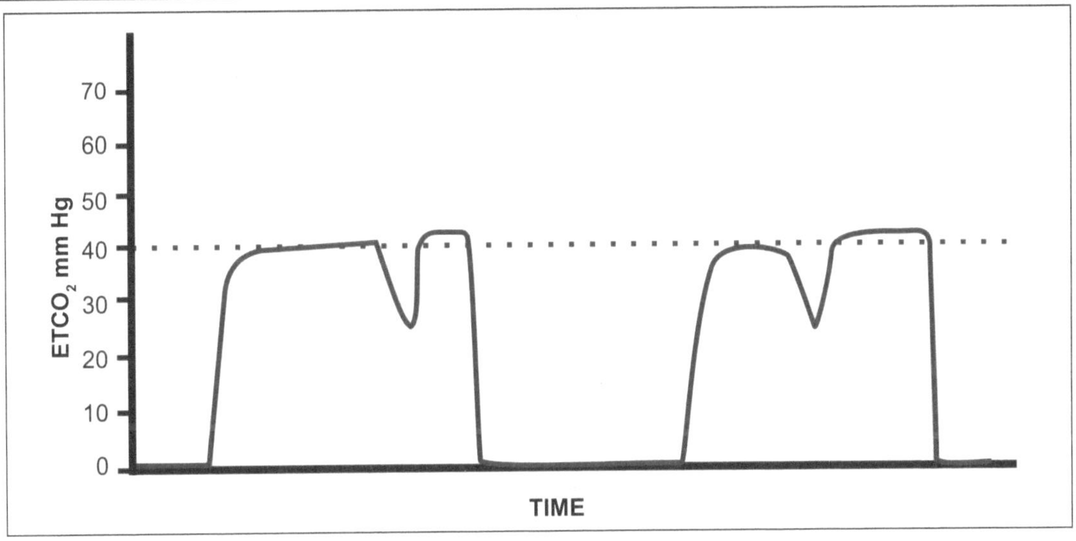

Explanation:

The Indian Society of Anaesthesiologists has designated capnography as a 'desirable' standard in its "Anaesthesia Monitoring Standards Recommended for India" with effect from 30th December 1999.

TERMINOLGY

- **Capnography** is the graphic display of instantaneous CO_2 concentration versus time (Time Capnogram) or expired volume (Volume Capnogram) during a respiratory cycle.
- **Capnograph** is the machine that generates a waveform and the capnogram is the actual waveform.

- **Capnometry** is the measurement and numerical display of maximum inspiratory and expiratory CO concentrations during a respiratory cycle 2.
- **Capnometer** is the device that performs the measurement and displays the reading.

1. **Normal Capnogram**

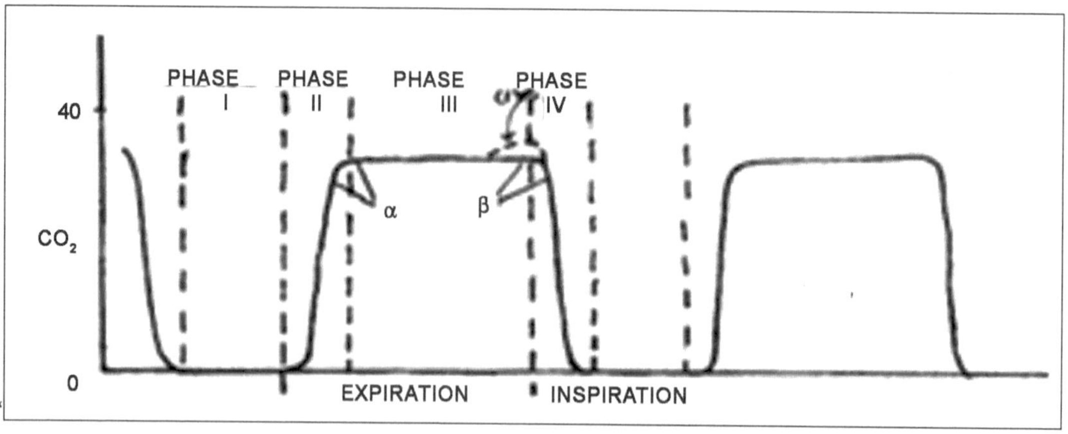

2. **Low end-tidal carbon dioxide with a good alveolar plateau may be the result of hyperventilation or an increase in dead space ventilation**

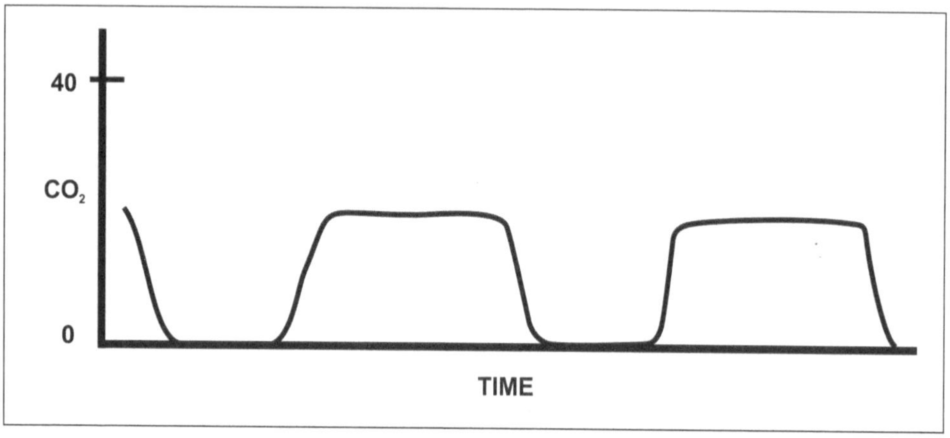

3. **Elevated end-tidal carbon dioxide with good alveolar plateau may be caused by hypoventilation**

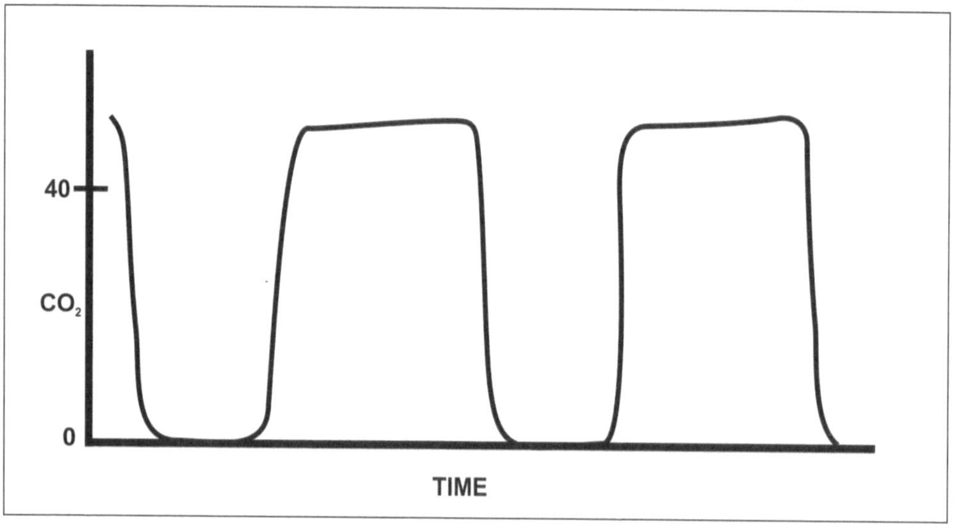

4. Events that cause an exponential decrease in end tidal CO_2 include sudden hypotension, circulatory arrest and pulmonary embolism

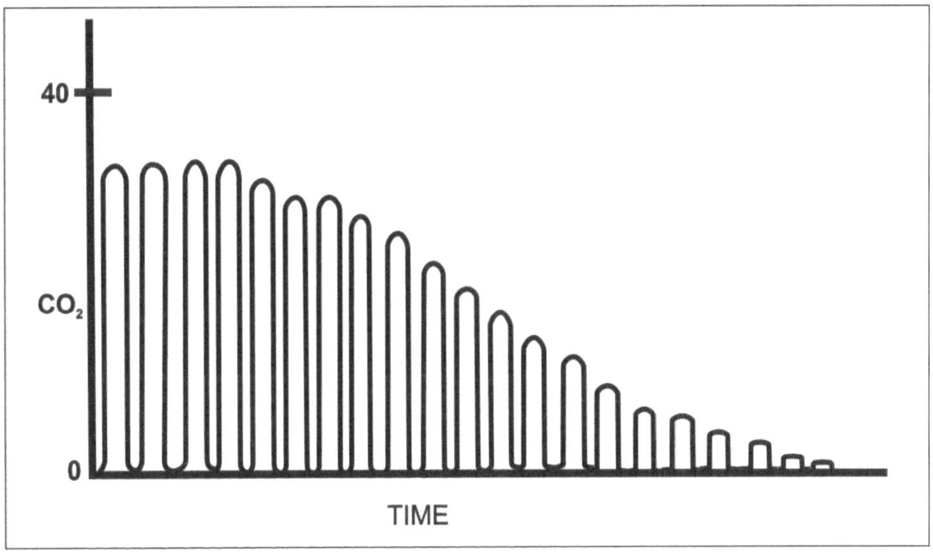

5. Small air embolus

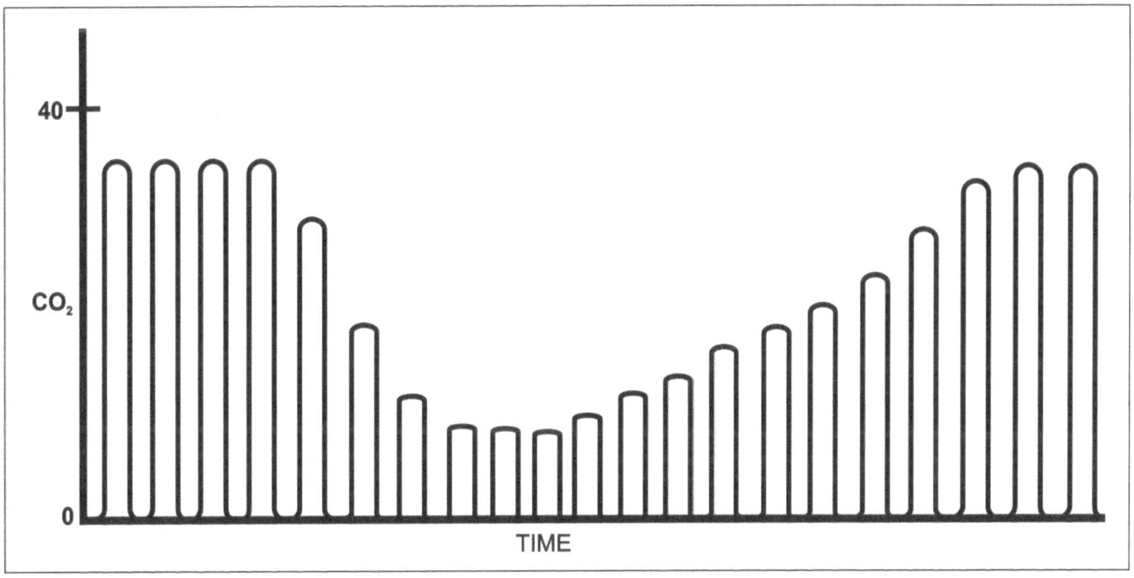

6. A leak in the sampling line during positive pressure ventilation

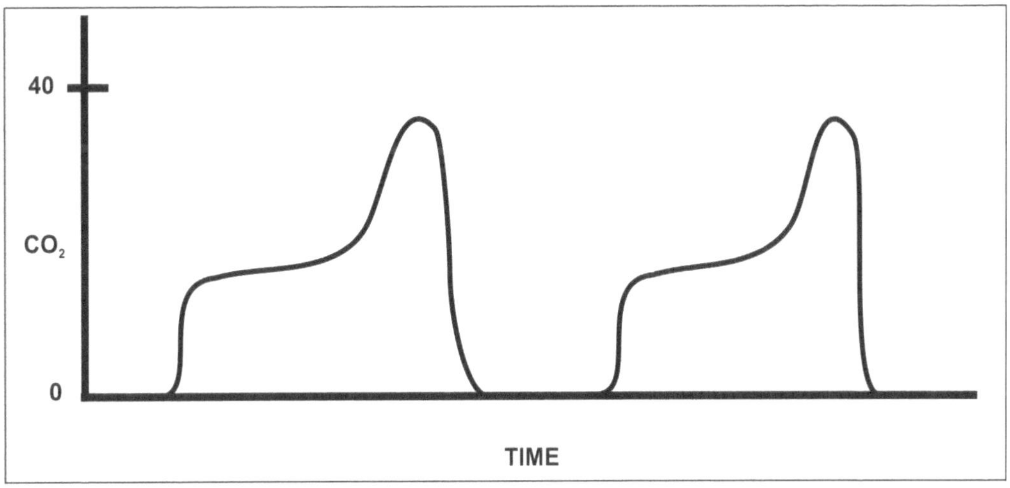

7. **Return to spontaneous ventilation**

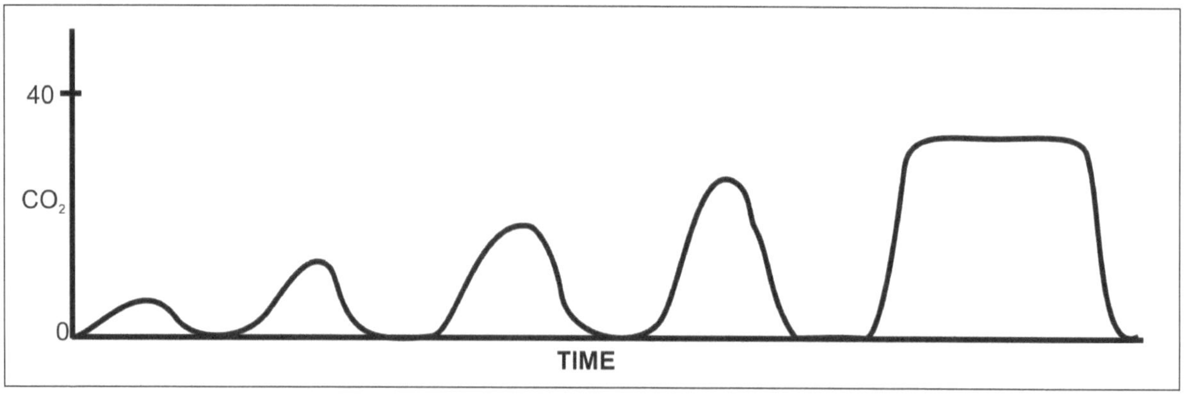

8. **Spontaneous respiratory efforts during mechanical ventilation**

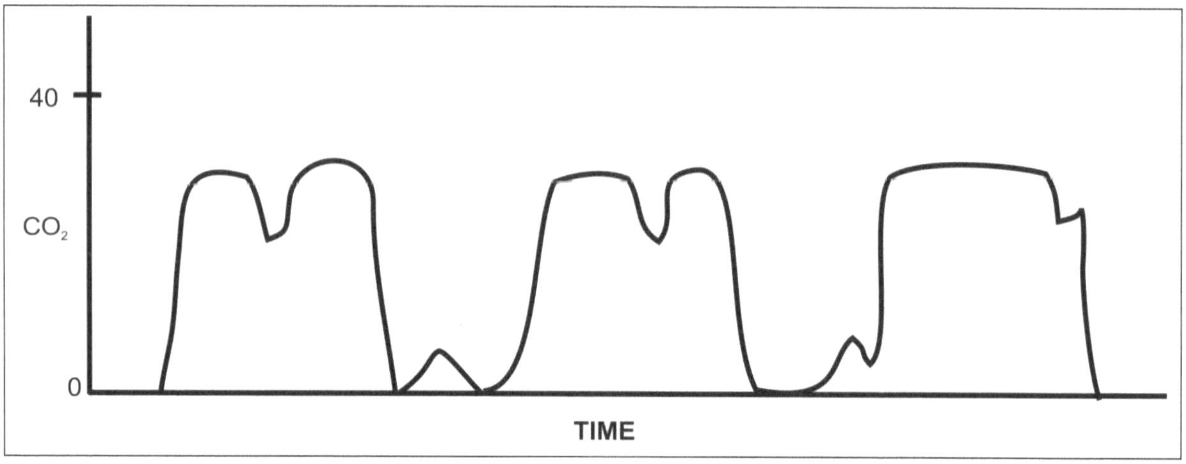

9. **Cardiogenic oscillations appear as small, regular, tooth like humps at the end of the expiratory phase**

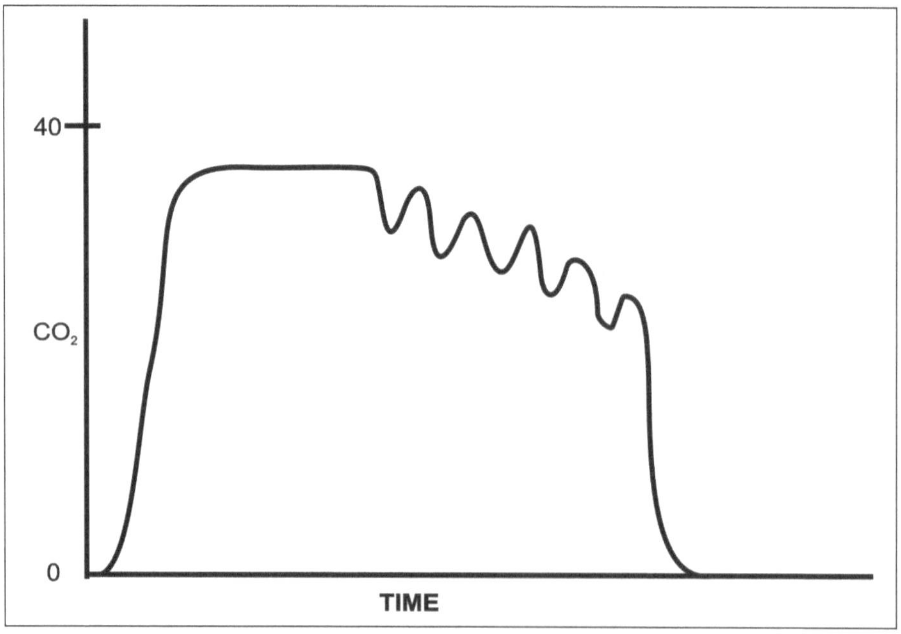

Ans: (b) Spontaneous efforts

Ref: *http://www.capnography.com*

5. A 60-year-old patient with history of hypertension and diabetes developed the following rhythm, BP was 80/60 mm of Hg and pulse was feeble. What is the next step of management?

(a) IV Diltiazem
(b) Ibutilide
(c) IV Adenosine
(d) DC cardioversion

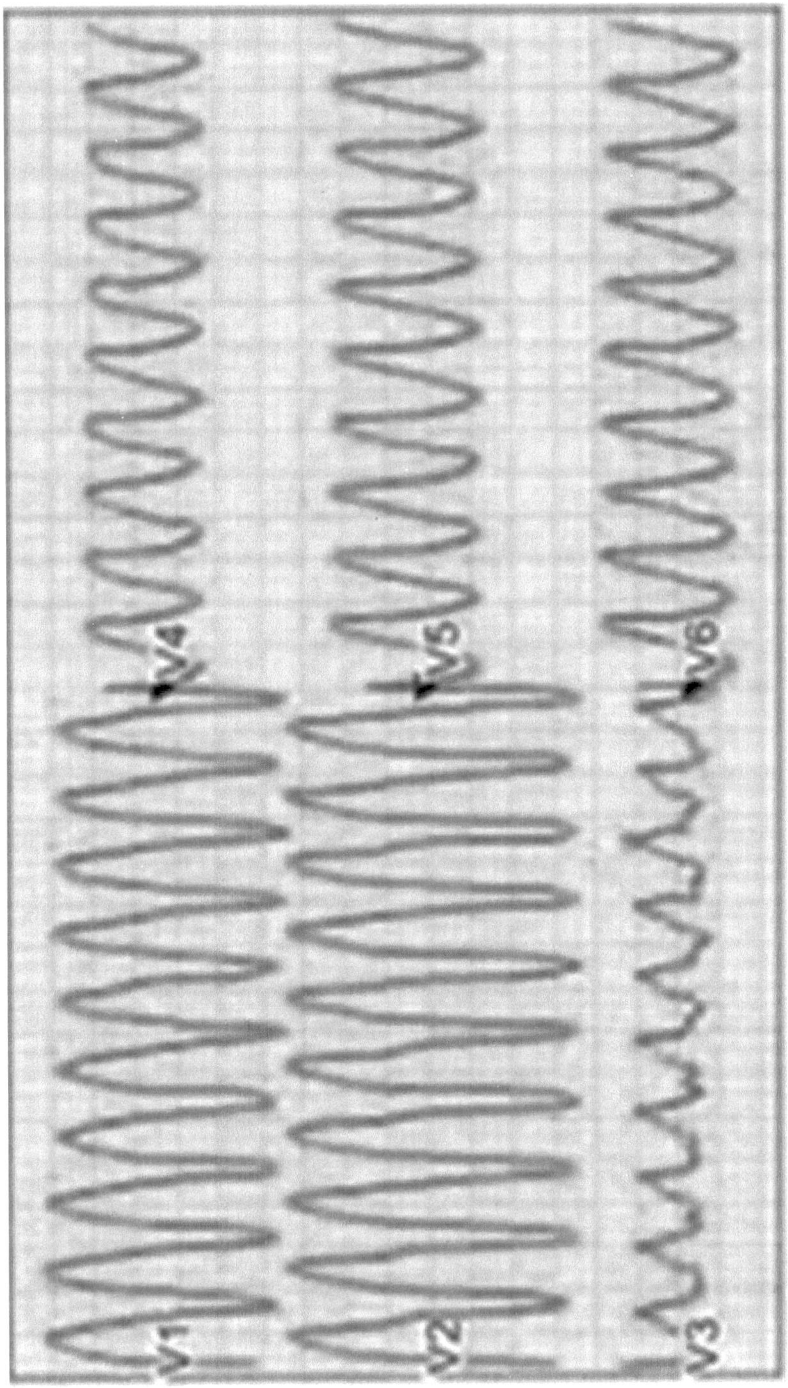

Explanation:

- This patient is clinically unstable (BP 80/60) and ECG is showing wide QRS complex (Monomorphic Venticular Tachycardia) Tachycardia. So the immediate treatment should be DC cardioversion to revert the rhythm to normal.

Adult Tachycardia with a Pulse Algorithm

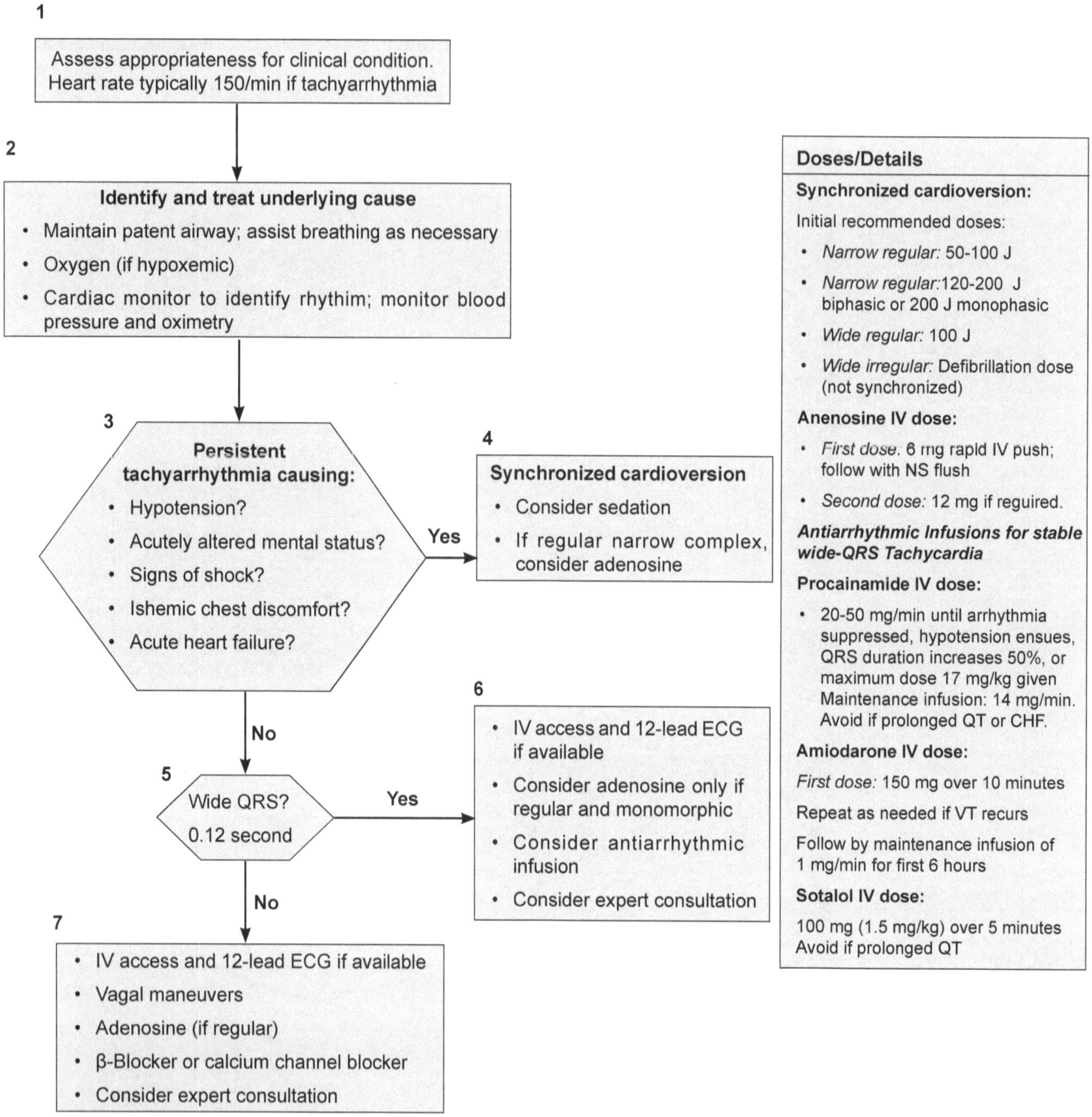

Ans: (d) DC cardioversion

Ref: *ACLS 2015, Guidelines by AHA*

RADIOLOGY

1. Pulmonary plethora is seen in:

(a) TAPVC
(b) TOF
(c) Right heart failure
(d) Ebstein anomaly

Explanation:

- **Pulmonary plethora (Increased pulmonary perfusion):** It is recognized by enlarged central and peripheral pulmonary arteries and veins in all zones, as occurs in situations with increased pulmonary blood flow: ASD, VSD and PDA with large left-to-right shunts.

Causes of Pulmonary Plethora and Oligemia in Chest Imaging

Causes of increased pulmonary flow–plethora (L to R shunt)	Reduced pulmonary flow–oligemia
• ASD • VSD • PDA • TGA • TAPVC • Vein of galen malformation • Truncus arteriosus	• Ebstein's anomaly • Triscupid atresia • Tetrology of Fallot • TGA with stenosis of pulmonary artery

Also Note:

- Common cause of **plethora without cyanosis: Partial anomalous pulmonary venous drainage**.
- Common cause of **plethora with cyanosis: Total anomalous pulmonary venous drainage**.

Ans: (a) TAPVC

Ref: *Grainger and Allison's Diagnostic Radiology, 6th Edition, Page 428*

2. A 20-year-old male with hypertension has the following chest X-ray with prominent aortic notch. What could be the likely cause?

(a) Aorto-arteritis
(b) Coarctation of aorta
(c) Aortic aneurysm
(d) Essential hypertension

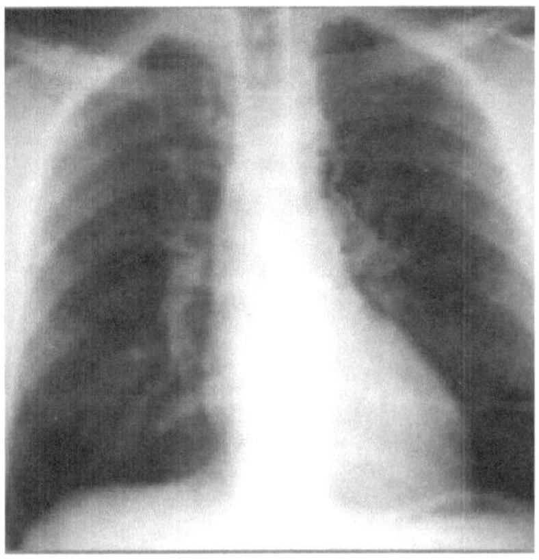

Explanation:

Coarctation of the Aorta

- Luminal narrowing of a short section of the aorta.
- It occurs most commonly at the site of insertion of the ductus arteriosus, and is thought to develop due to the presence of excessively integrated ductal tissue around the aortic isthmus.
- Patients may present with unexplained hypertension as a teenager or adult and are at increased risk of the attendant micro- and macrovascular complications.

- **X-ray Findings:**
  - Notching of the inferior ribs (**Dock sign**) by large intercostals arteries can be seen; and
    - Inferior rib notching of bilateral 3rd to 9th ribs due to dilated intercostals collateral vascular channels.
    - Inferior rib notching of right 3rd to 9th rib–if pre isthmic coarctation (before origin of left SCA).
    - Inferior rib notching of left 3rd to 9th rib–if aberrant origin of right SCA from post isthmic area.
  - **Reverse '3' sign** on X-ray due to impression by left SCA and post-stenotic dilatation.
  - A figure of 3 can be seen in Chest X-rays (CXR) because of prominence of aorta proximal to coarctation, indentation of aortic outline at coarctation and dilation of post-stenotic segment.
  - **Inverse figure of 3 or E sign** seen in barium meal.

Ans: (b) Coarctation of aorta

Ref: *Grainger and Allison's Diagnostic Radiology, 6th Edition, Page 434*

3. Examine the neuroimages given below. Cystic lesion in suprasellar region with calcification is seen in:

(a) Pituitary adenoma

(b) Meningioma

(c) Oligodendroglioma

(d) Craniopharyngioma

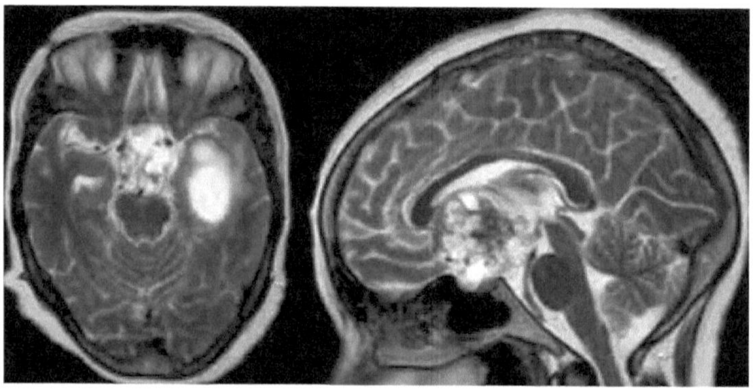

Explanation:

- **Craniopharyngioma** is the most likely diagnosis.

CRANIOPHARYNGIOMAS

- Craniopharyngiomas are **suprasellar tumors** which occur most frequently in childhood.
- They arise from **epithelial remnants of Rathke's pouch**, from which the anterior pituitary develops, and can be cystic, solid or mixed cystic/solid.
- Clinical symptoms are seen in craniopharyngioma due to compression of the optic chiasm or to raised intracranial pressure (ICP) secondary to obstruction of the foramen of Monro.
- **Diagnosis:**
  - The contrast-enhanced MRI demonstrated a heterogeneous enhancing sellar and suprasellar lesion with solid and cystic components.
  - In addition, CT images confirm the presence of calcification in the lesion, which are present in 80% of craniopharyngioma cases.

CRANIOPHARYNGIOMA

- There are two pathological type of craniopharyngioma. They are: adamantinomatous and squamous-papillary.
- **Adamantinomatous type:** Most commonly seen in children, which have large T1 hyperintense cystic components.
- **Squamous-papillary:** Most commonly seen in adults, is more likely to be predominantly solid and associated cysts return low signal on T1W images, similar to CSF.

- **Treatment:** Classic surgical approaches are:
  - Frontal interhemispheric and pterional transsylvian approaches.
  - Anterior interhemispheric approach with subsequent opening of the lamina terminalis.
  - Transcortical or transcallosal through a transchoroidal approach to the third ventricle.
- **Differential Diagnosis:**
  - Rathke's cleft cyst.
  - Gliomas.
  - Pituitary adenoma.
  - Meningioma.
  - Metastases.
  - Brain abscess.

Note:

- Pituitary adenoma is originated from Sella/pituitary, rest are Supra-sellar tumor, so pituitary can be seen separately.
- Pituitary adenoma Meningioma and Oligodendroglioma are solid tumors.
- Calcifications are generally not seen in pituitary adenoma.

Ans: (d) Craniopharyngioma

Ref: *Grainger and Allison's Diagnostic Radiology, 6th Edition, Page 1453*

4. Radiation dose monitoring in occupation of health care workers is done by:

(a) Linear accelerator (b) TLD badge

(c) Gamma camera (d) GM counters

Explanation:

- Thermoluminescent dosimeter (TLD) is a passive radiation detection device that is used for personal dose monitoring or to measure patient dose.
- TLD is used to measure external individual doses from x, β and γ radiation.
- It consists of TLD card loaded in a cassette having suitable metallic filters.
- It is based on the phenomenon of the imoluminescence, the emission of light when certain materials are heated after exposure to radiation. An RLD badge does not protect the worker from radiation. It detects and measures the radiation to which you have been exposed.

Ans: (b) TLD badge

Ref: *Christensen's Physics of Diagnostic Radiology, 4th Edition, Page 132*

5. A 24-year-old mother with 7-week of pregnancy presents to ANC OPD with history of exposed to chest X-ray in the hospital. What will you advise her regarding pregnancy management?

(a) Do chromosomal testing (b) Continue pregnancy

(c) Immediate termination of pregnancy (d) Do pre-invasive test

Explanation:

- Depending on radiation exposure dose in ascending order the investigations are: Radiography < Barium studies < Computed Tomography (CT) < Radioisotope scans < PETCT.

- Radiation exposure below 50 mGy at any stage of pregnancy is not an absolute contraindication.
- Even here, Radiography of chest which has less than 0.15 mGy dose.
- As pelvic radiography has more dose as compared to chest radiography.

Radiation exposure	Pregnancy risk factor
• < 5 rad or <50 mGy	• No risk factor at any stage of pregnancy
• 5-10 rad or >50-100 mGy	• Probably no, but there is no strong scientific evidence
• >10 rad or >100 mGy	• Usually spontaneous abortion is the fate in early pregnancy, later on there may be growth anomaly and CNS development

Ans: (b) Continue pregnancy

Ref: *International Commission on Radiological Protection (ICRP) guidelines (http://www.icrp.org/publication.asp?id=icrp%20publication%2084)*

6. Remote after loading dose used in:

(a) Brachytherapy (b) Electron beam

(c) Proton beam (d) Cyber knife therapy

Explanation:

- Remote after loading brachytherapy refers to a situation in which a radioisotope is placed onto or inside the patient.
- The radiation source is sealed in a protective capsule or wire which prevents the radioisotope from moving or dissolving in body fluids but allows the emission of ionizing radiation (in the form of α, β, γ or X-radiation) to the surrounding tissues.
- The source can be placed into the target tissues or tumor itself such as the prostate or breast (interstitial brachytherapy), into a body cavity such as the uterine cavity, oesophagus or bronchus (intracavitary/intraluminal brachytherapy) or onto the skin surface to treat a cutaneous malignancy.
- Brachytherapy applicators have been adapted to enable better imaging. For example, CT- and MRI-compatible intrauterine tubes have been developed for gynaecological treatments.
- Seeds containing 125 I are commonly used to treat prostate cancer.

Ans: (a) Brachytherapy

Ref: *Grainger and Allison's Diagnostic Radiology, 6th Edition, Page 1740*

7. Which of the following is the most likely diagnosis of the patient with the following chest X-ray?

(a) TGA

(b) TAPVC

(c) TOF

(d) Ebstein's anomaly

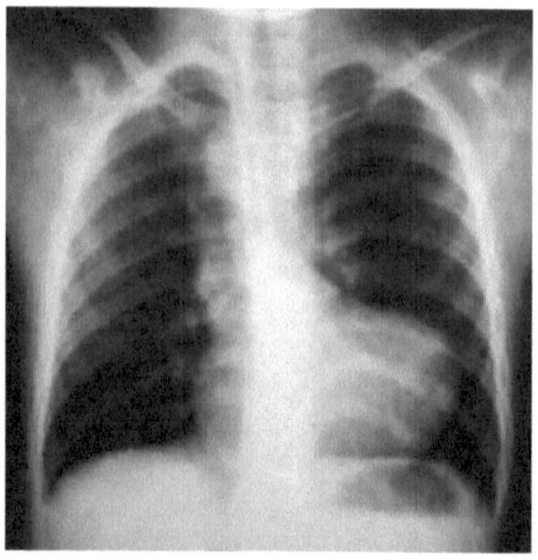

Explanation:

- CXR shows classic **boot shaped heart** seen in **TOF.**

Supracardiac Type Total Anomalous Pulmonary Venous Connection (TAPVC)

- It is the most common type of TAPVC, seen in 50% cases.
- Obstruction is quite in frequent, but when present it is most commonly caused by compression of left vertical artery by left pulmonary artery anteriorly and left bronchus posteriorly.

- **X-ray findings:** Enlarged heart termed as figure of 8/Snowman, which is caused by dilated left vertical vein, innominate vein, right superior vena cava along with dilated heart.

Obstructive Type TAPVC

- It occurs due to severe pulmonary congestion caused by obstruction the baby presents with very early onset dyspnea, intense cyanosis and right heart failure.
- A loud 2nd heart sound, gallop rhythm and systolic murmur of tricuspid regurgitation may be heard.
- **X-ray findings:** Small heart with ground glass appearance of lung.

Tetralogy of Fallot

- It is the only cyanotic heart disease that may present in adulthood.
- **X-ray findings:** Boot or wooden-shoe shaped heart (Coeur en sabot), clear hilar areas and lung field because of diminished pulmonary blood flow, large aorta and a right-sided aortic arch.
- ECG corresponds to right ventricular hypertrophy and right axis deviation.

Ebstein's Anomaly

- **X-ray findings:** Finding shows an important cardiomegaly with regards mainly to the right heart. The heart is shaped a little bit like a box, Box shaped heart.

Transposition of Great Arteries (TGA)

- **X-ray findings:** Egg on side/Egg on string appearance (Cardiomegaly with a narrow base and plethoric lung fields).

EXTRA EDGE

Radiological Appearance of Heart in Various Diseases

Cardiac Condition	Finding in CXR
Fallot's Tetralogy	Boot shaped heart
Tricuspid Atresia	Box shaped heart
TAPVC (total anomalus pulmonary venous connection)	Snow man appearance, 8 shaped heart, cottage loaf appearance
Constrictive pericarditis	Egg in cup appearance
Pericardial effusion	Water bottle, pear shaped appearance
Pulmonary hypertension	Jug handle appearance
Transposition of vessels	Egg shell cracking/egg on side appearance

Ans: (c) TOF

Ref: *Grainger and Allison's Diagnostic Radiology, 6th Edition, Page 428*

8. A 45-year-old female presents with sudden onset headache and neck rigidity. There is no history of trauma. What could be the likely diagnosis?

(a) Meningitis (b) Haemorrhagic stroke

(c) SAH (d) SDH

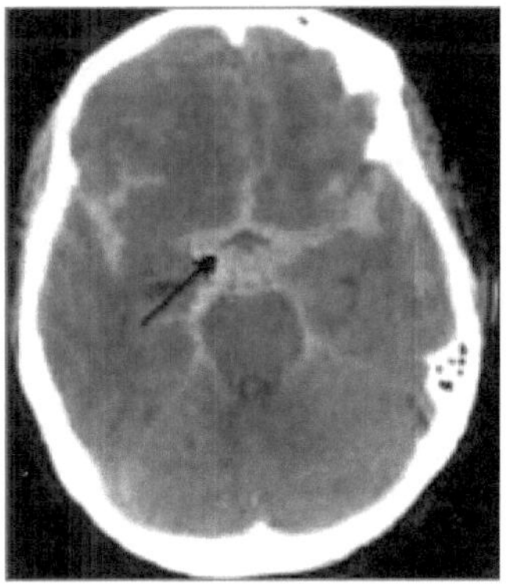

Explanation:

- The above clinical symptoms along with the radiological findings suggest it a case of subarachnoid hemorrhage.

Subarachnoid Hemorrhage (SAH)

- The age group of aneurysmal SAH is 40-60 years with M : F ratio is 1:2.
- **Etiologies:**
  - Berry aneurysms (Ruptured saccular aneurysms).
  - Trauma.
  - Arteriovenous malformation (AVM).
- **Clinical Features:**
  - Aneurysmal SAH presents with an abrupt-onset, intensely painful "thunderclap" headache, often followed by neck stiffness (Caused by meningeal irritation).
  - Other signs of meningeal irritation are photophobia, nausea/vomiting and meningeal stretch sign (Kerning and Brudzinski signs).
- **Diagnosis:**

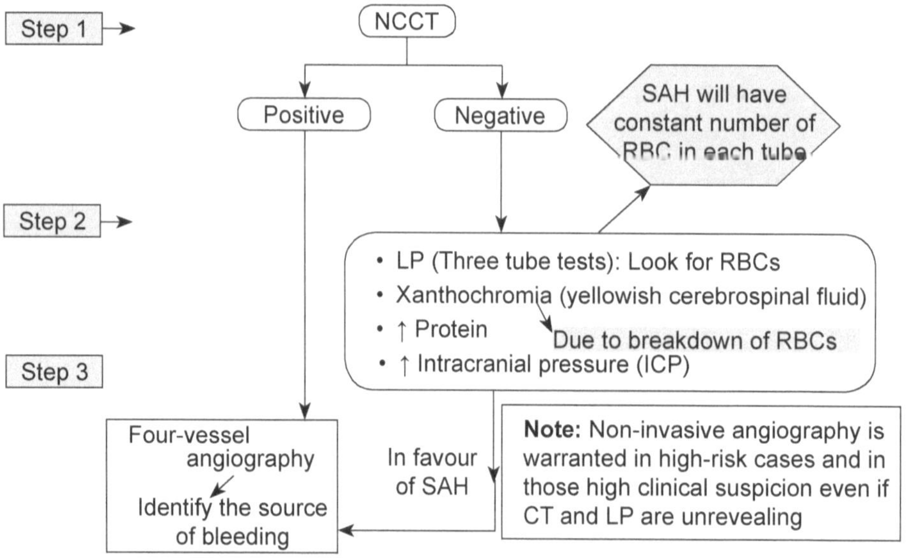

Contrast Computed Tomograph (NCCT); SAH, Subarachnoid hemorrhage; LP, lumbar puncture; CT, computed tomography

- **Treatment:**
  - **Most definitive treatment:** Neurosurgery. May perform angiographic coiling and/or stenting to stabilize aneurysm.
  - Rebleeding most commonly occurs in first 24 hours, so prevent the rebleeding by controlling the systolic BP < 150 mm Hg until the aneurysm has been clipped or coiled.
  - After 4-10 days of post-op subsequent ischemic stroke occurs, to avoid this situation nimodipine Calcium channel blockers (CCBs) are administered.

Subarachnoid Hemorrhage

- Bleeding due to trauma, or rupture of an aneurysm (such as a saccular aneurysm A) or arteriovenous malformation. Rapid time course. Patients complain of "worst headache of my life".
- Bloody or yellow (xanthochromic) spinal tap. 4–10 days after hemorrhage, vasospasm (narrowing of blood vessels) can occur due to blood breakdown or rebleed → ischemic infarct; nimodipine used to prevent/ reduce vasospasm. Increases risk of developing communicating and/or obstructive hydrocephalus.

Ans: (c) SAH

Ref: *Grainger and Allison's Diagnostic Radiology, 6th Edition, Page 1482*

9. Which sign is seen on USG when the femoral vein meets the great saphenous vein (GSV) and femoral artery at the saphenofemoral junction?

(a) Mickey mouse sign
(b) Tillaux sign
(c) Stemmers sign
(d) String sign

Explanation:

- **Mickey mouse sign:** It represents the normal anatomy of the common femoral artery, common femoral vein and great saphenous vein on ultrasound at the level just inferior to the inguinal crease.
- **Tillaux sign:** A clinical sign in which there is resonant area between the pubic bone and tumor indications the tumor to be mesenteric.
- **Stemmer's sign:** Stemmer's sign is seen in lymphoedema. Skin on the dorsum of the toes cannot be pinched due to subcutaneous fibrosis.
- **String sign:** Seen in Crohn's disease.

Ans: (a) Mickey mouse sign

Ref: *Bailey and Love Short Practice of Surgery, 27th Edition, Page 976*

10. A 35-year-old man presented with recurrent episodes of fever with chills and fatigue; Magnetic resonance cholangiopancreatography (MRCP) image is given below. What is your diagnosis?

(a) Primary biliary carcinoma
(b) Primary sclerosing cholangitis
(c) Caroli disease
(d) Oriental cholangitis

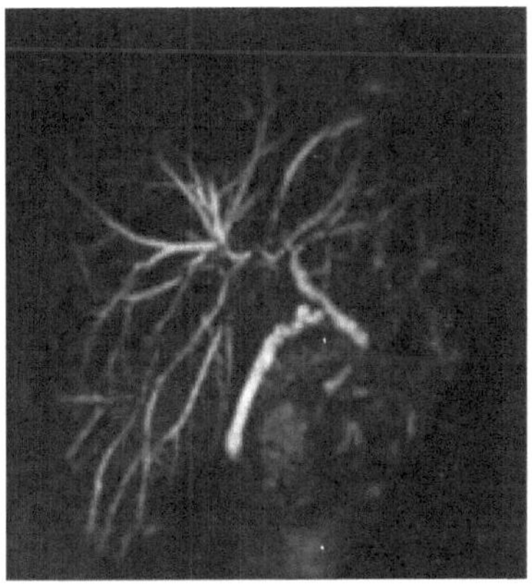

Explanation:

- Thick-slab oblique coronal MRCP shows multiple intrahepatic and extrahepatic segments of stricturing; which depicts it is a classic case of primary sclerosing cholangitis.

Primary Sclerosing Cholangitis

- MRCP shows beaded appearance of alternating strictures and dilatation of intra- and extrahepatic bile ducts.
- Primary sclerosing cholangitis is associated with ulcerative colitis in up to 80%.
- **ERCP Findings:** Strictures and characteristic diverticula-like outpouchings affecting the common duct.
- **USG:** Typical bile duct wall thickening on US.

Other Options

- **Primary Biliary Carcinoma:** MRI T2: If parenchymal lace-like fibrosis and periportal halo signs are seen together.
- **Caroli Disease:** CT scan shows "central dot" sign (enhancing dots within the dilated intrahepatic bile ducts, representing portal radicles).

Oriental Cholangitis

- **CT:** Focal areas of fibrosis with heterogeneous enhancement and focal steatosis.
- **MRCP.**

- Reduced arborization of peripheral ducts: "arrowhead sign".
- Multiple intra- and extra-hepatic biliary strictures.

Ans: (b) Primary sclerosing cholangitis

Ref: *Grainger and Allison's Diagnostic Radiology, 6th Edition, Page 1842*

11. A 30-year-old male presented with history of thickening of skin and shortness of breath and bilateral basal rales. Her CXR shows reticular opacities in bilateral basal fields. What should be the next step in this case?

(a) Do pulmonary function test
(b) Do CECT
(c) Do HRCT
(d) Echocardiography

Explanation:

- In patients with suspected chronic diffuse lung disease, HRCT is indicated in the following situations:
  - For detection in patients with normal or equivocal plain CXR appearances who have symptoms or pulmonary function tests suggestive of diffuse lung disease.
  - Where the symptoms and/or plain CXR findings are non-specific, to attempt a specific diagnosis.
  - To assess activity of disease.
  - To select an optimal biopsy site.
- In patients with suspected acute diffuse lung disease, HRCT is indicated in the following situations:
  - For detection in patients with normal or equivocal plain CXR appearances who have symptoms or pulmonary function tests suggestive of acute lung disease (especially in immunosuppressed patients).
  - For investigation of hemoptysis in selected patients.
  - To select an optimal biopsy site.

Ans: (c) Do HRCT

Ref: *Diagnostic Imaging Pathways–High Resolution Computed Tomography (HRCT) of the Lung Published; May 2011*

12. Identify the pathology in the image shown here:

(a) MCU showing Bulbar urethral stricture
(b) RGU showing Bulbar urethral stricture
(c) MCU showing Membranous urethral stricture
(d) RGU showing Membranous urethral stricture

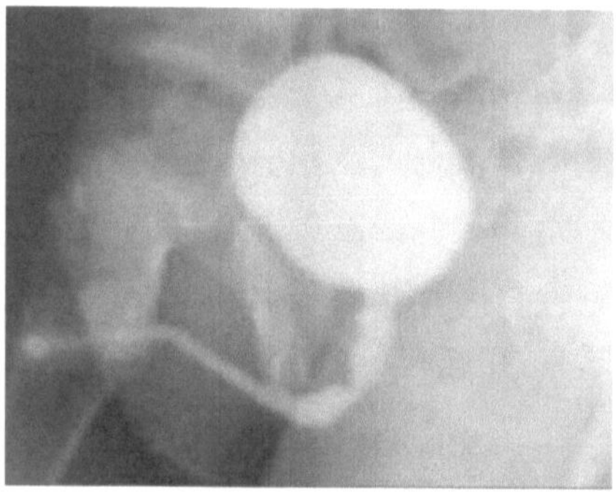

Explanation:

- To diagnose urethral strictures the investigations used are:
  - Retrograde (Ascending) urethrogram.
  - Descending Cystourethrogram or Micturating Cystourethrogram (MCU).
- The commonly used investigation to diagnose the Urethral strictures is to cannulate the penis and pass contrast upto bladder level and take X-ray known as **Retrograde urethrogram**.
- For understanding purpose in X-ray to say the image is RGU we will have:
  - Cannulated penis.
  - Incomplete bladder filling.

- **Types of Urthrography:**
  - **Retrograde urethrography (RGU):** Contrast is retrogradely injected with the urethral orifice occluded to prevent reflux of contrast.
  - **Antegrade (VCUG):** Bladder is filled with contrast via suprapubic or retrograde catheterization and the urethra is assessed during voiding.
- **Voiding cystourethrogram is mostly used to visualize and evaluate:** Prostatic urethra and changes in the bladder neck.
- **Retrograde urethrogram is mostly used to evaluate:** Membranous and anterior urethra, inflammatory lesions and diverticula.

Radiographic Anatomy on RGU

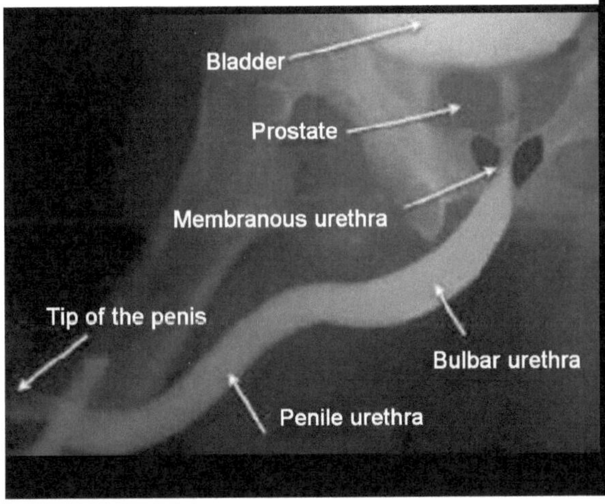

Radiographic Anatomy on MCU

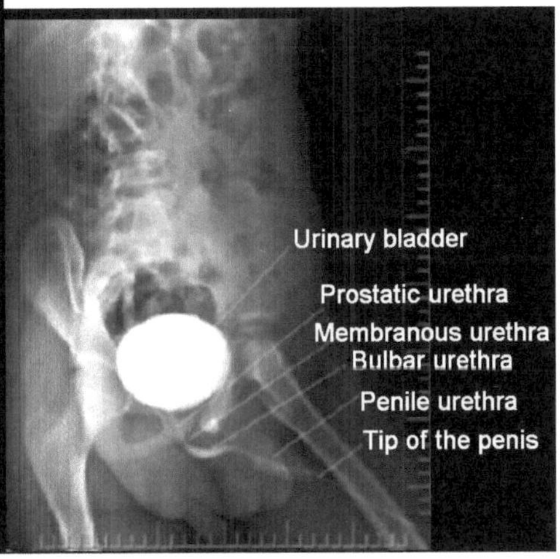

Ans: (a) MCU showing Bulbar urethral stricture

Ref: *Radiopedia*

PSYCHIATRY

1. An MBBS student girl comes to OPD complaining of intermittent episodes of feeling of impending doom, accompanied by intense perspiration. Usually the episodes occur prior to her exams. What is the most likely diagnosis?

(a) Panic attack
(b) Generalized anxiety disorder
(c) Phobia
(d) Schizophrenia

Explanation:

- Panic attack is a sudden period of intense fear or apprehension that may last from minutes or hours. Recurrent unexpected panic attacks are common in panic disorder.
- The major mental symptoms are extreme tear and a sense of impending doom with anticipatory anxiety.
- The other type of panic attack is situationally predisposed panic attack in response to a trigger.
- Panic attack inducing substances (panicogens): Carbon dioxide, yohimbine, cholecystokinin, caffeine.

Diagnostic Criteria for Panic Attack

A panic attack is an abrupt surge of intense fear or intense discomfort that reaches a peak within minutes, and during which time 4 (or more) of the following symptoms occur:

Note: The abrupt surge can occur from a calm state or an anxious state.

- Palpitations, pounding heart, or accelerated heart rate.
- Sweating.
- Trembling or shaking.
- Sensations of shortness of breath or smothering.
- Feelings of choking.
- Chest pain or discomfort.
- Nausea or abdominal distress.
- Feeling dizzy, unsteady, light-headed, or faint.
- Chills or heart sensations.
- Paresthesias (numbness or tingling sensations).
- Derealizations (feeling or unreality) or depersonalization (being detached from one-self).
- Fear of losing control or "going crazy".
- Fear of dying.

Note: Culture-specific symptoms (e.g., tinnitus, neck soreness, headache, uncontrollable screaming or crying) may be seen. Such symptoms should not count as 1 of the 4 required symptoms.

Ans: (a) Panic attack

Ref: *Niraj Ahuja, A Short Textbook of Psychiatry, 10th Edition, Page 90*